Eye Diseases in Hot Climates

Fifth Edition

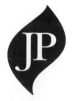

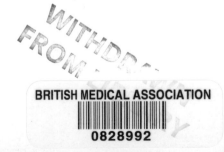

Eye Diseases in Hot Climates

Fifth Edition

Saul Rajak PhD FRCOphth
Honorary Lecturer, London School of Hygiene and
Tropical Medicine, London, UK

John Sandford-Smith FRCS FRCOphth
Emeritus Consultant Ophthalmologist
Leicester Royal Infirmary, Leicester, UK
Ophthalmologist, Christian Hospital
Quetta, Pakistan
Senior Lecturer in Ophthalmology
Ahmadu Bello University Hospital, Kaduna, Nigeria

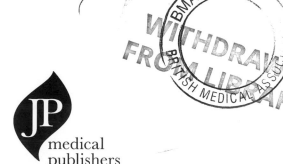

JP
medical
publishers

London • Philadelphia • Panama City • New Delhi

© 2015 Saul Rajak and John Sandford-Smith
Published by JP Medical Ltd, 83 Victoria Street, London, SW1H 0HW, UK
Tel: +44 (0)20 3170 8910   Fax: +44 (0)20 3008 6180
Email: info@jpmedpub.com   Web: www.jpmedpub.com

ISBN: 978-1-909836-22-8

British Library Cataloguing in Publication Data
A catalogue record for this book is available from the British Library

Library of Congress Cataloging in Publication Data
A catalog record for this book is available from the Library of Congress

Publisher: Richard Furn
Editorial Assistants: Sophie Woolven, Katie Pattullo
Design: Designers Collective Ltd

Indexed, typeset, printed and bound in India.

Preface

Around 250 million people worldwide are either blind or suffer serious visual impairment. Of these, 200 million have avoidable and preventable diseases and almost all live in poor countries. The goal of this book is to provide a practical guide for the healthcare professionals who look after these patients.

There are many excellent ophthalmology textbooks for those in the developed world, but hardly any books written specifically for those training or working in developing nations. *Eye Diseases in Hot Climates* aims to reach the areas that other books don't reach. It is a comprehensive guide to eye disease and eye care, but focuses on diseases such as cataract, vitamin A deficiency, trachoma and corneal infection, all of which are common, severe and potentially blinding in poor and tropical countries. In doing so the book supports the World Health Organization's VISION 2020 initiative in its goal of eliminating preventable and treatable blindness by 2020.

Much has changed in eye care since the publication of the fourth edition. Some diseases such as leprosy and onchocerciasis are less common thanks to effective treatment campaigns. Other diseases such as macular degeneration and diabetic retinopathy, which used to be a problem only in rich countries, are now widely seen throughout the world. Cataract remains widespread, but access to surgery and the range of treatment options are improving. HIV continues to have dramatic consequences in poor countries.

The Fifth Edition of *Eye Diseases in Hot Climates* has been comprehensively updated in response to these changes. Each chapter has been thoroughly revised and many new photos, tables and illustrations added. We hope the book continues to be not just the standard textbook for ophthalmic nurses, ophthalmic clinical officers, ophthalmic assistants and medical students in tropical and poor countries, but will also be an invaluable resource for ophthalmologists in any location. As flights get cheaper and the world gets smaller, patients and healthcare workers frequently travel from poorer countries to richer ones, and vice versa. Doctors and nurses working in rich countries need to know about the diseases of poorer countries, many of which have been labelled by the WHO as neglected tropical diseases.

We have written *Eye Diseases in Hot Climates* in a simple, direct style to help readers who may not use English as their first language. We have tried to make the book engaging and stimulating. Above all we have focussed on providing practical information and advice for those without ophthalmic training who nonetheless treat patients with only a limited range of diagnostic equipment and medications at their disposal.

Saul Rajak
John Sandford-Smith
June 2015

Contents

Dedications

To my wife Juliette and children, Eve and Florence.

SR

To Sheila my wife, who has brought up a family in three different continents and 12 different homes and hardly ever complained.

JSS

Acknowledgements

We would like to thank the Ulverscroft Foundation, Leicester, for their very generous financial support and encouragement for this and all the previous editions of the book.

Most of the illustrations have been prepared by either the staff of the Medical Illustration Department of Leicester Royal Infirmary (in particular, Georgean Lochead, Parul Desai and Jan Johnson) or by Juliette Rajak.

The clinical photos have come from a wide range of sources and people, to whom we are very grateful. We would particularly like to acknowledge Dr Edward Hughes, Dr Neil Rogers, Dr Margreet Hogeweg, Dr Andy Richards and Drs Michele and Ian Murdoch, for providing so many high quality images.

The International Centre for Eye Health, London, has been a constant source of encouragement and information. We would like to thank in particular Professor Allen Foster, Professor Clare Gilbert and Dr Matthew Burton.

Various friends and colleagues have offered us advice and help on this or previous editions. In particular, Dr Adrian Hopkins, Dr Astrid Leck, Dr Susan Lewallen, Dr Denise and Professor David Mabey, Mr Andy Richards, Dr Keith Waddell, Dr Martin Wiselka and, for indispensable advice on publishing, Michael Manson, Michael Leventhal, Harry and Tessa Rajak. We are very grateful to them all, but in the end we must take responsibility for any errors or mistakes.

It would not have been possible to write this book, or to live in the countries that this book is intended for, without the unfailing and wonderful support of our families. Saul would like to thank Tessa and Harry, Stella and Tony, Dinah, Sam, Rafi and Noa.

The authors thank the following for their generous contribution of figures to this edition:

Albert Lue Figure 20.7

Allen Foster Figures 10.11, 10.13

Allon Barsam Figures 9.21a–b, 9.26

Al Sommer Figure 10.9

Andre Curi Figure 16.17

Clare Gilbert Figure 10.7

David Mabey Figure 16.3b

Ed Hughes Figures 11.4, 11.8b, 11.12, 11.14, 11.15, 11.17, 11.18, 11.19, 11.20, 11.21, 11.24, 11.26, 11.29, 12.25a–b, 13.1, 13.4, 13.7, 13.10, 13.11, 13.12, 13.13, 13.14, 13.17, 13.22, 13.24a–b, 13.25, 13.28, 13.33, 13.34, 13.37, 13.40, 13.41, 13.44, 14.5a–b, 20.8, 20.9, 20.12 and Chapter 11 opening figure

Frank Green Figure 9.25

Ian and Michele Murdoch Figures 16.2, 16.3a, 16.3c, 16.4, 16.7, 16.11a

Ian Rennie Figures 11.2, 11.3

International Centre for Eye Health Figures 10.1, 10.10

Isabelle Schaeffers Chapter 5 opening figure

JE Marr Figures 7.13a–b

Justin O'Day Figures 16.2, 16.7

Laura Dunn Figure 9.1

Margreet Hogeweg Figures 17.1, 17.2, 17.3, 17.7a–b, 17.9, 17.11, 17.12 and Chapter 17 opening figure

Matthew Burton Figures 9.9a–b

Neil Rogers Figures 7.13a–b, 7.17 a–b, 9.14a–c, 11.5, 13.35, 13.36, 20.11, 21.11a

Paul Sullivan Figures 13.18, 13.19, 13.20a–c, 13.32, 21.11b

Peek Vision Figures 3.20, 15.4

Philippa Matthews Figure 9.1

Steve Tuft Figures 9.21a–b

Tom Lietman Figures 7.4, 8.2, 8.3, 8.4a
Timothy Featherstone Figures 15.22, 18.3, 20.4, 21.13
Vijay Shanmuganathan Figures 7.15, 7.18, 21.5a–c

Thanks to the organisations and people who kindly allowed us to reproduce their photographs
in previous editions:
The World Health Organization, Teaching Aids at Low Cost, Professor Alistair Fielder, Professor
Barrie Jones, Mr J Kanski, Mr E Rosen, Mr J Talbot, Mr M Kerr Muir, Dr E Wright, Andy Richards.

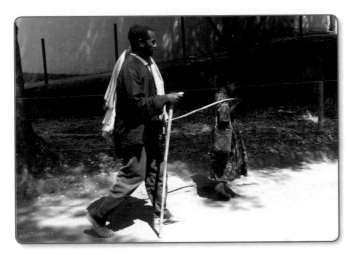

People don't go blind by the million; they go blind one by one, each with their own sadness and loss.

The eye is a truly amazing structure. Rays of light from the outside world enter the eye and are converted into electrical impulses that are transferred along visual pathways to the brain, which uses this information to generate a picture of the world – to allow us to see. The eyes provide about half the total sensory input from the entire body into the brain. There is, however, one small defect in the visual image produced by the healthy eye: the 'blind spot'. This is a small area in our field of vision where we are unable to see. It corresponds to where the optic nerve leaves the eye. Remarkably, our brain creates appropriate images to fill in the blind spot, so that we are not even aware of it. Unfortunately there is a very large 'blind-spot' in worldwide ophthalmology. This is the tragedy of avoidable blindness in poor countries. Approximately 285 million people worldwide are visually impaired. About three quarters of this is treatable or avoidable. And just as in the eye, we cover over this blind spot and ignore it. Medical science, governments and health care workers largely neglect the millions of blind and visually impaired people worldwide. Indeed, that is the only reason why they are blind.

The aim of this book is to focus on this 'blind spot'. It describes eye diseases and eye care in poor countries and in particular those diseases which cause treatable and preventable blindness.

What is special about eye diseases in hot climates?

The diseases of hot climates have traditionally been called 'tropical' diseases, although some hot countries are not exactly in the tropics, which is the region of the earth surrounding the equator. There are two important features about these areas with hotter climates. Firstly, some diseases may be influenced directly by the heat, humidity and solar radiation. For example, this climate encourages the growth and multiplication of bacteria, fungi and other micro-organisms that cause corneal infections and the insects and other carriers that cause many infective diseases. Secondly, and more importantly, a look at the world map will show that most hot countries are also poor (**Figure 1.1**). Poverty is associated with poor hygiene, poor nutrition, poor provision of and access to healthcare, civil wars and poor management of natural disasters, all of which are devastating for healthcare.

Terminology

In the last few decades, countries with poor economies have been referred to in several ways, such as the Third World, developing countries, resource poor countries/settings, low income countries/settings. Each of these terms has problems.

- The 'Third World' has complex political implications related to colonialism and the Cold War in the past. 'Third' is a rather derogatory term, which relates to 'third class' and 'third rate' and is therefore not a suitable description of poor countries.
- 'Developing countries' is complimentary and optimistic, but is sometimes simply not true. In many war torn or badly governed countries the economic and health situation is not improving or may even be getting worse.
- 'Resource poor countries/settings' is also often untrue, as some of the poorest countries have some of the highest levels of natural resources, but the money that they generate does not reach most of the population.

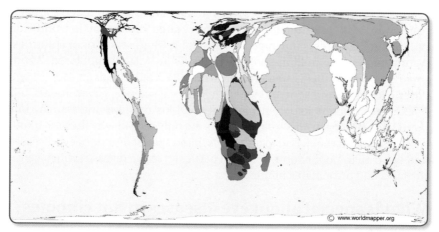

Figure 1.1 UN world poverty map. The size of each country is proportional to its poverty compared to the rest of the world. Therefore Africa and South Asia look much larger than other countries. © Copyright Sasi Group (University of Sheffield) and Mark Newman (University of Michigan).

- 'Low-income countries/settings' is the most accurate description of the sort of countries whose eye care we want to cover in this book, but it is a rather wordy and technical term.

We are therefore left doing a full circle back to the only phrase that accurately and honestly describes the economic situation in many areas: *poor countries*. We will therefore use this term throughout the book, although it must be emphasised that we are referring to the economic definition of the word 'poor' and it is not a reflection on other qualities in the many wonderful poor countries of the world. Also, these countries are often very rich in the culture and the resourcefulness of the people to overcome the difficulties and problems that are thrust on them.

Eye diseases that are more common in hot climates and poor countries

Some diseases, such as trachoma and xerophthalmia (vitamin A deficiency associated eye disease) are seen more frequently because they are caused or worsened by poverty, the heat or the endemic micro-organisms and vectors. Other diseases, such as cataract and glaucoma, are the same as those seen in rich countries, but are seen at a much more advanced stage because of the lack of access to healthcare. Sometimes, e.g. cataract, the disease can still be treated, but other times, e.g. glaucoma, the visual loss is irreversible. Finally, some diseases, such as age-related macular degeneration and retinopathy of prematurity are seen less frequently in poor countries, because the life expectancy of adults is shorter and very premature babies are unlikely to survive.

A summary of some of the ways in which a hot climate and poverty can cause serious and common eye diseases is shown in **Table 1.1**. However, it is important to remember that for a lot of these diseases many factors interact. For example, corneal ulcers and scars are often much worse in poor countries because of the micro-organisms that live in hot climates, the increased risk of agricultural eye trauma, malnutrition in children, the poor access to healthcare and immunisations and the poor availability of treatments when healthcare is sought. Therefore you will see that some diseases appear several times in **Table 1.1**.

Definitions of visual loss and visual impairment

The World Health Organization (WHO) defines blindness as 'visual acuity less than 3/60 in the better eye with the best possible spectacle correction or a corresponding visual field loss'. This degree of visual loss prevents the patient from walking about or navigating independently. In addition, the WHO has another category called 'low vision'. Low vision corresponds to a visual acuity of less than 6/18, but equal to or better than 3/60 in the better eye with the best possible spectacle correction. Such people have a significant visual impairment which often makes working difficult, but they can get around independently.

Table 1.1 Diseases associated with poverty and hot climates	
Risk factor	Disease caused or exacerbated by risk factor
Heat and solar radiation	Cataract Pterygium Solar keratopathy Eyelid tumours (e.g. basal cell carcinoma)
Insect and other disease vectors	Onchocerciasis Malaria retinopathy Trachoma Cutaneous leishmaniasis
Warm and humid climates	Fungal and bacterial keratitis Trachoma Allergic conjunctivitis
Malnutrition	Vitamin A deficiency associated eye disease
Poor hygiene	Trachoma Infective conjunctivitis Leprosy and tuberculosis
Poor access to vaccinations and widespread untreated disease putting others at risk	Vitamin A deficiency associated eye disease Congenital rubella Tuberculosis Trachoma
Increased risk of ocular trauma	Fungal and bacterial keratitis Penetrating eye injury
Poor access to healthcare	All diseases

The prevalence of visual loss and blindness: eye disease is very common

The most recent estimates are that worldwide 246 million people are visually impaired and 39 million blind. About 90% of them live in poor countries, 80% of it is avoidable and 60% are women. In fact, the proportion of women may be greater because women often have less opportunity to seek healthcare and be 'counted'. The prevalence figures for visual loss are very approximate estimates, as counting the number of blind and visually impaired people is extremely difficult for the following reasons:

- The majority of the world's eye disease is in poor countries. Many of these people live in remote, rural areas where they are not examined and their eye disease never 'counted'. Because of the cost and difficulty of reaching these people, the prevalence figures of eye disease and visual loss are all based on samples. These samples are of course all estimates and often underestimate the numbers in the most rural and deprived places, where the level of eye disease is often highest.
- Visually impaired people often hide their disease. There may be great social stigma attached to visual loss. Therefore, people with eye disease often do not inform their friends and relatives, let alone the health facilities or the researchers conducting prevalence surveys.
- Although the definition of blindness and visual impairment has been internationally agreed upon on paper, it is often difficult to translate

this to the 'real patient'. The classification of whether a person is visually impaired can vary greatly, e.g. in different lighting conditions and with different vision testing charts.

- Some people are continually becoming visually impaired as their disease progresses and some people's vision is being improved with treatment. The most dramatic example of this is cataract surgery in which a patient can change from being blind to having perfect vision almost immediately after a short operation.

The number of blind people in each region are shown in **Table 1.2**. Although the actual numbers of blind and visually impaired people are highest in Asia, this is because these are the most populous areas of the world. The highest prevalence of blind people are in some countries of sub-Saharan Africa (Niger, Mauritania, Mali, Chad, Somalia, Ethiopia and Burkina Faso).

Approximately 0.2% of the population in most rich countries are blind, but in poor countries the figure is between 0.5% and 1%. There are good reasons to believe that the difference between the two communities may be much greater than this:

- Blindness is such a significant handicap in poor and rural communities that blind people have a much shorter life expectancy. This is especially true for blindness starting in infancy, but it is also true for blindness starting at any age.
- In rich countries, many more people live into old age when the risk of visual loss increases. For example in England, three quarters of the people registered as blind each year are over 70 years. There are many

Table 1.2 Number of blind and visually impaired people in the world in 2010				
Region	Total population, millions (%)	Number of blind people, millions (%)	Number with Low vision millions (%)	Total number with blindness or low vision, millions (%)
Africa	805 (11.9%)	5.9 (15%)	20.4 (8.3%)	26.3 (9.2%)
The Americas	915 (13.6%)	3.2 (8%)	23.4 (9.5%)	26.6 (26.6%)
Eastern Mediterranean	580 (8.6%)	4.9 (12.5%)	18.6 (7.6%)	23.5 (23.5%)
European region	889 (13.2%)	2.7 (7%)	25.5 (10.4%)	28.2 (28.2%)
South East Asia (not including India)	579 (8.6%)	4.0 (10.1%)	23.9 (9.7%)	27.9 (9.8%)
Western Pacific (not including China)	442 (6.6%)	2.3 (6%)	12.4 (5%)	14.7 (5.2%)
India	1181 (17.5%)	8.1 (20.5%)	54.5 (22.2%)	62.6 (21.9%)
China	1345 (20.0%)	8.2 (20.9%)	67.3 (27.3%)	75.5 (26.5%)
Total	6738 (100%)	39.4 (100%)	246.0 (100%)	285.4 (100%)

Modified from Pascolini D, Mariotti SP. Global estimates of visual impairment: 2010. Br J Ophthalmol. 2012; 96:614–618.

fewer people over the age of 70 years in poor countries. Therefore, the difference in prevalence between rich and poor countries of visual loss in younger people is probably much greater than the overall difference.
- Blind and visually impaired people in rich countries are registered on national registers. This occurs because they receive social security benefits and additional support such as low vision aids and tools to help them in their home. On the other hand in poor countries, there are often economic and cultural reasons for people to hide their blindness. For example, one of the authors once examined a man who was totally blind. He requested a note to excuse his absence from work. He was employed as a night watchman and certainly did not want his employer knowing his visual acuity level.

Most blindness in poor countries is preventable or treatable

Over two thirds of worldwide visual impairment and blindness could be eliminated if the necessary treatment was provided for just refractive error and cataract. The major causes of preventable disease are listed in **Box 1.1**. There are also some causes of blindness that can neither be prevented nor treated. However, these are much less common in poor countries, either because they are rare, such as congenital abnormalities in children or because in many countries the life expectancy is not long enough for most people to develop these diseases such as degenerative and vascular diseases of the retina. Therefore, these diseases make up a much larger proportion of visual impairment in rich countries, where almost all people with refractive error are able to get glasses, those with cataract get cataract surgery before they are significantly impaired, glaucoma gets detected and treated early, and trachoma and onchocerciasis do not exist (**Figure 1.2**).

Inadequate healthcare resources

Eye diseases are a major health problem in most of the tropics and, in some places, may be the biggest community health problem of all. Yet there are not nearly enough trained medical staff to tackle this large and challenging problem. It has been said that there are more ophthalmologists in New York than in all of sub-Saharan Africa. In most African countries and in many rural areas of Asia there is less than one trained eye specialist for a million or more people compared to 81 per million in America.

Eye specialists are not only few in number, they are usually very unevenly distributed in most poor countries. They almost all work in the major cities and often treat mainly private and wealthier patients. Most poor countries have very small budgets for health care and very fragmented health systems, and therefore cannot offer attractive salaries or good working conditions to medical staff working in government hospitals. Therefore, most doctors are obliged or choose to work privately, and for specialists this nearly always means practising in the big cities or even leaving their home country to work in a richer country. They are therefore working far away from where most of the visually

Box 1.1 The major causes of preventable eye disease

- **Cataract**: this is the cause of almost half of the world's blindness. It is treatable with an operation. The overall cost of modern surgery including staff salaries can be less than 50 US dollars. The operation has extremely high success rates.
- **Trachoma**: over two million people are blind from trachoma and at least 50 million children are exposed to the eye infection that will put them at risk of blinding trachoma in later life. It is an infectious disease that is intimately associated with poverty and poor hygiene and disappears completely as living standards increase.
- **Glaucoma**: about six million people are blind from glaucoma. Glaucoma blindness is irreversible. However, if the disease is detected in its early stages, its progress can be arrested and in most cases the sight saved.
- **Xerophthalmia**: this is the result of vitamin A deficiency, which occurs because of poor nutrition and poverty. It only affects young children and it is thought that between one-quarter and half a million children a year go blind from xerophthalmia. Most of these children will die but many others will be left either blind or visually impaired.
- **Onchocerciasis**: this parasitic disease is only a problem in certain areas of the world, especially sub-Saharan Africa. However, between one-quarter and half a million people are blind from it and about 20 million significantly affected. Blindness from onchocerciasis has reduced substantially in recent years because of very effective drug treatment.
- **Uncorrected refractive error**: many millions of people require spectacles to see clearly but have never been given them. Patients with large uncorrected refractive errors can be functionally blind.
- **Diabetic retinopathy**. This is increasing in importance as the numbers of diabetics worldwide increases, especially in South Asia where dietary and lifestyle changes are probably responsible. Diabetic blindness from diabetic retinopathy can be prevented or delayed with education and careful control of blood sugars, but it sometimes also requires the use of expensive lasers to treat the eyes.
- **Wet age-related macular degeneration (AMD)**: until recently AMD was essentially untreatable. However, in recent years, drugs have become available that can be injected into the eye to slow down or even stop the progression of wet AMD. These drugs are widely used in rich countries, but they remain expensive, and prompt and skilled assessment and treatment is required when a patient starts to lose vision with AMD.

impaired people and the diseases of poverty are located. In some countries, there may be almost an excess of specialists in the capital cities, and competition for work, but hardly any specialists in the rural areas. Furthermore eye care

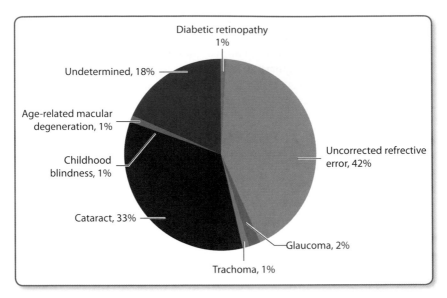

Figure 1.2 The major causes of visual impairment.

programmes have to compete with more serious life-threatening diseases for the small amount of money in health care budgets.

Plans and strategies for combating avoidable visual loss

There have been many large and small scale plans and strategies for addressing eye disease and visual impairment in poor countries. We will discuss the two major recent International Plans – VISION 2020 and Universal Eye Health – as well as a smaller and less prominent but potentially very effective strategy – institutional links between eye units in poor and rich countries.

VISION 2020

In 1999 the World Health Organisation (WHO) and the International Agency for the Prevention of Blindness (IAPB) launched a plan called 'VISION 2020 The Right to Sight'. IAPB is a coalition of many organisations involved in eye care, such as non-governmental organisations, eye care institutions and corporations, all of which are therefore involved in VISION 2020. The aim of VISION 2020 is to eliminate avoidable blindness, as a public health problem, by the year 2020 (as well as being the year 2020, it is also a reference to the assessment of vision, in feet rather than metres; 20/20 which is the same as 6/6 in metres, is 'normal' vision). The philosophy of VISION 2020 is that all people have the right to a basic level of healthcare, and this includes the right to sight and not to lose vision from treatable diseases. Therefore, the ultimate goal is that everyone has access to high-quality eye care that is part of a sustainable health system. VISION 2020 hopes to achieve this by providing guidance, support and advocacy for eye care. A summary of the original 1999 action plan is shown in **Box 1.2** and described in more detail in the following pages.

> **Box 1.2 Summary of VISION 2020 The Right to Sight**
> 1. To target certain diseases: Nearly all avoidable blindness is caused by a few diseases, and all the effort should be focused on these diseases:
>   - Cataract
>   - Trachoma
>   - Xerophthalmia
>   - Onchocerciasis
>   - Serious refractive errors
>   - Other causes of childhood blindness including measles, congenital rubella, retinopathy of prematurity and congenital cataract.
> 2. Human resource development: training and motivating people to do the work:
>   - Training for the surgical treatment of blinding cataract.
>   - Training in prevention and community eye health.
>   - Training in health education.
> 3. Infrastructure, and the development of appropriate technology: the development of systems and equipment to do the work cheaply and effectively:
>   - Cost effectiveness
>   - Cost recovery
>   - The need for appropriate technology
>   - Mobility
>   - Teamwork and co-operation

VISION 2020 Action Plan 2006–2011

The VISION 2020 plan was updated in 2006. This plan was based on the same three core principles in **Box 1.2**, but highlighted the importance of the following ideas:
- Effective and efficient comprehensive eye health-care needs to be integrated into well-managed national health systems.
- Human resource, infrastructure and technology must be scaled up in numbers and coverage.
- Additional activities that must be undertaken:
  - Advocacy and public relations
  - Information
  - Education and communication
  - Community participation.

VISION 2020, where are we now?

As we get closer to the year 2020, it is clear that the ambitious target of eliminating all avoidable blindness by 2020 will not be met. Worldwide, there are now thought to be 39 million blind people and 246 with low vision. In 1999, the estimated figures were 38 million blind and 110 million with low vision. There are probably several reasons for this apparent increase:
- The ageing population of the world: almost all the commonest causes of visual impairment become increasingly common with age. As the life

expectancy is increasing in most countries, there will be more visually impaired people.

- More complete and accurate surveys of eye disease: VISION 2020 has made visual loss a much more prominent issue, and therefore, many more surveys have been conducted. Therefore, the current figures are probably more accurate than the 1999 figures, which are likely to have been an underestimate.
- New cases: for some eye diseases, the number of cases being treated is little more than the number of new cases going blind, and therefore the overall number does not decrease.

Has VISION 2020 failed? The answer is of course a resounding 'no', as VISION 2020 has been responsible for raising the profile of visual loss, for treating many millions of people and for raising money for eye care and eye research. However, the original target of eliminating avoidable blindness by 2020 will not be achieved and there is still an enormous amount to be done.

Integrating eye care into general health services: Universal Eye Health

One of the possible shortcomings of the original VISION 2020 plan was its emphasis on eliminating certain specific diseases. A strategy that focuses on particular diseases is sometimes called a 'vertical' plan. In recent years, there has been increased emphasis on seeing eye care as part of general health care services. This is sometimes called a 'horizontal' health plan because it covers all aspects of health care.

The aim is still to prevent and treat avoidable blindness, but the method is more through improving eye services as part of the general health care system. The most recent WHO resolution is called 'Towards Universal Eye Health: A Global Action Plan, 2014–2019'. This WHO resolution, which has been endorsed by the World Health Assembly has the more realistic target for 2019 of aiming to reduce avoidable visual impairment by 25% from the 2010 levels. This plan has several principles, approaches and objectives, which are slightly different from the original 2020 approach. The major ones are:

1. Integrating eye care services into health care systems at all levels (primary, secondary and tertiary), i.e. a horizontal approach.
2. A goal of providing good access to rehabilitation services for the visually impaired. Providing rehabilitation services is almost impossible in a 'vertical' campaign and individual disease based approach to eye care, but can and should be achieved if patients are receiving eye care in an integrated health system.
3. Generating more evidence about visual impairment, i.e. the scale of the problem, the causes of visual impairment and what eye care services are available. This evidence can be used to push for greater political and financial commitments.
4. Addressing the global trend towards more chronic eye diseases related to ageing, which will become an increasingly large proportion of the causes of visual impairment.
5. The Global Action Plan specifically states that research is important and needs to be funded, because this is how new and more cost-effective

treatments are developed. Operational research is particularly useful for determining if treatment is actually reaching the people who need it. For example, one trachoma study found that although many hundreds of surgeons had been trained and equipped to do surgery, the majority were doing few or even no trachoma surgeries.

However, in the end, a 'plan' is only as good as the commitment and determination of us the eye care workers to put it into action.

Links between eye units in poor countries and rich countries

'Links' refers to partnerships between an eye department in a poor country and one in a rich country. Health institutions in rich countries should not think about just their own population's needs and there are numerous reasons for being involved in the health needs of poor countries. 'Links' are an excellent way of joining the respective health systems and should be seen as an obligation rather than a luxury for the following reasons:

- The ethical obligation: this is the most important reason. It is unacceptable for the wealthy nations to ignore the terrible healthcare provisions of a large proportion of the world's population and the needless visual loss that occurs throughout the poor countries of the world. Never has the phrase 'turning a blind eye' been more appropriate.
- The political obligation: poor countries are unstable and at much greater risk of civil war and extremism. Of course, we cannot prevent this, but assisting poor countries, with major needs such as healthcare and education, may help to create more stability.
- The 'brain-drain' obligation: many doctors and nurses from poor countries emigrate to rich countries. The health systems of rich countries have become dependent on these health care professionals and have not even paid for training them. This has decimated the number working in poor countries, despite the enormous need there and the cost of training them.
- The mutual benefit: these partnerships do not just benefit the institution in the poor country. It is of enormous value to individual health practitioners and the institutions they work in to see how healthcare is delivered in a poor country. There are some parts of healthcare that are done better in poor countries because of the enormous need. For example, it is normal to conduct 30 or more cataract operations in a day in some units in poor countries. In rich countries it can be a challenge to do more than 12.
- Personal learning: many health workers from a rich country on seeing the advanced pathology and needless visual loss that patients suffer in poor countries, find their attitudes are changed. They become more humble and understanding and learn the importance of setting priorities.
- Communicable diseases: the enormous migration around the world has facilitated the spread of diseases such as tuberculosis and 'flu viruses'. There are big increases in the incidence of some of these diseases in rich

countries. Treating and controlling them in the poor countries would minimise their spread.

The VISION 2020 LINKS programme is a UK programme that is designed to support the aims of Vision 2020 by setting up institution-to-institution partnerships, mainly in Africa. The programme is already seeing huge benefits to institutions and the people who work in them on both sides of the partnership. Informed partnerships have been established elsewhere in the world, but it hoped that other countries in the world will also set up more formalised partnerships.

The causes of blindness worldwide and the diseases targeted by VISION 2020

The major worldwide causes of blindness can be divided into four groups:

1.   Easily preventable diseases.
2.   Easily treatable diseases.
3.   Less easily preventable and treatable diseases.
4.   Untreatable or unpreventable diseases.

VISION 2020 is targeting the first two groups, although the increase in the ageing population has brought about greatly increased focus on the eye diseases of older people, some of which are untreatable. VISION 2020 has also made it a priority to target childhood blindness, because although often more difficult to prevent or treat, it has an enormous impact on the rest of the child's life and the community they live in.

Easily preventable diseases

This group consists of three diseases which are almost exclusively found in poor countries and particularly, poor countries with hot climates. These diseases are: trachoma, xerophthalmia (vitamin A deficiency associated eye disease) and onchocerciasis. They are all easily preventable, but once blindness has occurred, treatment or restoration of vision is difficult or impossible. Onchocerciasis occurs in just a few areas. Trachoma and xerophthalmia are more widespread in poor countries, although with great variation in prevalence. In the places where they are more prevalent, they can be major causes of blindness. Blinding trachoma can be prevented by improvements in hygiene and living conditions, and blinding xerophthalmia can be prevented by improvements in nutrition.

To prevent blindness from each of these three diseases, there is now also a 'magic bullet' treatment. A 'magic bullet' is a treatment, which is very effective, needs to be given only once or very infrequently, and has very few side effects. These magic bullets are:

- Trachoma: **azithromycin**, an antibiotic, which kills the Chlamydia bacteria which causes the disease.
- Xerophthalmia: **vitamin A capsules**, which almost immediately eliminate vitamin A deficiency.
- Onchocerciasis: **ivermectin**, a drug that kills filarial worms, which cause the disease.

Easily treatable diseases

Cataract and refractive error are found throughout the world. However, both of these conditions rarely cause severe visual impairment or blindness in rich countries but are by far the commonest causes of visual loss in poor countries where poor medical services simply cannot address the huge number of cases.

Refractive error

People with serious refractive errors need spectacles to see properly. Uncorrected refractive errors are a significant cause of visual impairment, and even 'blindness', in places where it is difficult to obtain spectacles. Refractive errors are particularly important because they usually develop in young children, and will therefore affect the education and development and therefore the entire future life of the child.

The surgical treatment of cataract and the cataract surgical rate

Cataracts are quickly and relatively cheaply eliminated with a surgical procedure. This procedure only needs to be done once for each patient. The results can be fantastic, but complications can also occur and the patient left with worse vision than before the operation. However, 'new' cataracts are continually developing in patients. This is illustrated in **Figure 1.3**. If more surgical procedures are being done than new cataracts developing, the number of people blind from cataracts will fall. But if more cataracts are developing than surgeries being conducted, the number of blind people will rise. The 'cataract surgical rate' (CSR) is the number of cataract surgeries performed per million people in the population. The CSR helps us to determine if the number of cataract surgeries being done is enough to keep up with new cataracts developing. For example, we know that when the CSR in rich countries was about 3500, surgical output kept up with new cases. However, there are issues that must be considered when targeting a particular CSR for a particular country:

1. When there is an enormous backlog of cataract – as there is in most poor countries – a very high CSR needs to be aimed for initially to get through the backlog and then the CSR can drop to a level that keeps up with new cases.
2. As cataract surgical technique and equipment have improved, patients and surgeons have desired cataract surgery at an earlier stage, i.e. when they are less visually impaired. Therefore, the CSR needs to rise unless these people are denied surgery, which practically and ethically is very difficult to do. Therefore, the CSR in rich countries has risen to approximately 5000 in recent years. If the CSR in a poor country is 3500, one might expect cataract blindness to be eliminated. However, it is possible and in fact likely that the less dense cataracts of richer people are being operated on, and poor people with dense, blinding cataracts are still struggling to receive surgery. This is probably the case in India where in the last 30 years the CSR has risen from 500 to approximately 5000, but many millions of poor people remain blind from cataract. Therefore, the CSR needs to be uniformly distributed throughout a

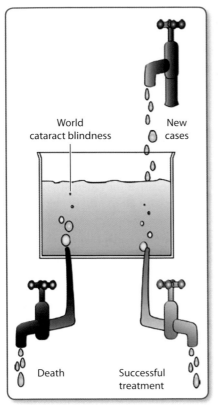

Figure 1.3 The size of the reservoir represents the number of people already blind with cataract (prevalence). The tap into the reservoir represents the extra number of people going blind each year from cataract (incidence). The taps out of the reservoir represent: (a) the people who have been successfully treated for cataract and recovered their sight, or (b) those who die of old age or disease while still blind.

World cataract blindness

New cases

Death

Successful treatment

country, so that there are not pockets of neglected blindness. This requires an even distribution of well-trained surgeons, and the teams and infrastructure that they require. This is rarely seen in poor countries, where many more eye surgeons are found in major cities.

3. A high CSR is only of benefit if the outcomes of cataract surgery are good. If there is a high level of complications, the vision of patients who are receiving cataract surgery will not improve and the number of visually impaired people will not reduce as expected.

4. The world's population is ageing. Therefore, the number of people with cataract is ever-increasing and the CSR must continue to increase with this.

As a result of these problems with the provision of cataract surgery, the prevalence of visually impaired people with cataract has remained fairly static, unlike the other WHO priority diseases, trachoma, xerophthalmia and onchocerciasis which have shown dramatic improvements in recent years.

Non-ophthalmologist cataract surgeons

Many African countries have 1 or less ophthalmologists per million people in the population. In these countries, it is entirely appropriate to train people who are not doctors to do cataract surgery, because otherwise many millions of people will continue to be needlessly blind. A good example of this is the Gambia, a small country in West Africa where the training of cataract surgeons who are not doctors is actively encouraged. The Gambia is also the only country in West Africa which is beginning to meet its target of eradicating cataract blindness. The surgical outcomes of well-trained high output nurse cataract surgeons are just as good as that of ophthalmologists. However, like all surgeons, their practice must continue to be periodically supervised and audited by others as well as auditing their own work.

Less easily preventable and treatable diseases

The most important of these are *glaucoma, diabetic retinopathy and wet macular degeneration.* They are all found throughout the world and in all communities. These are major causes of avoidable blindness but have not been given the same high priority in the VISION 2020 programme because blindness from these causes cannot be prevented quite so easily and they do not cause as much visual loss as cataract and refractive error in poor countries, where the life expectancy is shorter.

Glaucoma

About 6 million people are blind from glaucoma. Glaucoma is a disease that causes irreversible damage to the optic nerve (see Chapter 15). However, if the disease is detected in an early stage, surgical or medical treatment may be given to prevent blindness from developing.

Diabetic retinopathy

Diabetic retinopathy is the ophthalmic complication that commonly occurs with diabetes. Once the patient has gone blind, it is not possible to recover the vision. However, if the changes on the retina are detected at an early stage, education and interventions aimed at improving diabetic control as well as laser treatments for the eye can prevent the disease progressing, and even reverse some of the changes if done early enough. There has been an enormous increase in the number of diabetics worldwide, particularly in South Asia, probably because of dietary changes and increased life expectancy in this region. Therefore, diabetic retinopathy has become much more common. Unfortunately, patients need regular examinations to detect retinopathy, as well as good education and then lasers and possibly surgery for treatment. All of these are expensive and inaccessible for much of the world's population.

Age-related macular degeneration (AMD)

Until the last 10 years, AMD has been untreatable. However, the development of anti-vasoendothelial growth factor drugs, which are injected into the eye, has enabled one type – 'wet' – of AMD to be treated. The more common 'dry' type remains untreatable. The treatment does not reverse the damage, but can stop it progressing, and often needs to be repeated many times. The technology needed to assess the retina before and after treatment, as well as the regular eye examinations and the treatment itself, are unfortunately too expensive for most of the world's population.

Blindness from both glaucoma and diabetic retinopathy can be prevented, but requires screening and surveillance so that they can be detected at an early stage before there has been serious visual loss. Treating wet AMD requires urgent assessment and assessment as soon as the patient develops symptoms in order to be of benefit. Patients may go blind from these conditions even in rich countries. Blindness is much more likely in poor countries because of the lack of screening in primary health care and the lack of medical services in general and the lack of resources even when the diseases are detected.

Diseases that cannot be prevented or treated

There are numerous eye diseases that currently cannot be prevented or treated. The most important among these are degenerative and vascular retinal conditions, in particular dry AMD, and retinal vein and artery blockages, which are both relatively common in older people. There are also numerous inherited and congenital diseases of the retina, optic nerve and cornea, such as retinitis pigmentosa, hereditary optic atrophy and corneal dystrophies. Fortunately most of these are rare, but they usually occur in children or young adults and therefore will cause a whole life of visual loss. These diseases that cannot be treated or prevented are the main causes of blindness in rich countries. They are present just as much in poor countries but their significance is less because they are outnumbered by the treatable and preventable causes of blindness. The VISION 2020 programme was not originally focussing on these conditions, but Universal Eye Health has included the very important goal of providing visual aids and assistance to visually impaired people (see above).

The 'cost' of visual loss

Visual loss has enormous effects on home life, social life and working life. It is impossible to accurately calculate the true cost of this for the individual visually impaired person, their community and their country. However, it is clear that the 'cost' is enormous. A study in Australia highlighted some of the factors associated with visual loss that are particularly expensive:

Costs that affect rich and poor countries
- Loss of earnings
- The cost of people giving care to those with visual loss, and the loss of earnings of the caregivers
- The personal and emotional cost of suffering and premature death that is associated with visual impairment
- The medical costs of treating eye disease. For some diseases, the later the disease is detected and treated, the more expensive and less effective the treatment is

Costs that affect mainly rich countries
- The cost of low vision aids and equipment and home modifications.
- Welfare payments and taxation benefits.

There are several ways of estimating the precise economic benefits of treating eye disease, which are beyond the scope of this book. However, it is absolutely clear that the treatment of preventable eye disease, and particularly cataract and refractive error, which is relatively cheap and very effective, provides enormous economic benefits to the person, their community and their country. Cataract surgery is undoubtedly the single most cost-effective operation in the world.

Human resource development

There is an enormous shortage of ophthalmic care workers in poor countries. This limits the potential to roll out even the most carefully designed and run eye-care programmes. Human resource development involves training people to prevent and treat blinding diseases and also supporting them in their work once they are trained. The precise type of workers needed varies with each country, but typically they are:

- **Ophthalmologists**: doctors who have specialised in eye care and eye surgery. There are far too few in almost all poor areas of poor countries. Therefore, they may provide complex treatment and surgery and help run programmes, but cannot provide the huge amount of day-to-day care that is required in the community.
- **Optometrists and dispensing opticians**: these practitioners have been trained to assess refractive error and dispense appropriate spectacles. The burden of refractive error is huge, and therefore optometrists or eye care workers who have a basic training in this skill are crucial. Optometrists must also know how to detect the early signs of diseases such as glaucoma, diabetic retinopathy and cataract.
- **Ophthalmic nurses and nurses with eye care training**: although different countries have nurses with different levels of eye care training, in principle the bulk of eye care can and often is done by nurses. At one end of the spectrum some very specialised ophthalmic nurses are trained to perform cataract surgery and do this to a very high level, while at the other end of the spectrum, general nurses can be trained in some basic eye care and diagnostic skills, e.g. in treating trachomatous infection.
- **Orthoptists**: these practitioners have been trained to assess and treat squints and other defects of binocular vision and eye movements. Many of their patients are children, and they are therefore often skilled in measuring visual acuity in children. There are very few specialised orthoptists in most poor countries.
- **Community healthcare workers**: many countries train members of the community in specific tasks, e.g. dispensing vitamin A capsules and promotion of face washing and hygiene for trachoma control. These members of the community are a critical part of eye care and often provide a huge amount of eye care at a fraction of the cost of more highly trained professionals. Examples of these workers are health extension workers in Ethiopia, community distributors in onchocerciasis programmes and 'friends of the eyes' in The Gambia.
- **Traditional healers**: many communities in poor countries have minimal or no access to 'conventional' eye care workers. They are dependent on the traditional healers who have been practising long before VISION 2020 and other health plans. They are discussed in more detail on page 24.
- **Managers**: despite not being trained as eye care workers, managers are a critical part of an effective and efficient health system. Clinics,

hospitals and treatment campaigns do not run themselves, and require efficient managers or people delegated with this role. Without them, trained doctors and nurses may be sitting around without the correct equipment, or without the patients being directed to them; a sight seen far too often in poor countries.

The specific set-up of a country or a region's eye care health service will depend on their needs and resources. However, the fundamental principles are that the service should be able to assess and treat as many people as possible, as economically as possible and with an ultimately sustainable service that is part of a universal healthcare system. A critical requirement is that the many people involved in providing healthcare work together as a team. The management of most serious eye diseases of poor countries requires people with many different skills and training, all of whom depend on each other to do their job carefully and thoroughly.

Prevention, community health and health education

As discussed above, many blinding eye diseases that are common in poor countries are best managed with prevention rather than treatment. These include xerophthalmia, trachoma and onchocerciasis. Other diseases, such as diabetic retinopathy and glaucoma must be detected early in the community through community eye health programmes and then referred for treatment. Therefore, prevention and community health must play a major part in any eye care programme.

There are basic differences between the practice of clinical medicine and preventive medicine. In clinical medicine, the patient visits a health practitioner because they are sick (or concerned that they are sick). The doctor responds to the needs of the patient by trying to treat them and help them get better. Clinical medicine might be described as '*reactive*', because the patient initiates the process and the health practitioner reacts to this.

In preventive medicine, the medical profession takes the initiative and institutes measures in the community in order to make them healthy or prevent disease. Programmes of vaccination, clean water supply or insect vector control are prime examples. Community health could be described as '*proactive*'. The medical profession makes the first move and the community then makes a response. Curative medicine is almost always less cost effective than preventive medicine, because in curative medicine individual patients are treated, which is time-consuming and expensive, but for preventive medicine, whole communities can be treated, e.g. with clean water or health education. Unfortunately however, most government health spending is directed towards curative rather than preventive medicine and most health practitioners' time is spent on curative treatment. In poor countries particularly, there are few doctors. These doctors are often so busy treating patients in the big cities, that there is little interest in preventive medicine or community health, especially in rural areas.

Curative medicine attracts health practitioners for several reasons:
- Health practitioners get instant satisfaction from treating patients and making them better. For example, the results of a successful cataract operation are very rewarding, whereas preventive medicine is much more long-term and does not bring the thanks and joy of an individual patient.
- Health practitioners gain status in the community for providing treatment. However, the practitioners who plan and institute preventive medicine campaigns are rarely known by the community, despite saving the sight and even lives of enormous numbers of people.
- Treating patients gives financial rewards; individual patients will pay a lot of money to clinicians who are able to cure disease. Preventive medicine does not usually give great financial rewards.

Preventive medicine can seem much less attractive than curative medicine. The clinical work is often repetitive and boring, and administration takes up a lot of time. However, there is far more potential to make a major difference to the prevalence of blindness in a community.

Many people think that preventive medicine is the concern of governments and NGOs, and that individuals can do little or nothing to prevent disease. It is true that large preventive medicine campaigns require the involvement of health departments and/or NGOs. However, the individual medical worker can do a lot to help prevent some of the major causes of blindness. For example:
- Trachoma is a disease of poor hygiene, and health workers can teach and encourage good hygiene.
- Xerophthalmia is a disease of poor nutrition, and health workers can help to improve nutrition. They can also encourage measles vaccination schemes, which are an important way to prevent blindness from xerophthalmia.
- A good health practitioner can detect glaucoma or diabetic retinopathy early in the community before it has caused irreversible visual loss.

Health education

Health education forms a vital part of community health. Much eye disease and blindness is caused by poor hygiene or nutrition, or is related to the lifestyle of the community. The only real and lasting solution to these problems will come from within the community itself when people become aware of the importance of good nutrition and hygiene, and healthy living. Health education presents a very different sort of challenge – to win the confidence of communities and their leaders and persuade them to alter some of their traditional customs and ways of life. Health education is most effective when the stimulus for change comes from within the community itself rather than from outside it, i.e. when they understand the importance of the intervention for their own health and well-being. The key concept of health education is '*ownership*'. If the community feels that the health service in some way belongs to them and is for them and they have some part in being responsible for it, then they are much more likely to use it properly, and to respond to suggestions from health care professionals.

Hospitals, clinics and schools are traditionally used as places for health education. However, nowadays, much more imaginative ways of disseminating health education are being used, such as religious and cultural meetings and events, radio, television and newspapers and even mobile vans that stop in villages and perform educational theatre performances. An example of an increasingly successful health education message is 'clean faces' for trachoma control. It is now completely normal for children in the most rural villages to be cleaning their faces, from a newly installed water pump that has been provided in conjunction with the education. Whatever way the education is provided, it must be remembered that the closer any health worker is to the community the more effective they are likely to be. They are likely to be trusted to and listened to and they can repeat their message again and again, as is often required. Unfortunately, it is all too easy for a doctor or even a nurse to be seen as a superior and unapproachable person who dispenses injections and medicines and performs operations and leaves the rural community after just a short time.

Infrastructure and the development of appropriate technology

Infrastructure

This is the third main aim of the VISION 2020 plan; the aim is to provide universal coverage and access to eye care services that are required to prevent and treat visual loss. This requires suitably located primary, secondary and tertiary units for eye care. The infrastructure of eye care must have both a hospital base and a community base which support each other. The community health worker can identify and send the right patients to hospital for treatment. High quality, successful hospital treatment will then encourage and strengthen the acceptance of the community health worker within the community and encourage more patients to attend. There is little point in having lots of teaching hospital eye units in which complex surgery can be done, but no-one to dispense vitamin A capsules in the community and similarly there is little value in having lots of community screeners who can detect cataract, but no operating theatre in the region where cataract extraction surgery can be done. Infrastructure also includes some less obvious components, e.g. providing transport for people to reach eye units, or places for them to stay if they come for trachoma or cataract surgery. Infrastructure goes hand in hand with the human resources development discussed above, as sparkling new clinics and operating theatres are useless without healthcare professionals to work in them.

Mobile services: campaigns and outreach surgery

The infrastructure may also require the use of mobile eye care provision. This can take the form of specifically organised campaigns or outreach activity that comes from a larger clinic or health centre. It can be advantageous to take the service closer to the patient for several reasons:

- Some patients are unable to travel to the permanent clinic because of infirmity, illness, transport costs, lack of an accompanying person or responsibilities that they cannot leave such as childcare. Women particularly are often less able to access more distant healthcare.

- Providing intensive treatment can help to get the best use out of limited staff and resources, as it can allow a large number of people coming for treatment in a short period of time.

There are numerous examples of the success of taking the treatment to the community, e.g. the uptake of trachoma surgery is much higher if the surgery is taken to the villages than when it is done in health centres and hospitals. Similarly mass vaccinations or vitamin A supplement campaigns reach many more people when they are taken to the community. The vertical campaign model of healthcare is often not sustainable. However, outreach that is organised in a pre-existing health centre or hospital and uses the local staff, can be extremely effective, entirely sustainable and still fit within the 'normal health system'.

Technology

Eye care requires specific and sometimes expensive equipment. Good eye care planning and services depend on the appropriate equipment being supplied, serviced and kept up-to-date. This equipment needs to be of high quality, but affordable and durable. In a community clinic, torches, log books and simple stationary may be enough for some screening programmes, while in a hospital surgical equipment and even lasers may be required. Health care and medical treatment is becoming more and more sophisticated and tech nologically advanced. This is particularly true in ophthalmology where there have been major advances in technology in three particular areas:

- *Lasers:* many different lasers are used in ophthalmology. They are now used extensively to treat retinal disease, glaucoma, after cataract surgery and in corneal surgery.
- *Microsurgery:* since the widespread usage of the operating microscope and fibre optic illumination, intraocular surgery is now performed with much finer instruments and through small incisions. The equipment required for cataract and retinal surgery has changed dramatically, particularly if the phacoemulsification cataract extraction procedure is used, which uses a complicated, expensive machine that requires regular maintenance.
- *Diagnostic techniques:* the diagnosis of eye conditions has been revolutionised by new equipment, such as automated visual field screening for glaucoma, ocular coherence tomography for macular degeneration and diabetic macular disease, ultrasonography for intra-ocular disease and computerised tomography (CT) scanning and magnetic resonance imaging (MRI) for assessing the orbit, optic nerve and brain.

Unfortunately, all this technology is very expensive and even rich countries are finding that they must put cash limits on health care.

There is a difficult and sometimes insoluble balance to be found between the needs of individual patients and doctors, who want the very best and most modern equipment; and the cost of running a whole health system, which needs to provide care and preventive measures to as many people as possible. Apart from the cost, modern equipment has other disadvantages:

- It requires servicing, which can usually only be done by a specialist technician, who often works for the company that made or installed the equipment. Servicing is expensive and often difficult to access.
- Machines that break down are usually difficult to repair.
- Some machines require a lot of skill and training to use and then interpret the results.
- It is often doctors who are trained to do this, and therefore lots of modern equipment is very 'doctor intensive'.

Ophthalmologists are like all professional people, they want to be up-to-date with the most recent techniques and have the most modern equipment. However, this can make them 'blind' to the real needs of the community. Although this does happen in rich countries, it is a much bigger problem in poor countries where there is a huge gap between sophisticated care that is available in the big cities and the lack of access to care of many poor patients in rural areas.

Fortunately in some poor countries, low cost, high quality technology is being developed and produced locally. Perhaps the best example of this is intraocular lenses used during cataract surgery. Until recently, these were only made in factories in the Western World and were very expensive and therefore not accessible to the average citizen of a poor country. They are now made in factories in developing countries, where they cost a fraction of those made in the rich countries and are of similar quality. This has had the further benefit of forcing 'Western' manufacturers to reduce their prices. Other examples are eye drops and ointment which can be made in a small hospital pharmacy for a fraction of their commercial price.

Cost effectiveness

Any programme of health care must be cost effective to be of value to poor people. Reducing the cost while maintaining the quality is one of the biggest challenges of health care in poor countries. People often think that cheap medical care is bad medical care. There are indeed a few techniques which need expensive equipment and take a long time to perform. However, most eye problems can be treated simply, quickly and effectively using relatively unsophisticated equipment. It should be possible to provide an eye care service that even the poorest people can afford. Indeed, all the major causes of preventable world blindness, with the exception of diabetic retinopathy, are either treatable or preventable at very reasonable cost. Often the biggest challenge and greatest expense of healthcare in poor countries is not the cost of the actual treatment, but the cost of providing a nationwide service and reaching people in remote, rural areas.

There are now many excellent hospitals in the world which are outstanding examples of how to provide reasonable quality services at much reduced costs. There are various models of hospitals and programmes that are providing cost-effective care. Although each model is different they all seem to follow the same principles:

- They see large numbers of patients which lowers the unit cost for each patient, so that the more work that is done, the cheaper it becomes.
- They are not run for profit, and patients who can pay little or nothing are not discriminated against or turned away.
- All patients receive the same treatment. Some hospitals and clinics use a 'cost recovery' system in which patients who can afford to pay for some or all of their treatment, do pay. Although they receive the same treatment as other non-paying patients, they may receive some benefits such as better accommodation. Some units can be completely financially self-sufficient with this system.
- The cost of hospital equipment and medication has been greatly reduced by manufacturers based in poor countries, in particular, India and China.

Geographical variations in disease

In rich countries, there is a fairly similar pattern of eye disease throughout the country. There may be some racial differences but overall the blindness rates are fairly similar. However, in poor countries there may be quite marked differences in diseases between one area and another. The following are some examples of this:

- **Trachoma** is common all over the tropics. However, it is much more severe and disabling in dry, desert areas with many flies, than in the tropical rain forests. Some poor countries are almost free of trachoma, while others are seriously affected.
- **Xerophthalmia and corneal ulcers** in children varies widely depending on the local dietary habits and intake and even customs like how early babies are weaned.
- **Onchocerciasis** used to be very common in the Savannah Belt of West Africa with many people blind but was much less common in the coastal areas. Much of this has changed, thanks to the onchocerciasis control program, but there are still pockets of active disease, causing blindness throughout Africa.

Because eye diseases can vary so much from area to area, any plans for treatment and prevention must be carefully planned and flexible. For example, in xerophthalmia causing corneal ulceration and blindness in young children, it may be appropriate to solve this problem by nutritional advice in one area, adding vitamin A to the food in another and measles vaccination in yet another.

Rehabilitation

When a patient is visually impaired or blind and no treatment is possible, many health practitioners feel that this is the end of their responsibility and there is little more they can do. However, for the patient it means the beginning of a new and very difficult period in their life and they need all the help, support and encouragement that are available. With appropriate support and low vision aids, a severely visually impaired person can have a full working, home and social life. But without these, they can easily become a recluse. It is a responsibility of the health practitioner who sees the blind or visually impaired patient, to help them access any support that is available to them. Most countries have some sort of low vision and rehabilitation for blind or visually impaired people. These are usually run by appropriately trained staff. In rich countries, these services are usually very effective and allow the patient to get vision aids, improvements in their home, and social security benefits. However in poor countries there are many more blind people, a great shortage of trained rehabilitation care workers and of equipment for aiding people with sight loss.

There are three words with a slightly different meaning that are used to describe people who have difficulty in seeing well: visual impairment, disability and handicap.

- **Visual impairment** refers to the actual loss of vision that has happened to the patient.
- **Disability** refers to what a person is unable to do because they are visually impaired.
- **Handicap** is the personal, social and economic loss that comes because of the disability.

The purpose of rehabilitation is to help the patient to come to terms with their visual impairment, and to try to overcome and prevent as much as possible the disability and handicap.

Examples of aids and support for people with visual impairment

The United Nations has listed five principles in the care and rehabilitation of disabled people: independence, participation (in society), care, self-fulfilment and dignity. The following are a few examples of what can be done to help people with visual impairment to achieve these goals:

- Visual aids and magnifiers that can help make the best use of the patient's limited vision.
- Training in particular occupations or activities that may help the person become economically self-sufficient and may help them to be busy and engage with other people.
- Mobility training can help people to move around with confidence, and training in skills for living can increase their independence. Without this, one blind person sometimes means that two people are unable to be productive, if the blind person requires someone else in the family to lead him around and look after him.
- Special education can be given to children, even in a normal school. If blind children are educated, they can be expected to continue on to university.
- Social activities can help a blind person to feel valued rather than a helpless outcast.

Relationships with traditional healers

In all communities there are people who treat and attempt to heal patients by traditional methods. There are many different types of traditional healing, such as the use of herbs, homeopathy, or acupuncture or in some cases spiritual methods such as divination. There are also traditional methods of surgery, in particular, the operation of couching for cataract, or other techniques like applying cautery to the skin. Those of us trained in orthodox 'western' medicine tend to be dismissive of these alternative healers. If we have seen children's eyes destroyed by some toxic medication given for conjunctivitis or someone blinded after couching for cataract, we will probably feel both totally opposed to these methods and superior to the traditional healers, with some justification. Modern orthodox medicine is rightly proud of its rigorous training and scientific method. However, we need to look realistically at the whole situation.

- Traditional and alternative medical practice is carried out throughout the world including in rich countries, where there are many alternative types of healers. Many patients throughout the world therefore have great faith in traditional healers. For some traditional healers, their main motive may be to extract money from their patients. However, there are many more who have a genuine concern to help, and may feel a sense of vocation in their work. Remember, there are also quite a lot of orthodox medical practitioners whose main motive is also to extract money from their patients.
- The methods and principles used by different traditional healers are very varied. They range from barbaric and unsafe procedures, to innocuous but harmless procedures, to safe, sensible practices that may be better than anything that is locally available, particularly in places with no or very poor 'Western' medical services.
- Some traditional healers also dispense conventional 'Western' medicine. For example, there are many healers who sensibly use chloramphenicol ointment for conjunctivitis. Develop a good relationship with the local healer as early as possible and do not to ignore or oppose them. One example was when a doctor befriended some traditional healers, and gained their interest by showing them a cataract operation. He then tactfully explained to them what damage could happen to the eyes of young children, and then supplied them with unlabelled bottles of chloramphenicol drops to use instead of toxic herbs in sick children with bad eyes.
- There is often religious and spiritual significance to disease, particularly in Africa. Although some people may disapprove of this, it is very important to patients in many cultures.
- Most traditional medical practitioners are much closer to the community than the orthodox medical professionals, and they are much more readily available. For example, in India there are many homeopathic and Ayurveda practitioners in the villages and small towns, but doctors are usually only to be found in larger towns and cities. In Africa, the traditional healer is often the only source of any 'treatment' for many people. Furthermore they are usually very well respected in their communities, probably more so than visiting Western practitioners or those working a long way away. It is therefore very important to work with traditional healers and not against them or in competition with them.

- The only way of definitively overcoming the bad practices of the traditional healer is to provide an alternative service. It is therefore important to focus energy on providing a good, safe and available service in poor countries and not on fighting the traditional healers.
- Currently orthodox medicine has many failings and complications, and it must be acknowledged it too is far from perfect.

Increasingly, health workers have tried to encourage communication and co-operation with traditional healers rather than condemnation. One way has been to invite traditional healers into hospitals or clinics or even into operating theatres. The foundation for co-operation is *mutual respect*. Where this has occurred there have been opportunities to learn from traditional healers how local people think of disease and how they react to it. There have also been opportunities to teach traditional healers some of the ideas of modern medicine. Where there has been good co-operation, some traditional healers are happy to refer patients when the problem is beyond them, for instance a blind patient with cataract.

The 'traditional' treatment for cataract, couching, must be discouraged because the results are usually so bad and 'Western' cataract surgery has such successful outcomes. However, couching only persists in areas where modern medicine has been unable to deliver cataract surgery.

The human factor

This chapter is all about generalisations and ideas. It is important to finish by considering the individual blind person and his personal needs. The late founder of the International Agency for the Prevention of Blindness, Sir John Wilson, who was himself blind, said of blindness, 'Only in statistics do people go blind by the millions. Each person goes blind by himself.' Each unnecessarily blind person brings suffering and deprivation to himself or herself and their family. In addition, there is the frustration of being useless and totally dependent on others. It is harder being blind in those parts of the world where there is no education, rehabilitation or social welfare for blind people.

Those of us who care for blind people need to know what it is like to feel their limitations. One eye doctor who runs a training course for ophthalmic medical assistants in Africa makes half the students spend a day wearing blindfolds so as to experience being blind, and the other half to learn how to look after these 'blind' people. The next day, the roles are reversed. Several years ago, patients with certain diseases were treated with eye-pads applied to both eyes and strict bed-rest. Most doctors who tried it for themselves stopped recommending it for their patients, when they realised how unpleasant it was. To go blind may involve more than just loss of quality of life. It often involves loss of actual life itself. Most children who go blind from xerophthalmia do not live long, and it is probable that elderly people who go blind die sooner than those who can see. Occasionally, such patients can have their sight restored with surgery. A patient who has been blind for a year or so is delighted to receive their sight back, but interestingly those who have been blind most of their life often struggle more, often becoming confused and disturbed by the busy world of visual stimuli and some wish they had never had their sight back.

People who have been blind for many years usually adapt to it, and strengthen their other senses. They usually do so with great aptitude and dignity and it is our responsibility as health practitioners to treat them as people and not just as patients.

2

Basic anatomy and physiology of the eye

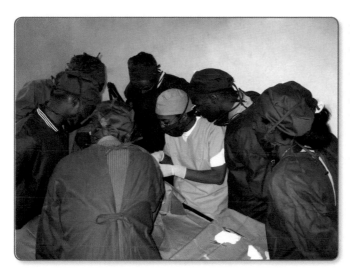

Anatomy is often taught in the classroom, but is best remembered when learnt in the clinic or the operating theatre where its importance and relevance can be appreciated.

The eye is a very complex and detailed organ. Its structure (anatomy) and how it works (physiology) can be divided into several parts:

1. The eyeball itself.
2. Its connection to the brain by the optic nerve.
3. The eyelids, conjunctiva and lacrimal (tear) system which together protect the eye.
4. The extraocular muscles, which control the eye movements.
5. The orbit, which contains and protects all the ocular structures.
6. The blood and nerve supply to all the eye structures.

The eyeball

The eyeball consists of three layers of tissue (**Figure 2.1**):

- An outer protective layer.
- A middle layer of blood vessels, pigment cells and muscle fibres.
- An inner, light-sensitive layer, called the retina.

The outer layer: the sclera and cornea

The outer layer is tough and thick, and is made of collagen fibres. Most of this layer is opaque, and is called the sclera (which means tough in Greek). The anterior part is transparent, so that light can enter the eye. This transparent 'window' is called the cornea.

The cornea itself consists of three main layers (**Figure 2.2**):

1. *The surface epithelium:* this outer layer is 5 or 6 cells thick, and is
    continuous with the epithelium of the conjunctiva at the limbus (the
    area where the cornea meets the sclera). The epithelium is extremely
    sensitive. Pain sensation is important for recovery (desensitised corneas

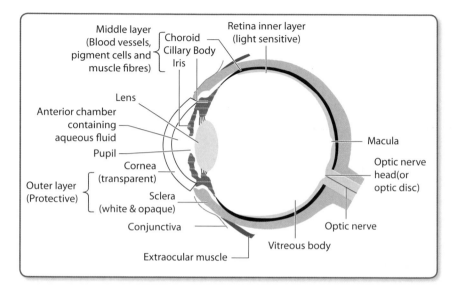

Figure 2.1 The basic structure of the eye, showing its three layers.

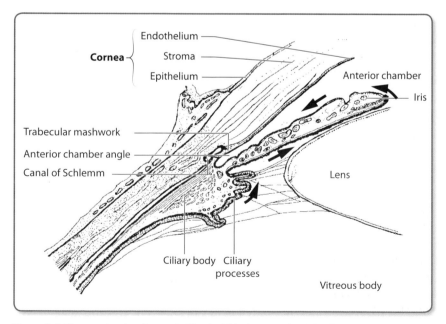

Figure 2.2 The anterior chamber angle. The thick black arrows show the direction of flow of the aqueous fluid.

do not recover well from injury or infection) and for warning that the eye has a problem and therefore protective action is required such as blinking, tear production or avoidance of the provoking agent. At the limbus there are special 'stem cells' from which new epithelial cells are generated. These epithelial cells spread and migrate on to the surface of the cornea where they are constantly being shed and replaced by new cells. The limbus is an important area in an eye that has had the epithelium damaged by a chemical injury; if the limbus is undamaged, the corneal epithelium will heal quickly, but if the limbus is badly damaged by the chemical, the corneal epithelium may not recover and the cornea may become opaque.

2. *The stroma:* this thick, tough layer forms the bulk of the cornea. The stroma consists of specialised collagen fibres, which are arranged in a regular pattern to make them transparent.
   i.   The anterior layer of the stroma is called 'Bowman's membrane' and is a special supporting membrane for the epithelium.
   ii. The posterior layer of the stroma is called 'Descemet's membrane', and is a tough supporting membrane for the endothelium.
3. *The endothelium:* lines the inner surface of the cornea. A single layer of very active cells which transfer fluid out of the stroma into the anterior chamber of the eye, keeping the cornea dehydrated. If these cells are not functioning properly, the cornea swells and becomes oedematous impairing vision.

The middle layer – the iris, ciliary body and choroid

If the outer layer of the eyeball is peeled away, the middle layer appears black, soft and round like a grape and is therefore also known as the uveal layer (uvea is from the Latin word for a grape). The uvea consists of three parts: the iris, the ciliary body, and the choroid. All three parts contain many pigment cells, which absorb light. The iris and ciliary body also contain smooth muscle fibres that are controlled by the autonomic (involuntary) nervous system. All of the uvea has a good blood supply, but particularly the choroid, which is made up almost entirely of blood vessels that supply the outer retina.

The iris

The iris is a ring of smooth muscle fibres with pigment cells (**Figure 2.1** and **2.2**). These form a circular sphincter muscle. When the muscle contracts the pupil constricts and when the muscle relaxes the pupil dilates. This allows the amount of light entering the eye to be controlled. The constrictor muscles are controlled by the parasympathetic system via the oculomotor nerve. Therefore, some very serious neurological problems such as an expanding cerebral aneurysm pressing on this nerve can present with a dilated pupil. The iris also has some dilator fibres, which are supplied by the sympathetic nervous system via the cervical sympathetic nerves and the carotid plexus. Therefore, if someone is excited or scared, their pupils dilate, because their sympathetic nervous system ('the flight or fight' system) is more active.

The ciliary body

The ciliary body is a ring of tissue around the eye (**Figure 2.1** and **2.2**). It contains smooth muscle and ciliary processes, and it is attached to the lens by numerous fine fibres (zonules), collectively called the suspensory ligament. The ciliary body has two main functions:

1. Accommodation: when the smooth muscle of ciliary body contracts, the lens becomes more round in shape and therefore increases its focusing power (see page 104).
2. Aqueous fluid production: the ciliary processes have a large surface area and are covered by ciliary epithelium, which produce aqueous fluid (this is traditionally called aqueous humour).

The choroid

The choroid consists mainly of blood vessels and pigment cells (**Figures 2.1** and **2.3**). It lies next to the retina and is separated from it by a thin elastic membrane called Bruch's membrane. The many blood vessels in the choroid form a fine capillary network called the choriocapillaris. The choroid has two main functions:

1. Blood supply to the outer retina. The choroid supplies two thirds of the retina's oxygen by diffusion across Bruch's membrane.

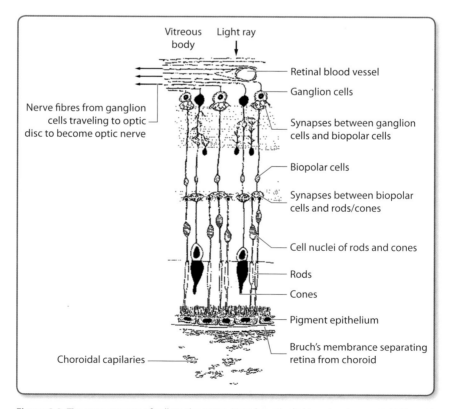

Figure 2.3 The arrangement of cells in the retina. Note how the light ray has to pass right through the entire retina before reaching the light-sensitive rods and cones.

2. The pigment cells absorb light inside the eye, which prevents unwanted reflections.

The inner layer – the retina

The retina is the light sensitive membrane at the back of the eye (**Figures 2.1 and 2.3**). The main function of the retina is to turn light into electrical impulses that go down the optic nerve to the visual centres in the brain where they are interpreted as the world we see. The cells of the retina are specialised, and have a very complex arrangement. On the outer surface, next to the choroid, is a single layer of pigment epithelial cells. The light sensitive cells, the rods and cones, rest on this layer. The rods are more sensitive in dim light, and these are more concentrated in the periphery of the retina. The cones are more sensitive in bright light, and these are more concentrated towards the centre of the retina. The central area of the retina is called the 'macula'. The macula consists of closely packed cone cells. The very centre of the macula is called the 'fovea'. The fovea is thinner than the rest of the retina, so that there are less layers of retina for light to pass through to reach the cones that are responsible for our central and sharpest vision (**Figure 2.4**).

The inner layers of the retina consist of the bipolar and ganglion cells, as well as their nerve fibres and synapses. The synapse is the name for the junction between one nerve cell and another. When light enters the eye it passes through the transparent layers of the retina to reach the rods and cones. These produce electrical impulses when they are exposed to light. This electrical impulse passes across a synapse to the bipolar cells, and from there it crosses another synapse to the ganglion cell. The bipolar and ganglion cells and their synapses relay and modify these electrical impulses.

The nerve fibres from the ganglion cells travel on the surface of the retina to the optic disc, where they acquire a myelin sheath and unite to form the optic nerve. The optic nerve then passes backwards through the sclera towards the brain. The retinal blood vessels also enter the eye at the optic disc and run on the surface of the nerve fibre layer. They provide oxygen for the inner layers of the retina.

The lens and the vitreous body

The lens consists of closely packed transparent cells enclosed in a capsule (**Figures 2.1 and 2.2**). The capsule is attached to the fibres of the suspensory ligament, which holds the lens in place. The lens and the cornea together

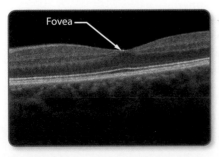

Figure 2.4 Ocular coherence scan of a normal macula and fovea. This is a very technologically advanced instrument that will not be available in many parts of the world. However, we have included this scan to show how the normal retina is very thin at the fovea to allow as much light as possible through.

focus the light on the retina. Four-fifths of the focussing power of the eye comes from the cornea and only one-fifth from the lens. Behind the lens is the vitreous body (**Figure 2.1**). This is an inert, transparent jelly, which fills most of the eye. The vitreous is adherent to the retina behind it for most of our life, but separates as we get older. However, if it is too adherent, this separation can cause a retinal tear or detachment if it fails to separate. The vitreous does not have any known function in the fully-grown eye and is frequently removed during retinal surgery without adverse effect.

The aqueous fluid and the intraocular pressure

The aqueous fluid is secreted by the epithelial cells of the ciliary processes on the surface of the ciliary body (**Figure 2.2**). This fluid passes between the iris and the lens, and enters the anterior chamber of the eye. It is absorbed from the angle of the anterior chamber where the iris meets the back of the cornea, where there is some complex, sponge-like tissue called the trabecular meshwork. The aqueous fluid passes through this meshwork by a mechanism called active transport into a collecting channel called the 'canal of Schlemm'. From here it passes into the small veins on the surface of the eye. The balance between the production and drainage of the aqueous controls the pressure in the eye. If the aqueous fluid does not drain away properly, there is a rise in the intraocular pressure. This can damage the optic nerve, i.e. glaucoma (see Chapter 15).

The visual pathways

The visual pathways connect the optic nerve with the part of the brain concerned with vision. This is the occipital part of the cerebral cortex (**Figure 2.5**). The optic nerve is not really a nerve, but a tract of the central nervous system. Therefore, a sheath of dura that contains cerebrospinal fluid surrounds it. It is also unable to regenerate after damage, because there are no Schwann cells (these are responsible for the regeneration of damaged nerves) or neurilemma around the individual fibres.

The optic nerve passes backwards from the eye to the apex of the orbit then through the optic foramen into the skull. Inside the skull, the two optic nerves meet at the optic chiasm, just above the pituitary fossa, to form the optic tracts. The optic tracts then pass round the brainstem to the lateral geniculate body, where all the fibres from the optic tract synapse with different nerve cells. The fibres from these cells then pass in the optic radiations to the occipital cortex at the posterior end of the cerebral hemisphere.

When both optic nerves meet at the chiasm, all the fibres from the nasal part of each retina cross over to the opposite side. In this way, everything in the left half of the field of vision in each eye is seen on the right side of each retina, and by the right side of the brain (blue lines in **Figure 2.5**). In the same way, everything in the right half of the field of vision in each eye is seen by the left side of the brain (red lines in **Figure 2.5**).

A few fibres in the optic nerve regulate the pupil size. After leaving the chiasm, they take a different route to the 'vision' fibres. They pass to the brain-

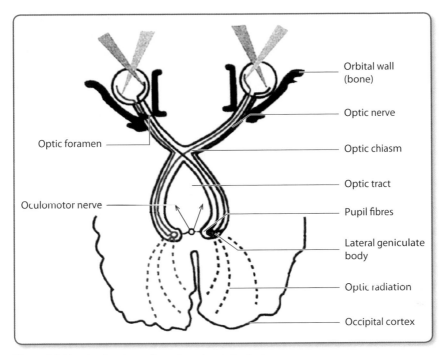

Figure 2.5 The visual pathways from the retina to the brain.

stem. Here they connect with the nucleus of the oculomotor nerve, which controls the size of the pupil and the process of accommodation. The pupil light reflexes are described on page 69.

The protection of the eyeball

The conjunctiva, the eyelids and the lacrimal apparatus protect the eye from injury and infection. They also keep the cornea healthy, moist and transparent.

The conjunctiva

The conjunctiva is a thin mucous membrane that lines the inner surface of the eyelids and the outer surface of the eyeball (**Figure 2.6**). The part lining the eyelids is called the 'tarsal conjunctiva', and it is firmly attached to the underlying tarsal plate. The part lining the eyeball is called the 'bulbar conjunctiva', but it is only loosely attached to the underlying sclera. The tarsal and bulbar conjunctiva are continuous with each other at the fornix.

The conjunctival epithelium is continuous with the corneal epithelium at the margin of the cornea (the limbus).

Beneath the epithelial surface, the conjunctiva contains many small islands of lymphoid tissue especially in the fornix, and many goblet cells, which secrete mucus. The main function of the conjunctiva is to protect the cornea. It does this in three ways:

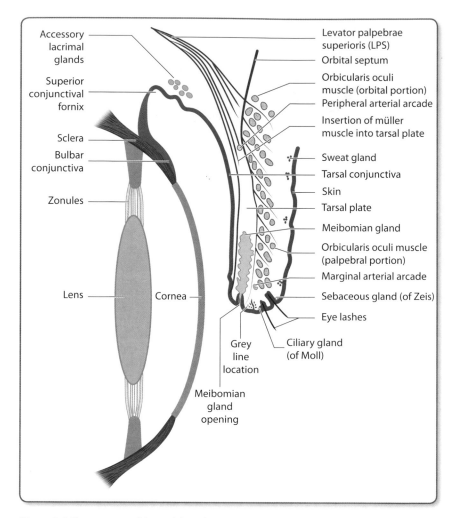

Figure 2.6 The structure of the eyelids and conjunctiva.

1. Supplying oxygen and other important substances to the cornea, particularly when the eyelids are shut.
2. Producing the mucin part of tears, which lubricate the cornea.
3. Helping to protect the cornea from infection. Conjunctival secretions contain antibodies and lymphocytes to fight against specific infections. The secretions also contain lysozyme, which is a nonspecific, antibacterial substance. For these reasons the conjunctiva has been described as a 'lymph node, cut open and lined with epithelium'.

The eyelids

The eyelids (**Figure 2.6**) protect the eye and keep the cornea healthy and moist. They work rather like car windscreen wipers: each time a person blinks, the tear film is spread across the surface of the cornea. The upper eyelid moves more than the lower eyelid and covers more of the cornea with each blink. Therefore diseases of the upper eyelid are more likely to affect the cornea.

The tarsal plate is a fibrous structure which keeps the eyelids rigid, and contains the Meibomian glands. These glands open out at the lid margin, and make a waxy, oily secretion which helps to form the corneal tear film. The conjunctiva lines the posterior surface of the tarsal plate. The orbicularis oculi muscle fibres are above and in front of the tarsal plate. The seventh cranial (or facial) nerve stimulates this muscle to close the eyelids. The levator muscle is also attached to the tarsal plate of the upper lid. This muscle opens the eyelids, and is supplied by the third cranial nerve. The eyelids have a very good blood supply, and the eyelid skin is very fine and very loose. There is a small muscle (Müller's muscle) behind the levator muscle that helps to lift the lid and is supplied by the sympathetic nervous system. The eyelashes are specialized hairs, and there are numerous sweat and sebaceous glands near their roots.

The lacrimal apparatus

The 'lacrimal apparatus' refers to all the structures around the eye that are required to produce and drain tears (**Figure 2.7**). The tears form a thin film of fluid on the surface of the conjunctiva and cornea. This tear film is vital for the health and transparency of the cornea. Tears are surprisingly complex and contain mucus (from the conjunctival goblet cells), fluid (from the lacrimal gland) and oil (from the Meibomian glands). If there is a problem

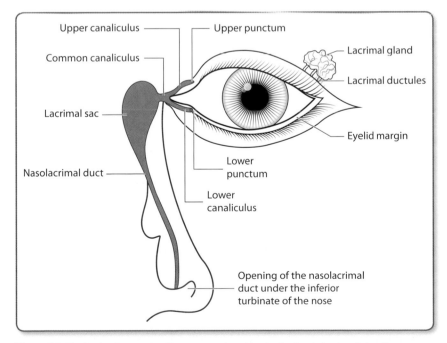

Figure 2.7 The lacrimal apparatus. Tears are produced by the lacrimal gland and they flow across the eye and drain through the puncti.

with any of these three production mechanisms, the tears will be of poor quality and may not protect the cornea adequately. Severe conjunctival scarring, such as in trachoma, damages conjunctival goblet cell mucin production, while autoimmune diseases, such as Sjögren syndrome, damage lacrimal gland aqueous production and severe rosacea and blepharitis affects Meibomian gland oil production.

The lacrimal gland only produces excessive tears in response to injury, inflammation or emotional stress. Normally, the resting production of tears comes mainly from the conjunctiva and small accessory lacrimal glands in the conjunctival fornix.

The tears drain into the nose through the nasolacrimal drainage system (**Figure 2.7**). The beginning of this is the punctum, which is a tiny opening at the inner end of each eyelid (i.e. there are two puncti on each eyelid). A narrow canaliculus passes from the punctum. The upper and lower canaliculi join to make the common canaliculus from where tears then drain into the lacrimal sac, and then down the nasolacrimal duct into the nose. Opening and closing the eyelids helps to 'milk' the tears through the system.

The extraocular muscles

There are six extraocular muscles, which control eye movement (**Figure 2.8**). They form a cone that passes backwards from the eye to the apex of the orbit. The actions of these muscles are rather complex, but do make sense if you think carefully about where the muscles comes from and goes to on the eyeball and what would happen if it contracts (shortens). There are four

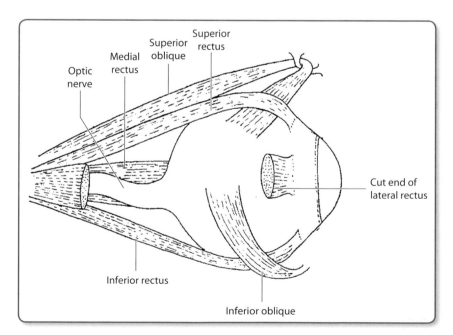

Figure 2.8 Lateral view of the extraocular muscles in the orbit. The lateral rectus muscle has been partly removed to show the optic nerve and the medial rectus muscle.

recti (lateral, medial, superior and inferior) and two oblique muscles (superior and inferior). The four recti muscles originate from the annulus of Zinn at the apex of the orbit around the optic nerve. The superior oblique muscle originates from the lesser wing of sphenoid in the posterior part of the roof of the orbit. The inferior oblique muscle originates from the antero-medial part of the maxillary bone in the floor of the orbit. All the muscles insert into the sclera of the globe, but the recti insert anterior to the equator while the obliques insert posterior to it.

The primary action of each of the recti muscles is straightforward, as they move the eyeball in the predicted direction (superior rectus moves the eye up, inferior down, etc.). However, the oblique muscles are more complicated. Remember that as they insert *posterior* to the equator, they will rotate the globe the opposite way to that which you would expect, i.e. superior oblique downwards, inferior oblique upwards. Secondly as they attach to the globe at an angle they have significant torsional effect, with the superior oblique turning the eye inwards (towards the nose, incyclotorsion) and the inferior oblique outwards (away from the nose, excyclotorsion). The main movements are discussed in Chapter 18 (page 436, Figure 18.1 and Table 18.1).

The orbit

The orbit is a bony cavity, which encloses the eye and its surrounding structures. The front of the orbit is thick, strong bone which protects the eye from injury. It is easy to feel this bone under the skin of the cheek and the eyebrow. The walls of the orbit that separate the orbital contents from the nasal sinuses are however, very thin bone (**Figure 2.9**). For this reason, nasal sinus disease occasionally spreads into the orbit, which can create severe and dangerous infections in the orbit. The floor of the orbit is also thinner, and is sometimes fractured by a punch to the eye (see Chapter 21).

The blood and nerve supply and lymphatic drainage of the eye and orbit

The blood supply to the eye and orbit comes from the ophthalmic artery. This is a branch of the internal carotid artery and enters the apex of the orbit through the superior orbital fissure. It breaks up into several branches, which supply the extraocular tissues. The blood supply to the eye itself comes from three sources:

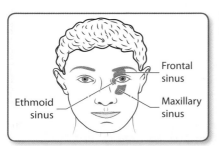

Figure 2.9 The position of the nasal sinuses in relation to the eye and orbit.

Frontal sinus

Ethmoid sinus

Maxillary sinus

1. A single retinal artery, which enters the eye with the optic nerve and supplies the inner retina.
2. The choroidal arteries, which pierce the sclera to supply the choroid and outer retina.
3. The anterior ciliary arteries, which come from the smaller arteries supplying the extraocular muscles. They enter the eye where the muscles are inserted into the sclera, and supply the iris and ciliary body.

The venous drainage from the retina passes into the retinal vein from the choroid and into the vortex veins. These drain into the orbital veins (superior and inferior ophthalmic veins), which go mostly through the superior orbital fissure to the cavernous sinus at the base of the brain.

There are no lymph vessels inside the eye. The lymphatic drainage of the eyelids and conjunctiva is mostly to the preauricular lymph node in front of the ear.

The sensory nerve supply to the eye and all the structures of the orbit comes from the ophthalmic division of the fifth (trigeminal) nerve. It enters the orbit through the superior orbital fissure and breaks up into branches that also supply sensation to the scalp and the side of the nose. The retina is, of course, connected to the optic nerve but there are no sensory or pain fibres in the retina. The extraocular muscles have their own motor nerve supply (see page 443).

3 Clinical methods: history taking and eye examination

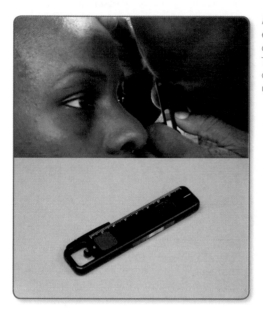

A careful and thorough history and examination is the key to making a diagnosis and treating your patient. This very low cost solar powered ophthalmoscope and loupe is being used to examine the retina.

The clinical assessment is fundamental for making the correct diagnosis and management plan. There are three major steps in assessing a patient:

1. **Take the patient's history.** This is the process of asking the patient about their symptoms and other issues that may be associated with the symptoms. Simple history-taking can be fairly straightforward, and you will learn how to ask the right questions with time and practice. Experienced eye care workers can often work out the diagnosis from just the history alone.

2. **Examine the patient.** There are several parts to an ophthalmic examination. Some are obligatory for all patients, others will depend on the symptoms and signs that are found:

    i.   *Test the vision:* this seems obvious and essential when assessing a patient with an eye problem. However, it is surprisingly frequently forgotten. The vision should be tested in both eyes with and without pinhole. Sometimes an assistant may test this, before the history is taken. Vision testing is fairly straightforward with a little bit of training and practice, except in young children which can be very challenging and skill and patience will make a great difference.

    ii. *Examine the eyes:* this is the most important part of the assessment. It is also the most difficult, and having good diagnostic equipment is essential for many eye conditions.

    iii. *Examine the rest of the patient:* in certain eye conditions it is very important to examine the rest of the patient. For example patients with tuberculous eye disease or inflammatory eye disease may have serious and even life-threatening disease elsewhere in their body.

3. **Special investigations.** The nature of the eye condition and the available resources determine what further investigations should or can be done. Investigations that might be appropriate include scans (e.g. X-rays, CT scans, MRI), blood tests and microbiological and histopathological examination of samples. Most diagnoses can be made without special investigations, which is a great advantage where good laboratory services are unavailable or very expensive. However for neurological disease or orbital disease imaging is often vital, and for infectious eye disease a good bacteriological laboratory will make a big difference in identifying the exact cause.

History-taking

History-taking is basically a conversation between the health worker and the patient. Good communication skills are needed to make the consultation as effective as possible. These skills should be taught to all health care students and assessed during the training and supervision of students and health care practitioners. If patients feel they can trust the person examining them and that they are really being heard sympathetically, they are much more likely to reveal all the facts and background about their complaint. Interestingly they are also more likely to be happy with the outcomes of any future treatment, even if the treatment is not successful. There are unfortunately many barriers to good communication with the patient:

- *Language:* The patient and health worker may not share a common language. Even if health-practitioners speak the same language, patients are often confused by the medical terminology, jargon and poor explanations.
- *Time:* There may not be time to allow the patient to say all he or she wants in order to feel respected and listened to.
- *Training:* Many healthcare workers are not adequately trained in communication skills and history-taking.
- *Culture and education:* The attitudes and understanding of the patient about symptoms and diseases may be very different from that of the doctor or nurse.
- *A superior attitude:* Sometimes health workers can adopt a superior attitude to the patient, who will then lose confidence and feel frightened or shy.
- *Misleading information:* Even in the best of circumstances, the patient may say what he or she thinks the health practitioner wants to hear rather than telling the truth, or they may be embarrassed about telling the truth.

Initially, health practitioners find that taking a full medical history can be a long and complicated procedure. A student should start by taking a full and detailed history, and with experience one learns what are the important questions to ask the patient and which questions need not be asked in every case. In a busy clinic there is often time for only a very short and simple history. However, in some cases the history is absolutely vital to understanding the case and making the right diagnosis. Good history-taking is an art that takes a long time to learn well. It requires three skills:

- Good communication skills.
- Asking the right questions to guide the patient to give informative answers.
- Listening carefully to the patient's answers, evaluating the answers to determine how reliable and significant they are, and then using the answers to guide the next question.

The structure of history-taking is given in **Box 3.1**. All of the stages of the history-taking aim to determine exactly what the patient is suffering from (the present complaint) and to find out other issues that may be relevant to this. When taking a history you should also be thinking about background information such as the patient's age, occupation and literacy. This information will indicate what vision and treatment the patient needs for work and activities of daily living. For example, a young person of working age is likely to be more affected by their cataract (and want earlier surgery) than an elderly retired person. The occupation is also important because some occupations are associated with specific diseases such as welders suffering corneal damage from the ultraviolet light ('arc eye') if they do not wear protective goggles.

Box 3.1 An outline of history-taking

1. Personal details
   a. Name
   b. Age
   c. Address
2. Present complaint, i.e. in one sentence, what has caused the patient to attend for consultation
3. History of the present complaint, i.e. details and background of the present complaint
4. Personal medical history
   a. Other current or previous medical conditions
   b. Current medication
5. Family history that is relevant to the present complaint.
6. Social history
   a. Occupation
   b. Smoking
   c. Alcohol
   d. Illegal drugs if relevant to the present complaint

Present complaint

There are many possible symptoms of eye disease, but the most important can be grouped under two headings: loss or alteration of vision, and discomfort or pain in the eye.

Loss or alteration of vision

Loss of vision is the most common visual symptom. Ask the patient if the onset was sudden or gradual, if there was any pain at first, and if there is any pain now. Visual loss is usually very obvious to the patient. However, the patient may not be aware of a gradual loss of vision in one eye only, or gradual constriction of the visual field. For example, patients with cataract occasionally present as an emergency with 'sudden loss of vision', but in fact have not noticed the gradual loss of vision until they happen to shut the other eye. Various alterations of vision may occur (**Figure 3.1**)

- *Dazzling or glare:* this is difficulty seeing in bright light. It may be caused by opacities in the cornea or lens.
- *Visual field defects:* these are areas of absent (absolute scotomas) or poor (relative scotomas) sight. They can be central or peripheral and may be caused by various disorders in the retina, optic nerve or visual pathways, especially glaucoma. Central visual field loss is much more likely to be noticed by the patient than peripheral loss. Some patients with severe

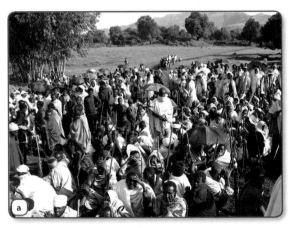

Figure 3.1 A crowd of patients waiting to be seen in a rural health centre. The picture shows how it appears to someone with (a) normal sight, (b) early cataract, (c) macular degeneration, (d) visual field loss from glaucoma

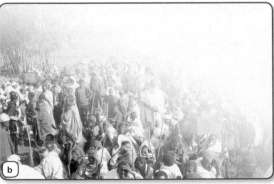

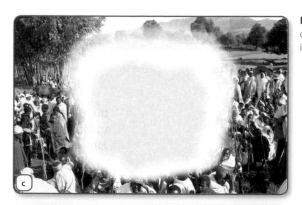

Figure 3.1 *Continued* A crowd of patients waiting to be seen in a rural health centre.

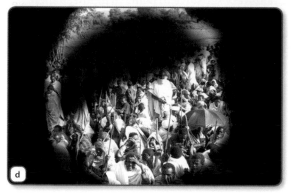

peripheral visual field loss may not complain of any problems but when you question them closely, they may say that they often bump into things or hit things with their shoulders or even with their bicycle handlebars.

- *Photophobia:* this is discomfort caused by bright light. It is usually a sign of inflammatory eye disease or corneal disease, especially corneal ulcer or anterior uveitis (inflammation in the front of the eye). It is sometimes a symptom of anxiety.
- *Distortion:* this is usually described as straight lines appearing to be bent or have a kink in them. It usually indicates a disturbance of the macula of the retina
- *Haloes or rainbow-coloured rings around lights:* these are caused either by early opacities in the lens, or by corneal oedema. Very small drops of fluid in the cornea split white light into the colours of the spectrum. Corneal oedema is usually caused by a rise in intraocular pressure.
- *Floaters:* these are spots or shadows which 'float' in front of the eyes and are usually caused by small opacities in the vitreous body, which cast a shadow on the retina. Patients often describe them as flies or hairs in their vision and that they have tried to wipe them away from in front of their eyes or clean them off their glasses.
- *Diplopia (double vision):* this usually occurs when the two eyes are not pointing in exactly the same direction, i.e. a squint. The squint may be very small and not easy to see without careful examination. This sort

of diplopia disappears when one eye is covered. Occasionally, the two images come from just one eye only (monocular diplopia), i.e. they are both still present when the good eye is shut. This is usually caused by irregularities in the cornea or the lens, which prevent light rays from focussing clearly on the retina.

Discomfort or pain in the eye

Discomfort or pain in the eye is usually a symptom of inflammation of the eye or of the structures surrounding it. The amount of pain can help determine the specific location of the eye problem:

- The conjunctiva is not very sensitive to pain. Typically, conjunctivitis presents with discomfort, irritation or grittiness rather than pain.
- The iris and cornea are both very sensitive to pain. Therefore, if there is moderate or severe pain, diagnoses such as iritis, corneal ulcers and acute glaucoma should be considered.
- Inflammation of the choroid (choroiditis) or optic nerve and other diseases behind the eyeball such as thyroid eye disease, usually produce a sensation of dull pain or ache behind the eye. This is sometimes severe, and is often worse with eye movement.

Eyestrain (asthenopia)

Eyestrain and tiredness of the eyes are common complaints, and the patient may complain of these symptoms on reading, working or studying. Eyestrain is often caused by psychological factors such as anxiety or worry. Eyestrain is very common among students facing difficulties with their studies. If there is an organic cause for eyestrain, it is usually one of the following:

- Poor vision: this causes the patient to struggle hard in order to see properly.
- Refractive error: this causes the image to be out of focus and in some types of refractive error (hypermetropia), the eye strains to try and overcome the blurring. Other refractive errors (typically myopia and astigmatism) cause blurring of vision rather than eyestrain.
- Squint: if the two eyes are not pointing in the same direction, the patient has to make a subconscious adjustment of the muscles moving the eye to avoid double vision. Continual efforts to move one of the eyes to join the images from the two eyes can cause eyestrain. If spectacles are badly fitted the optical centre of the lens may not be in the centre of the visual axis of the eye. This can cause the lens to also have a prismatic effect, causing similar problems to a squint.

Patients with eyestrain must be investigated fully to determine if it is psychological or organic. This can be very time consuming. A vision test and basic eye examination can exclude eye disease. A simple refraction (see chapter 5) can exclude a refractive error and a cover test (see page 445) can exclude an imbalance of the extraocular muscles. If no organic cause for the eyestrain can be found, in ideal circumstances the doctor can spend time trying to resolve the patient's anxieties and worries. A simpler and quicker solution is often to listen carefully to the patient and then reassure them. Some people give patients with eye strain plain spectacles with slightly tinted lenses.

Other symptoms

Discharge

Ocular discharge usually indicates conjunctivitis. The type of discharge can help determine the cause of the conjunctivitis. The following types of ocular discharge are commonly seen:

- Purulent (pus-like): this is suggestive of bacterial conjunctivitis.
- Serous (fluid-like): this is suggestive of viral conjunctivitis or irritation of the eye and conjunctiva.
- Stringy: long strands of white discharge usually occur in allergic eye disease.

Watering (epiphora)

The normal eye produces enough tears to keep it moist but not so wet that it overflows, except occasionally when there is rapid extra production, e.g. in windy, cold conditions, a foreign body in the eye or grief. If excess tearing is continually occurring, it indicates that either the tear drainage passages are blocked or that something is provoking continued excess tearing, e.g. irritation or pain in the eye. Both of these situations require further investigations, including syringing of the nasolacrimal drainage systems and close examination of the lids and conjunctiva to look, e.g. for inturning eyelashes or inflammation.

Headache

This is very common symptom and most people have headaches at times. A specific cause of the headache is not usually found. Migraine headaches are very common. These usually affect one side of the head and may also cause some visual disturbances and nausea during an attack. There are two important reasons for examining the eyes in people with headache:

1. Generalised headache is not usually caused by eye disease. However, pain in and around the eye is often described as headache. It can be caused by eye diseases such as inflammation in or around the eye (uveitis or scleritis), high pressure in the eye (acute glaucoma), or pressure behind the eye, e.g. from thyroid eye disease.
2. Eye examination can help to diagnose some serious brain conditions. Raised intracranial cerebrospinal fluid pressure in the brain causes severe headache. It causes optic nerve swelling (papilloedema), which can be seen on funduscopy and urgent further investigation is required to diagnose and treat this.

Personal medical history and medication

Some systemic diseases like diabetes and hypertension can affect the eyes, and many neurological diseases have ocular complications. You should also specifically ask about previous eye diseases, injuries or treatment. A complete list of the patient's medication (or other people's medication that has been used) including 'traditional medications' must be recorded, as some of these may affect the eyes or sight. For example, excessive quinine usage for malaria treatment can cause retinal damage and some traditional medicines cause serious chemical conjunctivitis and corneal damage.

Family history

Many eye diseases run in families, such as myopia and glaucoma. Members of the same family also share a common environment and are therefore much more likely to develop the same diseases, in particular, infectious eye disease such as tuberculosis and trachoma. In some cultures, consanguinity (both parents are close relatives of each other) is common. This increases the risk of the child having a genetic abnormality.

Social history: diet, alcohol, smoking and occupation

The patient's diet, drinking and smoking habits are sometimes relevant. For example, vitamin A deficiency is associated with severe eye disease (see Chapter 10) and heavy smoking and drinking combined with a poor diet is a cause of optic nerve damage (see Chapter 14).

Examination

Testing the vision

The human eye is an extremely complex organ, and there are many different ways to test the vision. In practice, however, only three types of test are regularly used:
- Visual acuity, which tests if the patient can see small objects or letters in good light directly ahead.
- The visual field, which tests the overall area of vision for each eye.
- Colour vision, which tests if the patient can discriminate between different colours.

All patients attending an eye clinic should have their visual acuity tested. Some patients with particularl clinical presentations will require either visual field or colour vision testing.

Visual acuity

The steps of visual acuity testing are shown in **Box 3.2**. It is important to test the visual acuity in each eye separately, if possible. This is usually measured with a Snellen chart (**Figure 3.2a**), showing either letters, or symbols/pictures for patients who cannot read (**Figure 3.2b**). In some countries, the LogMAR chart is preferred (**Figure 3.2c**). If the vision is very poor, and the patient cannot even see the largest letter on the Snellen chart, other tests can be done. Initially testing of visual acuity can seem a little complicated, but it becomes very quick and straightforward with a bit of practice.

The interpretation of the Snellen visual acuity chart

At the beginning or end of each line is a number, which are usually 60, 36, 24, 18, 12, 9, 6 and 5. This number is the distance (in metres) at which a person with normal sight should be able to see that line when standing at that distance from the chart. For example, if it is a 6 m chart, then a person with normal vision can see the top letter at 60 m, the second line at 36 m, the

Box 3.2a The steps of visual acuity testing in an adult, unaided or best corrected

1. Gently find out if the patient is literate or illiterate and use the appropriate testing chart. If the patient is literate the Snellen or LogMAR letter chart should be used. If the patient is illiterate, the 'tumbling E' chart should be used (**Figure 3.2 a–c**).*

2. Check the distance the chart should be used at and ensure that the patient is standing/sitting so that their head is the correct distance from the chart.

3. *Best corrected right vision*: if the patient has glasses to improve the distance vision, put these on. Cover the left eye. Then ask the patient to read the letters from the top of the chart until they are unable to read any further. Remember that sometimes a patient will make a mistake on one letter of a line, but will be able to continue reading the line beneath. Let them carry on reading, until you are sure they cannot read any more. Look at the reading on the smallest line that they have read. Record this reading. If they have read a letter or two from the line below, record this, as for example 6/9+2 (i.e. the 6/9 line, plus two letters from the line below), or if they read all except one letter of this line, record it as 6/9 – 1 (i.e. the 6/9 line, minus one letter of this line). If the patient is unable to read any of the letters on the chart, try the following tests for poor vision:

   a. Move the patient closer to the chart. For example if the chart is being tested at 6 m then move the patient to 3 m. If the patient can read this line, it is recorded as 3/60 (instead of 6/60 if the test had been done at 6 m)

   b. Counting fingers: ask the patient to tell you how many fingers you are holding up. Record this as CF at x metres (where x is the distance from the patient that you are holding up your fingers). Counting fingers at 1m is approximately equivalent to 1/60 vision.

   c. Hand movements: ask the patient to tell you when they can see you moving your hand and when they think it has stopped moving. Record this as HM at x metres (where x is the distance from the patient that you are moving your hand).

   d. Projection of light†: ask the patient to point to where the light is coming from when you hold up a bright light and direct it towards the patient's eye from each of the four quadrants of the patient's visual field (top right, top left, bottom right, bottom left). Record this as Perception of Light (PL) with projection.

   e. Perception of light†: ask the patient to tell you when you are turning on and off a light. Record this as PL without projection.

4. *Best corrected left vision*, using the same procedure as in (3)

Box 3.2b Testing pinhole vision

1. Hold up a pin-hole occluder which completely covers the left eye and has a cover with pinholes in it in front of the right eye (**Figure 3.3**). Continue testing with the same procedure as above.
2. Pinhole left vision, using the same procedure as above.
3. For people who can read or who do fine close work, the near vision should be tested as well. This is done with a reading chart with increasingly small print.

*The 'tumbling E' is used in the same way as the letter chart, but instead of asking the patient to read the letters, they are asked to point the fingers or sweep the arm in the direction that the horizontal sticks of the E are pointing, e.g. Ш: the patient should sweep their hands upwards, E: the patient should sweep their hands to the right (**Figure 3.2b**).

† Good projection of light indicates that the retina and optic nerve are functioning normally. Therefore, the defect is probably an opacity in the cornea, lens or vitreous body, and is treatable. Poor projection of light indicates retinal or optic nerve disease, and is probably untreatable. Poor projection of light is sometimes abbreviated as 'PL no P'.

---

third line at 24 m and so on. If the patient can only see the top line when they are standing at 6 m, their vision is 6/60. In America and some other countries, the distance is recorded in feet rather than metres; 6/6 is very similar to 20/20, 6/12 is 20/40 and 6/60 is 20/200.

The pinhole test

Any patient with defective visual acuity should be tested again through a pinhole (**Figure 3.3**). This minimises any refractive errors (page 105 explains how the pinhole test works).

- If the visual acuity improves when the patient looks through a pinhole, it usually indicates an error of refraction, which spectacles can correct. An exception to this is that if the patient has some irregularity in the cornea or an early cataract in the lens, the vision will often improve with the pinhole, but cannot be improved with spectacles. However, an improvement in vision with a pinhole does still tell you that the patient's retina and optic nerve are very likely to be healthy.
- If there is no improvement with the pinhole, then the loss of vision is very likely to be from eye disease.

Testing the visual acuity in children

Testing vision in children takes practice, experience and good interactions with the child and their parent. The exact type of test that should be used depends on the age of the child, but some approximate guidelines are given below:

Assessing vision in children from birth to 24 months

There are vision tests for infants (e.g. Keeler cards and Cardiff cards, **Figure 3.4a**). These assess 'preferential looking' in which an infant's gaze is drawn towards a particular image, if their vision is good enough to assess it.

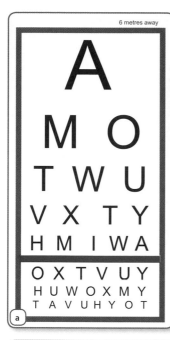

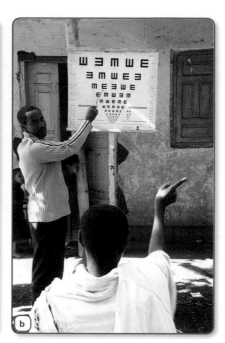

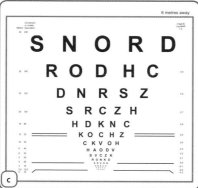

Figure 3.2 Visual acuity testing charts. (a) The Snellen chart. (b) The LogMAR chart for people who cannot read. The patient is asked to point or sweep their hands in the direction of the bars of the E. (c) The LogMAR chart.

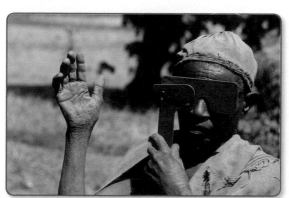

Figure 3.3 Testing the visual acuity through a pinhole. Lots of small pinholes can be seen covering the patient's right eye and the left eye is completely occluded.

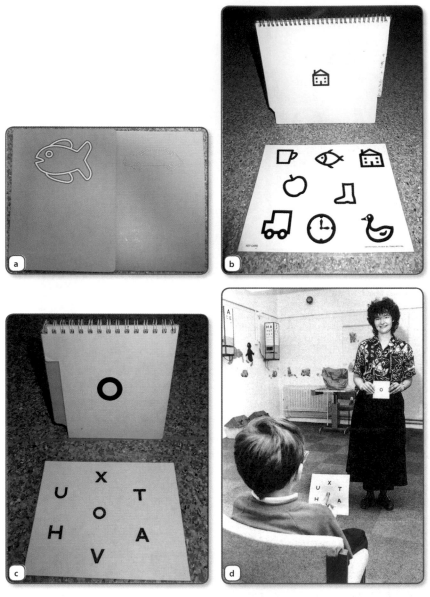

Figure 3.4 Testing children's vision. (a) Cardiff cards for testing children aged 1–3 years with preferential looking. (b) Kay picture cards for testing children aged 2–4 years with picture matching. (c) Sheridan-Gardner cards for testing children aged 3–5 years with letter matching. (d) The Sheridan-Gardner chart being used.

However, even if you do not have access to these tests, you can normally get a good idea about an infant's vision, just by looking at their behaviour and knowing the normal visual behaviour at different ages:

- Birth to 6 weeks: turns head and eyes towards lights.
- 6 weeks to 3 months: makes eye contact.
- 3–6 months: reaches out for large objects and watches moving objects.

- 6–12 months: picks up small objects, e.g. bread crumbs.
- 12–24 months: recognises people at a distance and can see and play with small parts of toys

Testing aged 2–3 years
Most people use Kay picture cards (**Figure 3.4b**). In this test, the child holds a card with pictures on it. The tester holds the test pictures up at the specified distance and the child has to point at the correct picture on their card. The test pictures get smaller and smaller until the child cannot see them.

Testing aged 3–5 years
Sheridan Gardiner cards have letters instead of pictures but are tested in the same way as Kay's picture cards, above (**Figure 3.4c** and **3.4d**).

'Normal' and driving vision
6/6 vision is considered normal. A visual acuity of 6/12 is generally good enough to hold a driving licence (although in some countries this has been converted to seeing a car licence plate at 20 m), and 6/18 or better is adequate for most ordinary tasks in life. A patient with less than 3/60 vision will have great difficulty doing any work which requires vision, and is usually considered 'blind'. However, if the visual field is good, he or she may still be able to get around and lead an independent life.

Blindness and low vision
The definitions of low vision and blindness are based on arbitrary cut offs. At present the WHO defines blindness as vision of less than 3/60 in the better eye and low vision of between 6/18 and 3/60 in the better eye. However, in reality, because other factors such as lighting and visual field are also so important for vision, some people can be virtually blind with 6/60 vision while other people can cope remarkably well.

The visual field
The visual field is not routinely tested in all patients. However, it is should be tested in any patient with suspected glaucoma, diseases of the optic nerves or visual pathways, and certain retinal diseases. Testing the visual field requires the patient to concentrate, and this is often difficult for children, and for some older or unwell people. In all visual field tests (except the field test for checking eligibility for driving), each eye is tested separately, while the other eye is covered. When covering the patient's eye, always use the palm of the hand, not the fingers because it is possible to see through gaps in between the fingers (**Figure 3.5**). If there is any doubt whether the patient might be looking through the other eye, an occlusive patch can be used to cover the eye.

There are several methods of testing the visual field. These are broadly divided into two types of test:
1. Kinetic tests in which a target is gradually moved from the peripheral visual field towards the centre. The most widely used kinetic tests are the basic confrontation visual field test, the Bjerrum screen and the Goldman visual field test.
2. Static tests in which the target appears in locations in the visual field and the patient has to indicate when they can see it. This testing is

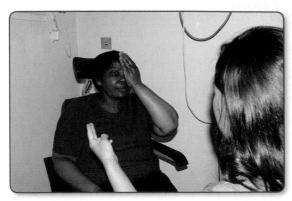

Figure 3.5 Testing the visual field by confrontation. The patient looks straight at the examiner with one eye and covers the other eye, indicating when she can see the examiner's fingers. Make sure your fingers are half way between your head and the patient's head.

usually done with expensive visual field machines, the most widely used of which is called the Humphrey visual field test.

Confrontation visual field testing (Figure 3.5)

Visual field testing machines will not be available in most clinics in poor countries. Therefore, you should know how to perform a good confrontation visual field test. This test does not require any special equipment. It is very simple to perform, but does require practice to be able to reliably detect visual field defects particularly in elderly or unwell patients. It will only detect large visual field defects. The basic principle of the test is to compare the patient's visual field with the examiner's. The steps of the test are given in **Box 3.3**.

Box 3.3 Confrontation visual field testing

1. The patient and examiner sit down facing each other. Their eyes should be at the same level and they should be close to each other, with knees almost touching.
2. Test the patient's right eye first; ask the patient to cover their left eye. The examiner must cover their right eye. Ask the patient to look straight into your left eye, and ensure that they continue to do this throughout the test.
3. Stretch your arm out to one of the four quadrants (top left, top right, bottom left, bottom right) and start wiggling your finger. Slowly move your hand diagonally inwards towards the centre and ask the patient to tell you when they can see your wiggling finger. Make sure your fingers are half way between your head and the patient's head. You must remember to move your hand slowly otherwise you will miss field defects. If you are unsure whether the patient understands and is complying with the test, you can also stop and start wiggling your finger and ask the patient to tell you when this happens. During this test you can compare the patient's visual field to your own.
4. Test the patient's left eye. Ask them to cover their right eye. You must cover your left eye and ask the patient to look straight at your right eye. Repeat the steps in (3).

The Bjerrum screen (Figure 3.6)

The Bjerrum screen is a calibrated black screen. The patient sits in front of it and looks at the centre of the screen. The examiner moves small white targets and is able to plot a much more accurate visual field than simple confrontation testing.

Automated tests

Various instruments are available which can give a very detailed assessment of the visual field. These are used in specialist units, where technicians and assistants can be trained to use them. The most modern ones are computerised and will do much of the work automatically. However, they are too expensive for general use.

Colour vision

The Ishihara chart is the most widely used test of colour vision (**Figure 3.7**). This is used particularly to detect congenital colour blindness. Colour blindness is not treatable and so detecting it is not often useful for eye care professionals. However, it is tested for certain occupations, which are not safe for colour blind people, such as some electrical jobs, which depend on clearly seeing the different wire colours.

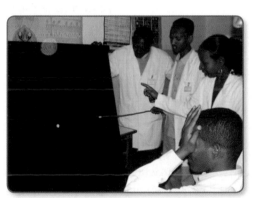

Figure 3.6 A Bjerrum screen. To do this test, the patient, with one eye covered, fixes their gaze on the central white target with the open eye. They have to say whether or not they can see a moving white target at the end of a black stick held by the examiner.

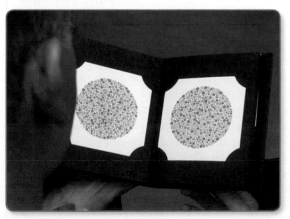

Figure 3.7 Two of the Ishihara colour vision testing cards.

If people develop colour vision impairment, it indicates the presence of disease, most likely of the optic nerve, e.g. optic neuritis or pressure on the optic nerve from orbital masses. The colour vision is often affected before the visual acuity, so it can be a very useful early sign of disease. You do not need to have an Ishihara book test to check for this; a useful and simple test is to compare the colour perception of one eye with another. Just hold a small red target in front of the patient and ask the patient to look at it first with one eye and then the other. If the red appears much less bright in one eye and there is no obvious defect in the ocular media in that eye, then it usually indicates optic nerve disease in that eye.

Examining the eye

Nearly all parts of the eye are visible either with the naked eye, or with an appropriate optical instrument. This is different to almost every other medical speciality, where it is not possible to actually see the places where the pathology occurs, and therefore depends on interpreting other signs or expensive scans. Anyone who cares for eye patients must know how to examine the eye. There is no pain or discomfort from examination and only a few basic instruments are needed. However, the examiner must get very close to the patient who needs to be reassured and relaxed. Ophthalmology, more than any other branch of medicine, depends upon good clinical skills to examine the patient. Good clinical skills depend upon having the right instruments. Some ophthalmic diagnostic instruments are very expensive, but a reasonable examination is possible with only a few simple instruments. There is indeed a great need for simple robust equipment, cheap to produce and distribute to small clinics in less developed countries all over the world. A very low cost, solar powered ophthalmoscope and magnifier has recently been designed and is shown in the picture on the first page of this chapter. **Table 3.1** gives a list of the basic and more advanced equipment used in eye examination. The two most important instruments are the direct ophthalmoscope and the slit lamp. Many readers of this book will not have a full range of instruments and must learn to make do with the limited equipment they possess. It is also very helpful to have a room that can be darkened for examining ophthalmic patients. Ordinary curtains are quite adequate, as the room does not have to be too dark.

Different equipment is required for examining the different parts of the eye:

- *Front of eye* (cornea, conjunctiva, iris, anterior chamber): this requires both a good light and magnification to see fine details. The cornea, conjunctiva and even iris can be clearly seen with a bright torch and loupes for magnification. A slit lamp is required to examine the anterior chamber for the inflammatory changes of uveitis.
- *Middle of eye* (lens and vitreous): the lens is initially examined using an ophthalmoscope, by assessing the red reflex. It can be examined with a slit lamp if available, which can also be used to assess the vitreous.
- *Back of eye* (retina and optic nerve): the standard instrument for this is called an ophthalmoscope. A slit lamp or indirect ophthalmoscope and condensing lens can be used in more specialist eye centres.

Table 3.1 A list of ophthalmic diagnostic equipment separated into those required by non-specialists in rural settings and those required in specialist eye clinics or hospitals	
Basic diagnostic equipment	**Purpose**
Visual acuity chart (Snellen/ LogMAR): letters and/or 'tumbling E'	Testing visual acuity
Children's vision testing chart, e.g. Sheridan Gardner or Kay's picture cards	Testing visual acuity in children
Pinhole viewer	Testing pinhole vision to help determine the cause of the visual loss
Hand torchlight	Examining the front of the eye and the pupil light reflexes
Magnification, e.g. loupes	Better view of the front of the eye
Ophthalmoscope	1. Examining the red reflex for cataracts and other diseases that obstruct light passage to the retina 2. Examining the retina and optic nerve 3. Examining the front of the eye with magnification
Tonometer, e.g. portable Goldman, Schiotz	Measuring the intra-ocular pressure
Bjerrum screen	Assessment of the visual field
Dark room	Most parts of the eye examination are best done with a bright light, but in a dark room
Drops	
Fluorescein dye	1. Examining corneal damage 2. Applanation intraocular pressure measurement
Mydriatic drops	Pupil dilation for examining the lens and the retina
Topical anaesthetic drops, e.g. proxymetacaine, tetracaine or amethocaine	Anaesthetising the surface of the eye for checking the intraocular pressure, performing minor procedures, e.g. removing foreign bodies, and to make examination of painful eyes easier
Advanced diagnostic equipment	**Purpose**
Slit lamp	Detailed examination of the front of the eye
Slit lamp and applanation tonometer	Intraocular pressure measurement
Slit lamp and condensing lens (e.g. 90 or 78 dioptre)	Examining the back of the eye. This gives a three-dimensional view of the optic nerve and retina
Slit lamp and gonioscopic lens	Examining the drainage angle of the anterior chamber and the peripheral retina
Indirect ophthalmoscope	Examining the retina with a three-dimensional view and indentation (pressing on the eye ball to bring the peripheral retina into view), especially for examining for retinal tears and detachment
Automated perimeter	Accurate assessment of the visual field
Retinoscope and trial lens set	Refraction and spectacle prescribing

The direct ophthalmoscope

An ophthalmoscope is a very useful tool (**Figure 3.8**) It is used for examining the back of the eye but can also be used to get a bright magnified view of

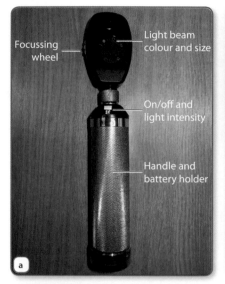
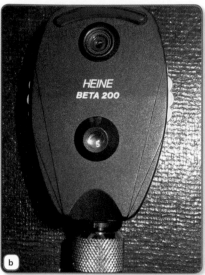

Focussing wheel

Light beam colour and size

On/off and light intensity

Handle and battery holder

HEINE
BETA 200

a

b

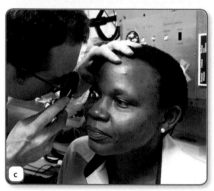

c

Figure 3.8 (a) Parts of the direct ophthalmoscope. (b) Close up of the refractive correction. This ophthalmoscope uses green to indicate a plus lens and red for a minus lens. Some instruments use red for plus and black for minus. (c) Using the ophthalmoscope: the right hand and right eye are used to examine the patient's right eye.

the front of the eye, i.e. *every part of the eye from the front to the back can be examined with an ophthalmoscope.* Even if an ophthalmoscope is not available, do not despair completely. Much useful information can be gained just from examination with a torch, particularly examination of the pupil light responses and examination of the eyelashes and eyelids for diseases such as trachoma.

The principle of the ophthalmoscope is that it illuminates the eye and allows the examiner to look down the same axis as the rays of light entering the patient's eye. In this way, the examiner can see the retina and optic nerve at the back of the patient's eye (the fundus, from the Latin for 'deep'). The patient's own cornea and lens act as a magnifying lens to anyone looking into the eye, and so no extra magnification is necessary. To see the fundus clearly, the ocular media must be transparent, and therefore if there is opacity of the cornea or lens it will not be possible. It is also necessary to dilate the pupil with mydriatic drops. Although with a lot of practice, the fundus will be visible through a constricted pupil, you will get a much clearer and wider view through a dilated pupil. The image of the fundus through the ophthalmoscope is about 15 times larger than its actual size. In a myopic patient, the magnification is greater, and in a hypermetropic patient it is less.

How to use the ophthalmoscope

If the patient wears spectacles, it is best to remove them, and to use a correcting lens in the ophthalmoscope instead. If the examiner wears spectacles, he or she can either keep them on or use a lens of equal power in the ophthalmoscope. The ophthalmoscope must be held very close to the patient's eye, as well as the examiner's. Remember to warn the patient that you will be coming very close to them. The procedure is described in **Box 3.4**.

Box 3.4 How to use an ophthalmoscope

1. Prepare the ophthalmoscope.
a. Start with the focussing wheel (**Figure 3.8a**) at 0. However, if you are wearing spectacles you can take them off and instead put a similar lens in the focussing wheel. If you know the patient's prescription include this as well; this is particularly important if they are aphakic or very myopic. For example, if you are +5 and the patient aphakic, start at approximately + (or green) 15.
b. Check that the size of the light is correct. For a normal dilated examination, this should be the largest circle (without the cross in it).
c. Check that there is no filter, i.e. the light is yellow, not blue or green.
2. Assess the red reflex. Look through the ophthalmoscope at the right eye and then the left eye from approximately 30 cm away. Check that you can see a clear, bright red reflex in both eyes (see Chapter 12 for more information about the red reflex).
3. Examine the patient's right fundus: hold the ophthalmoscope in your right hand, and hold the patient's head still with your left hand (**Figure 3.8c**). Start slightly to the right side of the patient (about 30 degrees) and looking through the ophthalmoscope gradually move closer to the patient's eye, until your right hand is gently touching the patient's cheek, but you are not touching the patient's eye with the ophthalmoscope*. When you can see blood vessels, use your index finger to dial the focussing wheel until the blood vessels are completely in focus, making sure that as you do this, you are not moving away from the patient. Then, look all around the fundus and especially the optic disc. If you are not sure where the optic disc is, remember the branches of the blood vessels point towards the optic disc (**Figure 3.9**).
4. Examine the patient's left eye: repeat step (3), but this time using your left eye and your left hand to hold the ophthalmoscope and your right hand to hold the patient's head.

*An alternative method is to put the ophthalmoscope in approximately the correct position, just in front of the patient's eye with your hand gently resting on their forehead to hold it steady. Then move your eye to the ophthalmoscope and you will only need to make small adjustments in position to see the fundus.

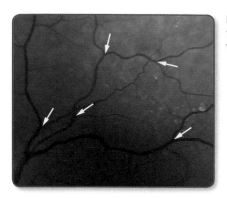

Figure 3.9 By following the retinal vessels in the direction of the white arrows, the optic disc will be reached.

Normally you should be able to see the patient's fundus clearly, with just a few small rotations of the focussing wheel. If you do not get a clear view, it is usually for one of two reasons:

1. The patient has a very large refractive error. Try dialling up a much larger plus or minus lenses in the ophthalmoscope to bring the fundus into focus. If the patient is very myopic it can be particularly difficult to see the fundus clearly. For a myopic patient you must hold the ophthalmoscope very close to the patient's eye as well as using a strong minus lens in the ophthalmoscope.
2. The patient has some opacities in the transparent parts of the eye, i.e. the cornea, lens or vitreous. These should have already been detected when testing for the red reflex (**Box 3.4**).

Other filters and light beams on the ophthalmoscope

Apart from the use of different lenses to focus on the patient's retina, many ophthalmoscopes have various filters that will change the colour or size of the light beam.

- A narrow beam is useful for looking through a small pupil, as it cuts down on the dazzling reflection from the patient's cornea.
- A green (red free) light helps to highlight the retinal blood vessels and any retinal haemorrhages. This can be particularly useful for examination of diabetic retinopathy and retinopathy of prematurity.
- A blue light can be used to show up any staining of the cornea with fluorescein dye.
- Some ophthalmoscopes can project a star or a cross on to the retina, which can help the examiner to see the macula, and to check that the eye is fixing properly.

The indirect ophthalmoscope

Specialists sometimes use a different type of ophthalmoscope, called an 'indirect ophthalmoscope' (**Figure 3.10**). This is a special headlight, which is used with a condensing lens of 20, 28 or 30 dioptres in front of the patient's eye. An indirect ophthalmoscope produces a very clear three-dimensional inverted view of a large area of the fundus, but it takes skill and practice to use it well. It is especially useful in assessing retinal detachments, examining myopic patients and children and for looking through opacities in the ocular media.

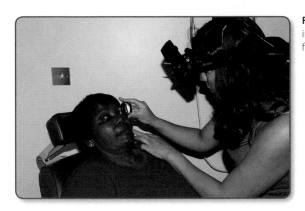

Figure 3.10 The use of the indirect ophthalmoscope for fundus examination.

The slit lamp

The slit lamp is a binocular microscope with an adjustable bright beam of light (**Figure 3.11**). The main uses of the slit lamp are:

- *High magnification of the front of the eye:* the slit lamp is essentially being used as a microscope.
- *Fundus examination:* for this a small, strong lens of 78 or 90 dioptres is held in front of the eye. This allows a very clear, detailed and three-dimensional image of the fundus to be viewed through the slit lamp.
- *Drainage angle and peripheral retinal examination:* a lens, called a gonioscope, with mirrors built into it is placed on the eye. This allows the anterior drainage angle (where the peripheral iris meets the posterior surface of the cornea) and the peripheral retina to be examined.
- *Intraocular pressure measurement:* applanation (touch) tonometry is the most accurate technique for pressure measurement (**Figure 3.11**). An applanation tonometer can be fitted to the slit lamp to measure the eye pressure.

Methods of magnification for examining the front of the eye

Examination of the front of the eye requires magnification and illumination. The best instrument for this is the slit lamp. The disadvantage of the slit

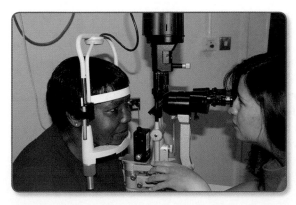

Figure 3.11 A slit lamp being used with an applanation tonometer.

lamp is that it is expensive and not portable. Fortunately, there are simpler ways to provide magnification and illumination (**Box 3.5**).

The ophthalmoscope

The ophthalmoscope can also be used as a magnifying lens with a built-in light source, although many people do not realise this. This can be very useful for examining the cornea, conjunctiva, lids and eyelashes. Hold the ophthalmoscope very close to the patient's eye, as in fundus examination, but using a very strong positive lens, e.g. +15 or +20 dioptres in the ophthalmoscope. It is now focused on the front part of the eye, and will give a clear, enlarged view of the conjunctiva, cornea, iris or lens. The focus can be adjusted either by moving it slightly nearer or further from the eye, or by using a different positive lens in the ophthalmoscope.

Handheld magnifying lens

A hand-held magnifying lens (often called a 'loupe') is basically a strong convex lens that is held just in front of the eye. The examiner will need to hold some sort of light source with his other hand.

Binocular telescopic spectacles (Figure 3.12a and b)

Having the magnification on or over the spectacles allows both hands to be free for conducting the examination (or surgery). Various types of spectacles are available. A cheap, robust and widely available type of spectacle is particularly useful in rural clinics and is worn as a headband over the top of the observer's regular glasses (**Figure 3.12a**). Other types include ones that clip onto a normal pair of glasses, or ones that are made readily attached to the specially made prescription glasses of the observer (**Figure 3.12b**).

Principles of illumination

Good illumination is also necessary to see many of the subtle pathological changes in the front of the eye and the transparent ocular media. Three different types of illumination are used to examine the eye (**Figue 3.13**).

1. *Diffuse illumination (**Figure 3.13a**):* the rays of light are travelling in all directions. Normal daylight, electric light and torchlight are examples of diffuse illumination.

Box 3.5 Methods of magnification and illumination

1. Getting close and using the accommodation of the observer and a torch.
2. A handheld magnifier (a 'loupe') and torch or magnifier with a built in light source
3. Wearing ordinary near vision spectacles (e.g. +3 lenses) and torch.
4. Telescopic magnifying lenses ('spectacle loupes') or telescopic spectacles and torch.
5. Ophthalmoscope with high plus correction.
6. Binocular microscope, i.e. the slit lamp.

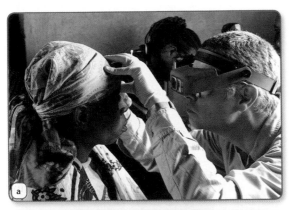

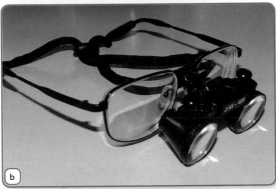

Figure 3.12 Magnifying loupes. (a) Cheap, robust magnifying spectacle loupes that are very useful for use in rural areas. (b) Expensive loupes with the owner's glasses prescription built into the spectacle lens so that they can be worn when doing surgery.

2. *Focal illumination (**Figure 3.13b**):* a small beam of light rays converges upon a point. The best example of focal illumination is the slit lamp. There are some hand torches for examining the eye which give a converging beam of light.
3. *Coaxial illumination (**Figure 3.13c**):* the examiner looks down the same direction (or axis) as the light rays lighting up the eye. An ophthalmoscope has this type of illumination but the slit lamp can also be adjusted so that the light beam is coaxial with the microscope.

Focal illumination shows up any tiny defect or opacity that is not visible with diffuse illumination. An example of this is a room containing some smoke or dust. The smoke or dust is difficult to see with normal illumination. However, if a ray of sunlight enters the room through one small window, it will highlight the particles of smoke or dust. In the same way, focal illumination shows up cells or protein exudate in the anterior chamber, which occur in intraocular inflammation. Focal illumination also shows up the structure of the cornea and the lens much more clearly. By looking at **Figure 3.13b(right hand image)**, it is possible to assess the thickness of the cornea and the lens, and also the depth of the anterior chamber. This is not possible with other types of illumination.

Coaxial illumination from an ophthalmoscope can also be used to examine the *red reflex*. This is a method for detecting any defects or opacities – even

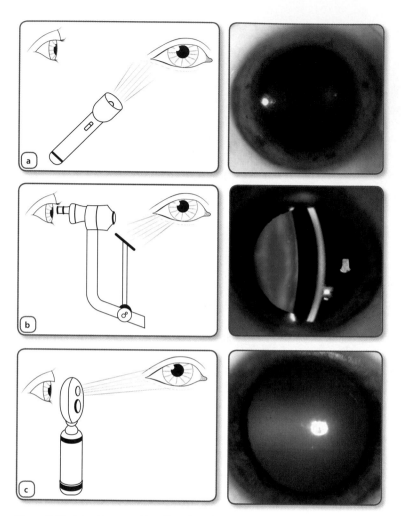

Figure 3.13 A healthy eye with a dilated pupil seen with the three different types of illumination. The healthy clear lens looks different with the three types of lighting. (a) Diffuse illumination: the lens looks black. (b) Focal illumination: the layers of the lens can be seen. (c) Coaxial illumination: the lens looks red because of the red reflex from the retina behind it.

very small ones – in the ocular media. It is necessary to dilate the pupil, to allow a red glow of reflected light from the fundus to be seen in the pupil (**Figure 3.13c-right hand image**). This is called the 'red reflex'. Against this red glow, any small opacity in the ocular media stands out as a small shadow. There are two ways of bringing these opacities into focus:

1. To get a general view of the cornea, lens and vitreous, use a weak positive lens (about +5 dioptres or less) in the ophthalmoscope.
    Hold it close to your own eye, but about 20 cm from the patient's eye. Then bring it slowly closer to the patient's eye looking through the ophthalmoscope all the time. In this way, first the cornea, then the lens and then the vitreous will come into focus, and any opacity in them can be seen.

2. To get a magnified view of the cornea and lens, use a strong positive
   lens (about +20 dioptres) in the ophthalmoscope. Hold it very close
   to your own and the patient's eye. The cornea and lens will come into
   focus and opacities will be seen. This is one way of seeing even tiny
   opacities in the cornea, such as keratic precipitates, and even the
   microfilaria of onchocerciasis, when a slit lamp is not available.

If the ocular media are completely opaque, then of course, no red reflex at all
can be seen coming from the pupil. An absent red reflex is a very important
sign, particularly in children when it is very likely to indicate serious disease
in the eye such as retinoblastoma.

Systematic examination of the eyes

It is not necessary to examine every part of the eye in detail in every patient.
However, it is best to start with a routine system, so that nothing is left out.
The usual method is to start at the front with the eyelids, and pass backwards
finishing with the fundus.

The eyelids

Most eyelid disorders are fairly obvious, and so do not require any special
techniques to observe them. However, two particular disorders are not always obvious and should be specifically looked for: facial palsy and ingrow-
ing eyelashes:

- Facial palsy: observe the patient blinking and ask the patient to gently
  close their eyes and assess if they close completely. Poor eyelid closure
  is a serious defect (see Figures 17.3 and 17.4).
- Inturning (trichiatic) eyelashes: lift up and slightly evert (turn-out) the
  upper eyelid. Any inturning eyelashes, or areas where inturning lashes
  have been epilated, will then become visible (see Figures 8.6–8.8).

The conjunctiva

Diseases of the conjunctiva are so common that examination is essential.
Most of the pathological changes in the conjunctiva are visible, either to the
naked eye or with a simple magnifying lens. The bulbar conjunctiva (which
lines the eyeball) is easy to see. Hold the eyelids open and ask the patient to
look in different directions. The lower fornix and the conjunctiva that lines
the lower eyelid are also easily examined, by pulling down the lower lid.

The upper tarsal conjunctiva (which lines the upper lid) is more difficult to
examine. However, it is a common site for foreign bodies, and for pathological changes, especially in trachoma. With a little practice, the upper lid can
be easily flipped over (everted) without causing any discomfort to the patient
(**Figure 3.14** and **3.15, Box 3.6**). This will make it easy to examine. As you get
better at this technique you will find that with a co-operative patient the upper eyelid can be everted with just the thumb and forefinger of one hand.

The upper fornix is inaccessible, and so very difficult to examine. It is possible to evert the upper lid over a retractor to see the upper fornix.

The cornea

Diseases of the cornea are very common in hot countries. Therefore, careful corneal examination is essential. In theory, this should be easy, because

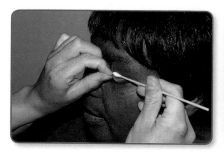

Figure 3.14 The patient looks down and the eyelid is stretched gently away from the patient.

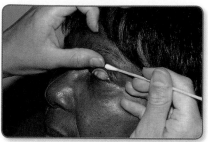

Figure 3.15 Gentle pressure on the back of the tarsal plate allows the lid to be everted and held in position whilst it is examined.

Box 3.6 Everting the upper eyelid
1. Ask the patient to look down, without squeezing the eyes shut.
2. Hold the upper lid eyelashes between the finger and thumb of one hand, and gently stretch the eyelid away from the patient.
3. With the other hand, rest a cottonwool bud or glass rod towards the back of the upper margin of the tarsal plate, so that there is very slight pressure.
4. Push down, to flick the tarsal plate inside out.
5. At the end of the examination ask the patient to look up and the lid will return to its normal position.

---

the cornea is right at the front of the eye. Indeed, severe corneal disorders are usually obvious. However, many diseases produce changes in the cornea that are small and faint, and so more difficult to detect. The slit lamp is the best way of examining the cornea, but most significant pathology can be detected with simple magnification and a light or with an ophthalmoscope. Some common corneal disease changes that should be looked for include:

- *Ulcer:* a corneal ulcer is a common and important condition. A shallow epithelial ulcer can be difficult to detect, but stains very clearly with fluorescein dye. It is therefore essential to put a drop of fluorescein into the conjunctival sac and examine the cornea with a blue light in any patient with a painful red eye (Figures 9.2 and 9.7b).
- *Scars and blood vessels:* these may occur in previously damaged or infected areas of the stroma (central tissue of the cornea).
- *Collections of inflammatory cells and other debris:* these may collect on the endothelium (the posterior surface of the cornea). They are called 'keratic precipitates' (Figures 11.4 and 11.5), and indicate inflammation inside the eye.
- *Corneal oedema:* this makes the cornea appear hazy rather than transparent. It is an important sign of potentially serious corneal disease.
- *Loss of corneal sensation:* the cornea is very sensitive to touch. A loss of sensation is therefore an important finding. It usually indicates

either a lesion of the ophthalmic branch of the fifth (trigeminal) nerve, or a present or past viral infection in the cornea. To check for loss of sensation, touch the cornea lightly with a tiny piece of clean cottonwool, and note if the patient can feel it or not. It is helpful to compare the sensation in the two eyes, if only one eye is affected.

- *Irregularities of corneal shape:* the cornea is a bit like a glass window. It allows most of the light to pass through, and helps focus it on the retina. However, its shiny outer surface also reflects some light. It is possible to use this fact to detect any irregularities in the shape of the cornea. Hold a patterned disc, called a Placido's disc or a keratoscope, just in front of the cornea and observe the reflection. Irregularities in the shape of the cornea will also cause distortion in the red reflex seen with an ophthalmoscope.

The anterior chamber

The normal anterior chamber contains only aqueous fluid, which is optically clear. Therefore, the examination should assess if there are any visible particles or fluids in the anterior chamber, which should not be there, such as white blood cells, protein exudate, red blood cells and microfilariae:

- *White blood cells and protein exudate:* these are the most common abnormalities to occur in the aqueous fluid. They are both found in inflammatory eye disease. It is hard to see the white blood cells and the protein exudates with the naked eye but they show up in the beam of the slit lamp (see focal illumination above) (Figure 11.2). It is called aqueous flare. In the same way, white blood cells in the slit lamp beam twinkle like dust particles in a beam of sunlight.
- *Red blood cells:* these are found less commonly. They may be present after an injury.
- *Microfilaria:* these may be seen in patients with onchocerciasis.

Very large numbers of red or white blood cells will be visible to the naked eye. They fall to the bottom of the anterior chamber, and form either a hyphaema (red blood cells) or a hypopyon (white blood cells) (Figure 9.7 and Figure 21.9). If there are only a few cells in the anterior chamber, they will only be visible with a slit lamp.

The depth of the anterior chamber should be estimated. This is only possible with focal illumination, by comparing reflections from the cornea, iris and lens (**Figure 3.13b**). A simple method of measuring the anterior chamber depth with an ordinary torchlight is described on page 389.

The iris

The iris can be seen without any special instruments, but magnification obviously helps to see its details. In particular the pupil margin should be carefully examined for any irregularity or any adhesion between the iris and the surface of the lens. These are called 'posterior synechiae'. These adhesions become much more obvious on dilating the pupil with mydriatic drops (Figures 11.1 and 11.6).

Adhesions can also develop between the front of the iris and the back of the cornea. These are called *anterior synechiae*. A penetrating ulcer or penetrating injury to the cornea can cause them. Narrow angle glaucoma can also cause them, but in this case they are very peripheral at the drainage angle and can only be seen with a slit lamp and a special (gonioscopic) lens.

The pupil

The pupil is simply the space surrounded by the iris. However, assessing the pupil size and its variation in size with light is one of the most important parts of the eye examination.

Pupil size

Many factors can affect the size of the pupil:

- The amount of light. The pupil will be smaller in the light and larger in the dark.
- The age of the patient. The pupil becomes smaller with age.
- Emotions: excitement causes the pupil to dilate. Anxiety sometimes makes the pupils constrict.
- Drugs and diseases can also affect the pupil size (**Table 3.2**). Remember that sometimes the patient will either not know that they have accidentally rubbed their eye with a substance that can cause pupil dilatation, or not admit that they have taken something, e.g. an illegal drug, that can cause pupils to change in size.

The pupil reactions

A careful examination of the pupils can be done with just a torch in a room which is not too bright. The pupil reactions are not easy to understand but once they have been understood, they are a simple and extremely valuable test. The reaction of the pupil happens automatically and is called a reflex. There are two pupil reflexes:

1. The **light reflex** in which the pupil reacts (constricts) when light is shone in the eye and then dilates again when the light is removed.
2. The **accommodation or near reflex**, in which the pupil constricts when the eye looks at a near object, e.g. when reading.

Except in a few rare neurological conditions the accommodation reflex is not of any significance. However, the light reflex is extremely important.

Table 3.2 The common causes of dilated or constricted pupils	
Causes of dilated pupil	**Causes of constricted pupil**
Drugs: Topical, e.g. dilating (mydriatic) drops, some plants substances, e.g. Belladonna (deadly nightshade) Systemic, e.g. some antidepressants, some illegal/recreational drugs, e.g. cocaine, amphetamines	Drugs: Topical, e.g. pilocarpine Systemic, e.g. opiates, some pesticides, some illegal/recreational drugs, e.g. heroin
Mechanical: ocular trauma	Iritis: current episode causes poor dilatation, previous episode causes adhesions between iris and lens preventing dilation
Glaucoma: acute glaucoma, severe chronic glaucoma	Paralysis of sympathetic nerve supply to the iris, (Horner's syndrome)
Nerve supply to the iris, i.e. any lesion of the 3rd (oculomotor) cranial nerve	

The normal pupil light reflexes: The two pupils should be equal in size, and when a light is shone into the eye the pupil constricts. This is because the light stimulates a few of the nerve fibres in the retina and optic nerve that are not concerned with vision, but instead are concerned with regulating the pupil size in response to light. The reflex path is as follows (Figure 2.5):

1. When light is shone in the eye, electrical impulses pass down the 'light fibres' in the optic nerve to the nucleus of the oculomotor nerve in the mid-brain.
2. The fibres synapse (relay) with fibres going in the oculomotor nerve back to **both** eyes, because some fibres cross in the midbrain to the nucleus on the other side. The oculomotor nerve supplies the iris sphincter muscle.
3. The iris sphincter muscle of **both eyes** contracts causing both pupils to constrict. The constriction of the same eye that the light was shone into is called the direct light reflex. The constriction of the pupil of the other eye is called the consensual light reflex. Both pupils should constrict equally to the light being shone in one eye.

Therefore, in a person with a normal light reflex, both pupils are always the same size as each other and both always react in the same way as each other. The light reflex is divided into two parts:

1. The *afferent* part. The passage of the electrical impulse from the retina and along the optic nerve to the mid brain is called the afferent part of the reflex ('a' in afferent is from the Latin for 'to' because the pathway is going to the brain).
2. The *efferent* part. The passage of the electrical impulse from the mid brain along the oculomotor nerve to the pupil constrictor muscle is called the efferent part of the reflex ('e' in efferent is from the Latin for 'from' because the pathway is coming from the brain).

If the pupils are not reacting normally the defect may be in the afferent or the efferent part of the reflex. A defect in the efferent part (something wrong with the oculomotor nerve or the sphincter muscle) will nearly always cause the affected pupil to be dilated. If the defect is in the afferent part, then both pupils will be equal in size and will both change size in the same way as each other, except when very rarely there may be both an afferent and an efferent defect in the same eye.

Afferent pupil lary defect and relative afferent pupillary defect: An afferent pupillary defect (APD) is a sign of optic nerve or extensive retinal disease. It is a very important sign, because although optic nerve disease is common it is not always easy to detect. There may be a total APD if the optic nerve is completely destroyed. However, often the nerve is partially affected. This will cause a relative afferent pupil lary defect (RAPD), i.e. the APD is relative to the other (normal) eye. The pupil motor fibres in the optic nerve are smaller and often more sensitive to damage than most of the other fibres which transmit the visual image to the brain. This is what makes the RAPD such a good sign of damage to the optic nerve. It is tested with the swinging light test in which the light reactions in the two eyes are compared, in order to detect the abnormal eye. The swinging light test will detect a fairly slight RAPD in one eye that would not be detected by just observing the direct pupil light reflex. However, it is important to remember that if both optic nerves are equally diseased, then the swinging light test is not helpful, because one will not be relatively worse than the other. If a patient has poor vision in one eye and there is no afferent pupil defect, there must be some other cause of the poor vision such as cataract or amblyopia.

Testing the pupil light reflexes: The steps of pupil reflex testing are described in **Box 3.7**. **Table 3.3** describes the pupil reflex tests in three situations: (1) a person with normal light reflexes, (2) a person with a total afferent pupil defect, and (3) a person with a relative afferent pupil defect.

Detecting an APD when there is only one functioning pupil

An APD can even be demonstrated when there is only one functioning pupil (an afferent and an efferent pupil defect in the same eye). This is best understood by giving a practical example. Consider a patient whose right eye has been injured causing traumatic cataract and traumatic paralysis of the pupil so it will not constrict (traumatic mydriasis). If the optic nerve is also damaged, there is no point in removing the cataract but if the optic nerve is healthy, then

---

Box 3.7 The steps for testing the pupil reflexes

1. Prepare the room lighting: not too bright, but not too dark either, so that the pupils can be clearly seen.
2. Examine and record the resting size of both pupils. It is sometimes important to do this both in a very light room and in a dark room.
3. Ask the patient to focus on an object in the distance. Ensure the patient keeps focussing on this object throughout the test, to prevent them accommodating on a near object, as accommodation causes the pupils to constrict.
4. Use a bright torch with a focused beam of light that will shine into one eye only.
5. Shine the torch at the right eye and assess the reaction of the right pupil.
6. Remove the light from the eye for a few seconds and then shine it at the right eye again and assess the reaction of the left pupil.
7. Shine the torch at the left eye and assess the reaction of the left pupil.
8. Remove the light from the eye for a few seconds and then shine it at the left eye again and assess the reaction of the right pupil.
9. The *swinging light test*:
   a. Shine the torch at the right eye for approximately 4 seconds.
   b. Move ('swing') the light suddenly and quickly to the left eye and assess the immediate pupil response of the left eye.
   c. After the light has been on the left eye for approximately 4 seconds, swing the light suddenly and quickly back to the right eye and assess the immediate pupil response of the right eye.

an operation will help the patient. **Table 3.4** shows the examination findings in the two situations, i.e. a healthy and an unhealthy optic nerve.

Table 3.3 Pupil reactions in three situations			
	Normal pupil reactions	**Complete afferent pupil defect, e.g. advanced optic atrophy in right eye**	**Relative afferent pupil defect, e.g. optic neuritis in right eye**
Resting pupil size	Pupils are equal in size and appear normal	Pupils are usually equal in size. Sometimes the eye with the APD has a large pupil	Pupils are equal in size and appear normal
Light shining in right eye	1. Direct response (right pupil): The pupil constricts. After approximately 1 second, the intensity of the constriction reduces a little, but it remains constricted, because the eye has adapted to the light. 2. Consensual response (left pupil). The pupil constricts in the same way as the right	1. Direct response (right pupil): The right pupil does not constrict. 2. Consensual response (left pupil). The left pupil also does not constrict.	1. Direct response (right pupil): The right pupil constricts, although you might note that it does this rather slowly. 2. Consensual response (left pupil). The left pupil constricts.
Light shining in left eye	1. Direct response (left pupil): The pupil constricts. After approximately 1 second, the intensity of the constriction reduces a little, but it remains constricted. 2. Consensual response (right pupil). The pupil constricts	1. Direct response (left pupil): The pupil constricts. After approximately 1 second, the intensity of the constriction reduces a little, but it remains constricted. 2. Consensual response (right pupil). The pupil constricts	1. Direct response (left pupil): The pupil constricts. After approximately 1 second, the intensity of the constriction reduces a little, but it remains constricted. 2. Consensual response (right pupil). The pupil constricts
Swinging light test	1. Light shining in right: the right pupil constricts to the bright light. 2. Light swinging to left: the left pupil's first reaction is to constrict slightly and then will dilate a bit*. 3. Light swinging back to right eye: it does the same as left, i.e. the immediate response is to constrict a bit more and then it dilates a bit.	1. Light shining in right: the right pupil does not constrict to the bright light. 2. Light swinging to left: the left pupil's first reaction is to constrict slightly and then will dilate a bit*. 3. Light swinging back to right eye: the right eye dilates despite having a bright light shining at it.	1. Light shining in right: the right pupil constricts to the bright light. 2. Light swinging to left: the left pupil's first reaction is to constrict slightly and then will dilate a bit*. 3. Light swinging back to right eye: the right eye initially dilates despite having a bright light shining at it. The pupil then starts to constrict.

*You may be wondering, if the light shining in the right eye has made both the right and the left pupils constrict, then how can moving the light to the left eye make the pupil again constrict? There are two reasons for this: (1) when the light is being moved from the right eye to the left eye, the light will be on neither pupil for a very short time. In this time both pupils will dilate slightly, (2) during the 4 seconds in the bright light, the right eye becomes adapted to the bright light and both eyes dilate slightly. The left eye is not adapted to the bright light and therefore when the torch is shone on it, it constricts a little more until it adapts.

Table 3.4 Testing for an APD when there is only one functioning pupil*		
	Situation A: a healthy optic nerve	**Situation B: optic nerve injury**
Light shining in right eye	1. Direct response (right pupil): the pupil does not constrict because of the traumatic mydriasis 2. Consensual response (left pupil): the pupil reacts because the right afferent pathway is intact	1. Direct response (right pupil): the pupil does not constrict because of the traumatic mydriasis 2. Consensual response (left pupil): the pupil does not react because the right afferent pathway is damaged
Light swung to shine into left eye	3. Direct response (left pupil): the pupil remains constricted 4. Consensual response (right pupil): absent because of the traumatic mydriasis	3. Direct response (left pupil): the pupil will start dilated and quickly constrict 4. Consensual response (right pupil): absent because of the traumatic mydriasis
Light swung back to right eye	If you keep watching the left eye, it will remain constricted because of the intact consensual response	If you keep watching the left eye, you will see it dilate, because of the absent consensual reflex

* Consider a patient with eye trauma who has a right traumatic cataract and traumatic mydriasis and you want to use the pupil reflexes to determine if the trauma has also caused optic nerve damage.

Efferent pupil defect

If the light pathway from the brain to the eye is affected, the effect on the pupillary light reflex is fairly straightforward. Let's consider an example: right oculomotor nerve palsy. The following will be seen on examination:

1. The pupils will be unequal, the right pupil being larger than the left (compare this to an afferent pupil defect when they are the same size).
2. When the light is shone in the right eye, the right pupil will not constrict because it is paralysed, i.e. negative direct response. However, the left pupil will constrict because the right afferent pathway is intact (normal consensual response).
3. When light is shone in the left eye, the left pupil will constrict (normal direct response), but the right pupil will not constrict (negative consensual response).

The pupil light responses are difficult to understand and some practice is needed to perform them correctly. However, it is probably the most useful single test in deciding how serious the eye disease is and what the likelihood is of the patient ending up with good vision at the end of treatment. An afferent pupil defect nearly always means permanent visual loss with little hope of the patient recovering the lost vision. The only exception to this is optic neuritis, in which the vision may recover.

The lens

The lens is best examined with the red reflex from an ophthalmoscope and/or with a slit lamp. Like all transparent structures, it looks very different under diffuse, focal and coaxial illumination (**Figure 3.13a and b**) and one can learn different things about the opacity with these different forms of illumination. Lens opacities are very common, and it can sometimes be difficult to make an accurate assessment of lens opacity. Chapter 12 describes in detail the appearance of lens opacities.

The vitreous body

The vitreous body is not an easy part of the eye to examine. Fortunately, it is not a very common site for significant pathological changes. A good way of detecting opacities in the vitreous is to use a direct ophthalmoscope looking through the +4 or +5 dioptre lens. It is possible to focus on the different layers of the vitreous body by gradually bringing the ophthalmoscope nearer to the patient's eye. The opacity is then seen against the red reflex. A large opacity, such as an extensive vitreous haemorrhage, will completely obscure the red reflex. The vitreous body can also be examined more thoroughly with either the indirect ophthalmoscope or the slit lamp. This can be important when looking for inflammatory, blood or pigment cells in the vitreous or congenital vitreous abnormalities.

The fundus

The use of the ophthalmoscope has already been described (see above). Some parts of the fundus can be examined through a normal constricted pupil, in particular the optic nerve head and the retinal blood vessels emerging from it. However, for a full fundus examination, the pupil must first be dilated with mydriatic drops. This reduces dazzle from reflected light and brings the macular area and periphery of the fundus into view. It also allows a much better view of the optic disc area.

It is convenient to divide fundus examination into three parts:

- The optic nerve head and the retinal blood vessels emerging from it. The optic nerve head is slightly nasal to the centre of the eye. The examiner must therefore hold the ophthalmoscope slightly temporal to the patient's visual axis, while the patient looks straight ahead. Another way to locate the optic nerve head is to follow one of the retinal blood vessels back to its origin (**Figure 3.9**).
- The macula is examined by asking the patient (with a dilated pupil) to look straight ahead at the ophthalmoscope light. You may find that the bright reflex from the fovea disturbs your view. However, if you practise examining the macula you will soon learn how to overcome this.
- The periphery of the fundus is examined by asking the patient to look in 8 different directions (up, up and right, right, down and right, etc.).

Examining the eyes of young children

Examining the eyes of babies and young children is often very difficult. It requires patience and encouragement to gain the confidence of the child. Eye examination is not painful and hopefully there will be no need to restrain the child. Sometimes pretending first to examine the eyes of the parent or an older sibling may help the child to cooperate. If it is still difficult to get a good view, the following techniques may be helpful:

- Seat the baby on his parent's lap, so that you can ask the parent to put one hand across the forehead to steady the head and one hand restraining the arms (**Figure 3.16a**).
- Lay the baby with his head on the examiner's lap, and his body on his parent's lap. Gently hold open his lids with the fingers and thumb of one

hand (**Figure 3.16b**). The other hand is then free to instil any eye drops, or hold a torch or condensing lens.

- If the baby is very upset it is usually better to wait until they have calmed down and try again then. However, occasionally it is essential to examine the baby immediately, for example if a penetrating injury or corneal ulcer is suspected. The best way to restrain an upset baby is to wrap them up in a blanket, ensuring that the baby's arms are inside the blanket (**Figure 3.16c**). This is probably the best way to get a satisfactory view of the eye, but it also usually causes the baby to become most upset.
- In very difficult cases, it may be necessary to instil a drop of local anaesthetic, and use a speculum to hold open the eyelids. However, any type of speculum can seriously damage the cornea. It must be used with the greatest of care, and only by a person with the relevant experience.
- The last resort is to give a general anaesthetic. If examination is urgent and essential but not possible, e.g. for suspected non-accidental

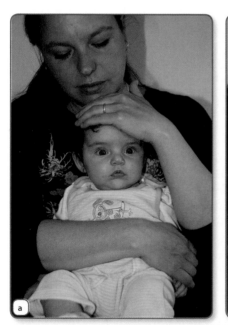

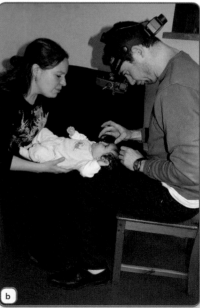

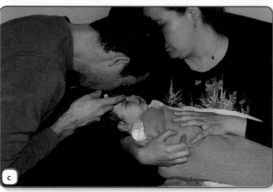

Figure 3.16 Techniques for examining babies. (a) Holding position: the parent places one hand across the forehead and the other hand across the body with the baby's arms held down. (b) Indirect: the baby is laid down with their head on the lap of the examiner and the body and legs on the parent's lap. (c) Swaddle: the baby is wrapped up in a blanket with their arms inside the blanket.

injury (see Chapter 22), or possible penetrating trauma, then general anaesthetic must be done.

The intraocular pressure

The risk of glaucoma increases in middle age. Therefore ideally, this should be part of a routine eye examination in anyone over 40 years. The intraocular pressure certainly should be measured in any patient with suspected glaucoma. Measuring the intraocular pressure is called tonometry. There are three methods commonly used: digital tonometry, Schiotz tonometry and applanation tonometry.

Digital tonometry

A very simple method of assessing the intraocular pressure is to place two fingers on the closed eyelid, and gently push on the eyeball to try and 'feel' the pressure. This is not at all accurate. It is only really possible to feel the difference between a hard and a soft eye, and to compare the two eyes to determine if one eye has a very different pressure from the other.

The Schiotz tonometer (Figures 3.17 and 3.18)

This measures the intraocular pressure from the resistance of the cornea to indentation; the higher the pressure, the greater the resistance. The Schiotz tonometer is reasonably cheap and robust. It is not used anymore in rich countries, but is still widely used in poor countries. It is fairly accurate (to about 3 mm of mercury) but it must be used correctly (**Box 3.8**).

Unfortunately, a rise in intraocular pressure is not the only thing which helps the cornea to resist indentation. The rigidity of the cornea and sclera

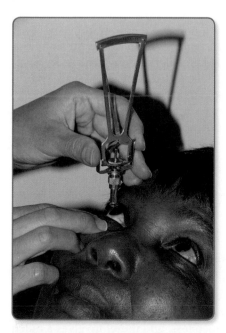

Figure 3.17 The Schiotz tonometer.

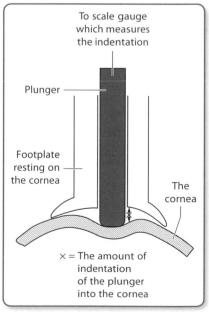

To scale gauge which measures the indentation

Plunger

Footplate resting on the cornea

The cornea

x = The amount of indentation of the plunger into the cornea

Figure 3.18 The principle of the Schiotz tonometer.

Box 3.8
Schiotz tonometry

1. Make sure the tonometer is very clean and dry. Even a tiny speck of dirt, or grease or moisture can cause friction in the plunger, causing a very inaccurate reading. Each day the tonometer should be taken apart and the cylinder cleaned and dried with ether. Additionally, before each use, test the tonometer on the little convex metal disc to ensure it registers at zero.
2. Instil local anaesthetic drops into the patient's eye.
3. Lay the patient flat, and ask him to look straight up, relax and not squeeze his eyes. If the patient has difficulty in looking straight up, it is helpful to hold his own hand outstretched above his face and tell him to look at his own hand with the other eye.
4. Add the lightest weight to the plunger.
5. Hold the tonometer so that the footplate rests on the centre of the cornea.
6. Look at the scale of the tonometer to find out the degree of indentation. If the weight is not enough to indent the cornea, use a heavier weight. Use the chart to calculate the intraocular pressure for that particular weight, and that degree of indentation.
7. To check the accuracy of the tonometer, put a slightly heavier weight on the plunger. The indentation will increase, but the intraocular pressure (as calculated by the chart) should remain the same.

Applanation tonometry

1. Apply local anaesthetic drops and fluorescein dye.
2. Press the head of the applanation tonometer lightly on the cornea.
3. The fluorescein dye collects at the edge of the flattened area of the cornea. When this is viewed with a blue light through the transparent applanation tonometer head, it looks like a green circle.
4. The applanation tonometer head contains a prism which changes the circle into two half circles.
5. These half circles get bigger as the tonometer head presses harder on to the eye.
6. When the inside edges of these overlap (Figure 3.19), the intraocular pressure is recorded.

also affect the amount of indentation. Occasionally, patients have abnormal rigidity of the cornea and sclera, and this gives an inaccurate reading.

The applanation tonometer

This is a more accurate instrument. It works by pressing a flat, round surface against the cornea, and measuring the size of the circle it flattens (**Figure 3.19**). This method deforms the eye much less, and therefore gives a much more accurate result. The technique is given in **Box 3.8**. Unfortunately, the standard applanation tonometer is expensive and must be used with a slit

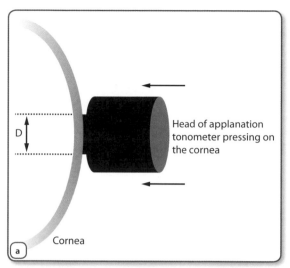

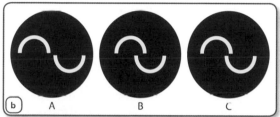

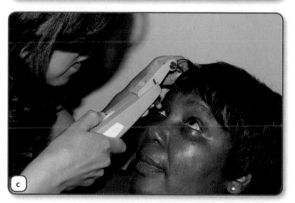

Figure 3.19 Applanation tonometry. (a) The principle of the applanation tonometer. 'D' is the diameter of the flattened part of the cornea. When the rings are in the correct position, the diameter is 3.06 mm. At this external diameter, the grams of force used to flatten the cornea, multiplied by 10, can be directly converted to mmHg. (b) The view through the applanation tonometer. (c) The intraocular pressure is measured correctly.

lamp (**Figure 3.11**). However, the 'Perkins' applanation tonometer (**Figure 3.19c**) can be used without a slit lamp, and the 'Glaucotest' is a simple, cheap and portable type of applanation tonometer.

Other types of tonometer

These include the 'puff' non-contact air tonometer, which blows a puff of air into the eye and the 'i-care' tonometer, which fires a tiny, painless probe at the cornea and automatically measures the pressure.

Other parts of the examination

A full eye examination also includes the eye movements, the orbit and the lacrimal apparatus. These are all described in their specific chapters.

Mobile phone technology

The widespread availability and rapid and extraordinary development of phone technology is quickly making mobile phones and their applications ('apps') an essential part of eye care. It is now possible to use them for many parts of the examination, such as visual acuity, colour vision and visual field testing and even retinal examination (**Figure 3.20**). Also, eye care workers can now carry whole text books of ophthalmology and medicine on their phones giving them instant access to information about their patients and their diseases and they can store patient information for clinical work and research studies. However, despite having the assistance of this spectacular technology, the underlying principles of careful patient examination, making a differential diagnosis and then a diagnosis and treating safely and sensibly have and probably always will remain fundamental to seeing patients.

Other tests

In specialised units, it is possible to do other more sophisticated tests to examine the eye in further detail.

Fundus fluorescein angiogram (FFA) (Figure 13.11)

In this investigation serial pictures of the retina are taken following an intravenous injection of fluorescein, usually into a vein in the arm. It provides a greater understanding of vascular diseases of the retina, and in some specific diseases it can help guide treatment. It is particularly useful in assessing macular degeneration as it can identify if there is 'wet macular degeneration' (see page 337).

Ocular coherence tomography (OCT) (Figure 2.4)

OCT has only become widely used in recent years. Perhaps more than any other instrument, this has changed ophthalmic investigation. It is a scanning machine that uses a near infra-red light to capture multiple cross-sectional images of the retina in just a few seconds. The cross-sections of the macula and fovea are very useful for assessing diseases like macular degeneration and diabetic macular oedema and the images of the optic disc can be very helpful for monitoring the progression of glaucoma.

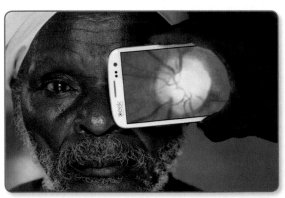

Figure 3.20 Peek vision: mobile phone technology being used for patient examination.

However, OCT machines remain prohibitively expensive for most parts of the world where eye care professionals, must still depend on very accurate clinical assessment of the retina and optic disc with an ophthalmoscope or slit lamp.

Ocular ultrasound scan

Sometimes opacities in the cornea or lens prevent the vitreous and retina from being viewed with an ophthalmoscope or slit lamp. In this situation, ocular ultrasound can be used to 'view' behind the opacity or obstruction and get helpful information about the state of the vitreous or the retina. However, simple tests of retinal function like the pupil light reaction and the projection of light are usually more helpful and of course free and easily available, unlike ultrasound machines which are very expensive and scarce.

Electroretinograms and electro-oculograms

These tests record the electrical potential of the eye when light is shone into it and provide information as to how the retina is functioning.

Visual evoked response

This test records the activity in the brain following light shone into the eye and can give some indication of the health of the optic nerve.

CT scan and MRI (Figure 21.18)

CT scan and MRI can detect disease in the brain, the soft tissues of the orbit, and in the bony skeleton, the orbit or the skull.

Most of the above investigations require very expensive equipment and are not usually essential for diagnosing and treating most common eye disease. One piece of equipment that is extremely useful is a laboratory microscope. With this, bacterial or fungal infections of the cornea can be identified and treated more appropriately. These are common conditions and giving the correct treatment can make a lot of difference.

Appropriate management of the patient

At the end of history-taking and examination, the clinician should come to one of four conclusions:
1. Nothing seriously wrong can be seen with the patient's eyes. This requires *reassurance*. However, the clinician must always remember that they may be wrong and so consider a further opinion or advise the patient to come back if the complaint does not improve.
2. There is something wrong, which the person carrying out the examination can treat. This requires giving the appropriate *treatment.*
3. There is something wrong, but either the examiner is uncertain exactly what it is, or it is beyond his abilities to treat correctly. The patient should be *referred* to someone who is better trained or better equipped.
4. The patient has a refractive error and needs glasses. The patient should be *refracted* (this may require a referral to an optician).

The management options can be remembered with the 'four R's': **Reassurance**, **Rx** (this is a widely used abbreviation for treatment), **Referral** or **Refraction**.

Principles of treatment

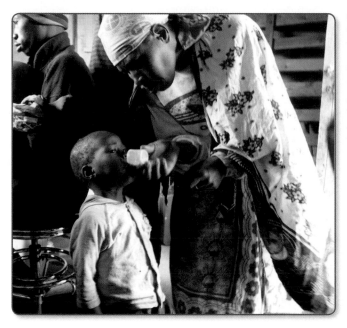

Often the simplest treatments are the best and most effective. This young boy is receiving an azithromycin tablet to treat and to prevent trachoma.

There are various ways of treating patients with disorders of the eye:

- Medical and surgical treatment: these are the two 'conventional' ways of treating illness. Anyone seeing eye patients must have a basic understanding of the medical and surgical treatment of eye disease.
- Correction of refractive error (see Chapter 5): this is mainly done with spectacles and is very important in poor countries, where there are few opticians and many people with untreated refractive error. Sometimes refractive error is also treated with contact lenses or surgery.
- Community health and preventive treatment: this is a crucial part of the management of some diseases, such as trachoma, onchocerciasis and vitamin A deficiency. These diseases are discussed in the relevant chapters.
- Traditional medicines: these are widely used in many countries with variable safety and success (see Chapter 1).

Medical treatment and ocular pharmacology

Medication can be applied to the eyes in several ways:

1. Topically: the drug is applied directly on the eye.

2. Systemically: the drug is given by mouth or injection and reaches the eye through the bloodstream.
3. Injections in or around the eye: medication can be given under the conjunctiva (sub-conjunctival), into the Tenon's space (sub-Tenon's), beneath the eyeball (orbital floor), around or behind the eye (peri- or retrobulbar) or even into the eye (intravitreal).

Topical treatment

Topical treatment can be given as drops or ointment. This form of treatment is more effective for treating the front of the eye, i.e. disease of the conjunctiva, cornea, anterior chamber and iris. Drops and ointments have different advantages and disadvantages:

Drops

Drops are the most convenient and common way of giving topical treatment to the eye. However, the active drug is only in contact with the conjunctiva and cornea for a short time. If it is necessary to maintain high levels of the drug, the drops must be applied frequently, e.g. every hour or half hour. Some drops also contain substances such as methylcellulose to make them more viscous, so that they stay in contact with the eye for longer.

Ointments

Ointments stay in contact with the eye for longer and are often used at night just before sleep. Some patients also find ointments easier to apply than drops. However, ointments blur the vision temporarily and are messier than drops. Another disadvantage is that the active drug is usually dissolved in the oily part of the ointment. It is not always predictable how quickly the active drug will pass out of the ointment into the tears, and then into the tissues.

Many patients need simple instructions on how to apply drops or ointment. **Figures 4.1 and 4.2** are examples of leaflets given out to patients with their eye medicines. You might like to photocopy these and give them to the patient. However, it always better to explain and demonstrate how to use the treatment to the patient and their accompanying person. Most patients can apply their own drops or ointment with a little practice, but it is easier if someone else does this for them. Also, remember to tell patients, that if they are not sure if the drop went into the eye, they can try again, as a second drop is very unlikely to be harmful, whereas not getting the drop in at all may be unsafe.

Side effects of topical treatment

Topical treatment is generally very safe. Side effects are not common or severe but they can occur.

*   *Stinging or burning sensation on application*: this usually occurs because the pH (acid/base level) of the drop is different from that of tears. The pH level may be necessary to keep the active ingredient stable and dissolved.
*   *Allergic reactions* (Figure 7.22): This will cause redness and irritation of the conjunctiva and surrounding skin. Allergic reactions are most

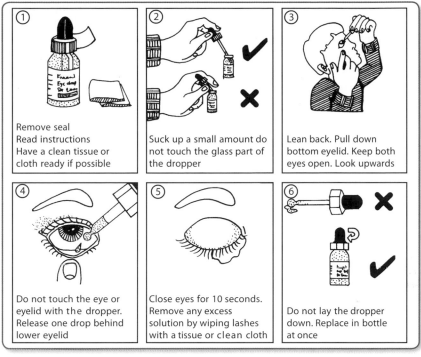

Figure 4.1 A leaflet explaining how to use eye drops.

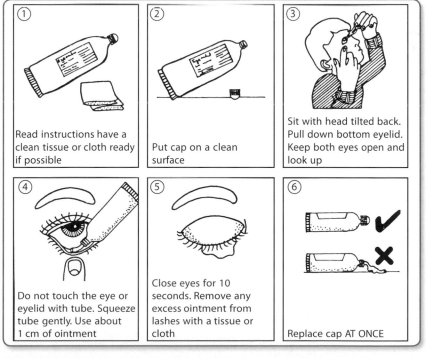

Figure 4.2 A leaflet explaining how to use eye ointment.

common with antibiotics, but may occur with almost any drug. Patients are sometimes allergic or intolerant to the preservative in the drops rather than the active ingredient. Preservative free drops can be used to avoid this, but they are much less widely available, more expensive and often need to be kept in the fridge.

- *Toxic reactions.* If a drug is being applied very frequently it may be toxic to the cornea and conjunctiva. For example, a patient may have an infected corneal ulcer and be treated with hourly antibiotic drops. These will kill the bacteria and sterilise the eye, but may affect the corneal epithelium, which might not heal until the drug is stopped or given less frequently.
- *Systemic reactions.* These are rare and one of the great advantages of topical treatment is that systemic reactions in the rest of the body are rare. Atropine (for dilatation of the pupil) and the beta-blockers (for glaucoma) are the main exception to this. Both of these can very occasionally cause serious and even life-threatening side-effects (see below).

Systemic treatment

Systemic treatment means that the drug is given by mouth or injection, and reaches the eye through the bloodstream. Systemic treatment is more effective for the back of the eye – the choroid, sclera, retina and optic nerve – as well as for the lacrimal passages and the orbit. It may be used in very severe cases of conjunctivitis.

Injections in and around the eye

Subconjunctival injections

Subconjunctival injection is a good way of quickly giving a high concentration to the front of the eye. The medication will be very active for about a day and may continue to have some effect for a few days. Subconjunctival injections may be helpful in the following situations:

- more serious or severe disease where a higher concentration of the drug is required
- to give a more continuous effect than intermittent drops
- if there is doubt that the patient will be able to administer drops frequently
- a subconjunctival injection of steroid (to suppress inflammation) and a mydriatic (to dilate the pupil) can be effective for treating acute anterior uveitis.

The technique for giving subconjunctival injections is given in **Box 4.1**. Not all antibiotics are suitable for subconjunctival injection. However, **Table 4.1** has a list of some antibiotics and other medications that can be used. The usual dose for a subconjunctival injection of antibiotic is 100 mg except for gentamicin for which the dose is 20 mg.

Intravitreal injections

Intravitreal injections are increasingly frequently used (**Figure 4.3**). They are used in two main situations:

> **Box 4.1 Subconjunctival injection technique (Figure 4.3)**
> Subconjunctival injections do not need to be painful if they are given with care. The technique for a subconjunctival injection is as follows:
> 1. Anaesthetise the conjunctiva with local anaesthetic drops. It is best to soak a tiny swab in local anaesthetic and leave it in the lower fornix for 1 minute, rather than just giving drops. This gives much better anaesthesia. A small injection of local anaesthetic first will lessen the pain of a subconjunctival injection, but if a local anaesthetic swab has been left in the conjunctiva for a minute this should not be necessary.
> 2. Ask the patient to look up and then insert a small hypodermic needle through the conjunctiva in the lower fornix.
> 3. Advance the needle a few millimetres just under the conjunctiva, and inject about 0.5 mL of the appropriate drug.

Table 4.1 Medicines that can be used for subconjunctival injection

Antibiotics (all 100 mg, except gentamicin)	Steroids
Gentamicin (20 mg)	Cortisone or hydrocortisone 20 mg
Penicillins: *Methicillin, Carbenicillin, Cloxacillin, Ampicillin, Crystalline penicillin*	Betamethasone 2–4 mg
Cephalosporins: *Cefuroxime, Cephazolin*	Depomedrone 20–40 mg (depomedrone is a prednisolon preparation which dissolves very slowly over a few weeks and gives long lasting treatment)
Chloramphenicol	

1. Antibiotics for endophthalmitis: this usually occurs post-operatively (mainly cataract surgery) and after a penetrating injury. Intravitreal treatment reduces the risk of blindness from endophthalmitis.
2. Anti-VEGF drugs for wet macular degeneration: these are used to suppress macular degeneration (see Chapter 13).

Intravitreal injections must be given in exactly the right amount and in the right way. Otherwise, they can cause great damage and even sight loss.

Endophthalmitis: choice of medication

Ideally, two antibiotics should be used, one for gram-negative bacteria, and one for gram-positive bacteria. The recommended antibiotics for gram-negative bacteria are either ceftazidime 2.0 mg or amikacin 0.4 mg. As both of these may be difficult to obtain gentamicin 0.1 mg can also be used. The recommended antibiotics for gram-positive bacteria are either vancomycin or cephazolin 2 mg. The exact choice of antibiotics depends on what is available and what is recommended locally, however some possibilities are:
- Amikacin and vancomycin.
- Gentamycin and vancomycin.
- Ceftazidime and vancomycin.

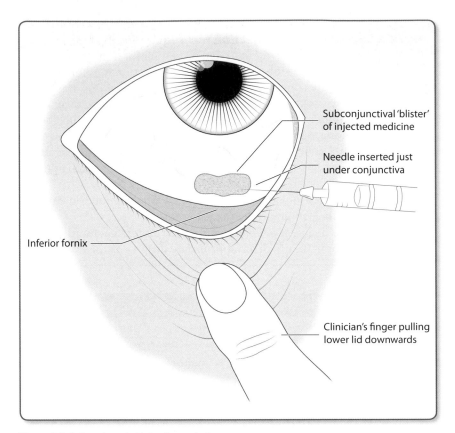

Subconjunctival 'blister' of injected medicine

Needle inserted just under conjunctiva

Inferior fornix

Clinician's finger pulling lower lid downwards

Figure 4.3 Subconjunctival injection technique.

Endophthalmitis: method of injection

The injections are made up in a 1.0 mL syringe; 0.9 mL is discarded leaving the last 0.1 mL to be injected. Therefore, the way to calculate how to make the injection is to put ten times the dose to be given in a 1.0 mL syringe and discard 9/10 of it. Make sure there is no 'dead space' in the needle when using such tiny amounts. Sterile preservative-free saline for injections must be used to dilute the active antibiotic. A 10 mL syringe is also needed to help dilute the antibiotic. **Table 4.2** explains how to make up the above medications. **Box 4.2** and **Figure 4.4** shows the technique of injection.

Endophthalmitis: vitreous samples

If good laboratory services are available then it is very important to aspirate a tiny amount of the vitreous for bacteriological examination and culture in an empty 1.0 mL syringe before making the injection.

Injections into the eye are upsetting both for the patient and the doctor and risk damaging the eye. If they are given carefully they should not cause too much pain and they are the best hope (almost the only hope) of saving the eye if there is established endophthalmitis.

Table 4.2 How to prepare intravitreal injections for endophthalmitis treatment

BACTERIAL INFECTIONS

Gentamicin. Dose 0.1 mg in 0.1 mL (prepare 1.0 mg in 1.0 mL)	Vancomycin. Dose 2 mg in 0.1 mL (prepare 20 mg in 1.0 mL)
1. An ampoule of gentamicin contains 40 mg/ml. Take 0.25 mL (i.e. 10 mg of gentamicin) from this and make up to 10 mL with normal saline in the 10.0 ml syringe (i.e. 10 mg in 10 mL =1.0 mg/mL) 2. Draw up 1.0 ml of this in a 10 ml syringe (i.e. 1 mg in 1.0 mL). 3. Discard 0.9 mL (i.e. 0.1 mg in 0.1 ml remains)	1. Dissolve 500 mg of powder in 10 mL of normal saline (concentration = 50 mg/mL) 2. Discard 8 ml, leaving 2 mL (i.e. 100 mg in 2 mL remains). 3. Add 3 ml of normal saline (i.e. 100 mg in 5mL, concentration = 20 mg/mL) 4. Draw up 1.0 ml of this in a 1.0 mL syringe (i.e. 20 mg in 1 mL) 5. Discard 0.9 ml leaving 0.1 mL (i.e. 2 mg in 0.1 mL remains)
Amikacin. Dose 0.4 mg in 0.1 ml (prepare 4 mg in 1 ml)	**Cephazolin and ceftazidime. Dose for both: 2 mg in 0.1 mL (prepare 20 mg in 1.0 mL)**
1. A vial of amikacin contains 500 mg in 2 mL (250 mg/mL). Take 1.6 mL (i.e. 400 mg in 1.6 mL) 2. Make up to 10 ml with normal saline (i.e. 400 mg in 10 mL = 40 mg/mL) 3. Discard 9 ml leaving 1 mL (i.e. 40 mg in 1 mL) 4. Make up to 10 ml with normal saline (i.e. 40mg in 10 mL = 4 mg/ mL). 5. Draw up 1.0 mL of this in a 1.0 mL syringe (i.e. 4 mg in 1 mL) 6. Discard 0.9 ml. The remaining 0.1 mL = 0.4 mg.	1. Dissolve 500 mg of powder in 10 ml of normal saline (concentration = 50 mg/mL). 2. Discard 8ml, leaving 2mL (i.e. 100 mg in 2 mL remains). 3. Add 3 ml of normal saline (i.e. 100 mg in 5 mL, concentration = 20 mg/mL) 4. Draw up 1.0 mL of this in a 1.0 ml syringe (i.e. 20 mg in 1 mL) Discard 0.9 ml leaving 0.1mL (i.e. 2 mg in 0.1 mL remains)

FUNGAL INFECTIONS

Amphoteracin (prepare 5 µg in 0.1mL)
1. Dissolve 50 mg of powder in 10 mL of normal saline (concentration = 5 mg/mL) 2. Withdraw 0.1 mL and discard the rest (i.e. 0.5 mg in 0.1 mL). 3. Make up to 10 mL with normal saline (i.e. 0.5 mg in 10 mL) Discard 9.9 mL. The remaining 0.1 mL = 5 microgram.

Box 4.2 Technique for giving intravitreal injections in endophthalmitis treatment

1. Insert a sterile speculum to hold open the eyelids. Apply local anaesthetic drops to the conjunctiva, and then leave a small sponge swab soaked in local anaesthetic on the surface of the conjunctiva for at least a minute. This greatly increases the anaesthesia. A small amount of local anaesthetic can be injected under the conjunctiva but this should not be necessary. If the topical anaesthetic is given time to work intravitreal injections should not normally be painful.
2. Put a few drops of iodine or betadine 5% in the eye
3. Use a fine (e.g. 25 gauge orange needle), short hypodermic needle on the 1.0 mL syringe containing the antibiotic. Make sure there is no dead space containing air in the needle. Insert the needle 4 mm

Box 4.2 Continued

back from the limbus in the outer and upper quadrant of the eye, aim the point of the needle towards the centre of the eye and do not insert it more than 1 cm into the eye. (Most needles with 1.0 mL syringes are only 1 cm long). You can ask the patient to look towards their nose to help expose an optimal area to insert the needle.

4. Hold the needle steady with the same hand that you used to insert the needle into the eye and use the other hand to press the plunger of the syringe to inject the antibiotic. If as recommended, two different antibiotics are used, the needle can be left in place while the syringe is delicately removed and replaced with the syringe with the second antibiotic. However, you may find it easier to make two separate injections.

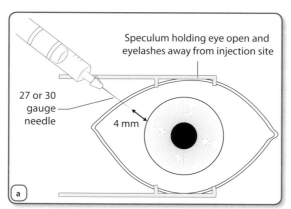

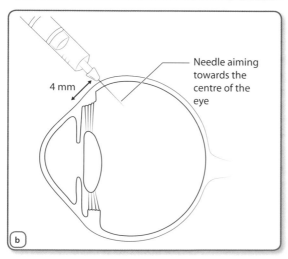

Figure 4.4 The location of an intravitreal injection.

Commonly used drugs in ophthalmology

Antibiotics

Antibiotics are used for treating bacteria. Most eye infections from bacteria occur in the conjunctiva or cornea. Therefore, antibiotics are usually applied topically to the eye. This avoids the possible side effects of giving them systemically and a very wide range of antibiotics to be used for eye treatment.

Chloramphenicol is the most popular antibiotic for topical use in the eye. It has a wide range of activity, good penetration, and it is cheap. Systemic chloramphenicol has a risk of causing aplastic anaemia, but this is not thought to occur following topical use. It is sometimes avoided in younger children because of this theoretical risk, and *fucithalmic* (fusidic acid) is often used instead. It is widely available as a drop and an ointment.

Tetracycline ointment is widely used in poor countries, because it is effective against *Chlamydia trachomatis,* which causes trachoma (see Chapter 8).

Other topical antibiotics that are particularly useful for treating corneal ulcers include penicillin, neomycin, gentamicin, polymyxin, framycetin, ciprofloxacin, ofloxacin, tobramycin, and sulphacetamide (or mixtures of these).

If the antibiotic is only available as powder for injection, it is possible in an emergency to dilute it to make a 1% solution in water. This can be used as eye drops (see also page 204).

Antiviral and antifungal drugs

Antiviral drops and ointments are available to treat viral infections of the cornea (see page 194), but they are quite expensive. Antifungal drops and ointment are needed to treat fungal infections of the cornea (see page 207). These are available in a few countries but may be very difficult to obtain. This is a pity because fungal corneal ulcers are common in tropical climates. Systemic antiviral and antifungal drugs are now available. They are used mostly in patients with AIDS and unfortunately are currently very expensive.

In patients with acute eye infections, topical treatment with antibiotics, antiviral or antifungal drugs should be given frequently, especially if the cornea is involved. This means that drops should be applied at least every hour and ointments every 2 hours. Antibiotic drops and ointments are also widely used to prevent conjunctival and corneal infections. These treatments are also used to prevent eye infections after minor eye injuries, corneal foreign bodies and eye surgery. When given to prevent infection rather than to treat it, the drops or ointment need only be applied three or four times a day.

Anti-inflammatory agents

Steroids

Corticosteroids are the most powerful anti-inflammatory drugs that are widely available. Hydrocortisone, prednisolone, betamethasone and dexamethasone are all used extensively for both topical and systemic eye treatment.

Topical and subconjunctival steroids

Topical steroid treatment is used frequently for keratitis, anterior uveitis, allergic types of conjunctivitis and after surgery. There are no significant systemic side effects, but unfortunately topical steroids quite often cause serious side effects in the eye. Steroids can also be given by subconjunctival injection (see above).

The side effects of topical and subconjunctival steroids

1. *Infection risk:* steroids act by suppressing the inflammatory response in the tissues, but they also suppress the defences of the body to infection. Topical steroid treatment therefore encourages any micro-organisms in the conjunctiva and cornea to multiply. The infection may continue to spread, but because the inflammatory responses are suppressed the patient's symptoms improve. This complication is especially serious if there is a herpes simplex viral infection of the cornea (see page 192). The wrong treatment with topical steroids will make a herpes simplex corneal ulcer very severe and persistent.

2. *Cataracts and glaucoma:* patients who receive topical steroid treatment over a long period of time are at risk of cataract (particularly posterior subcapsular) and glaucoma (these patients are called 'steroid responders'). The stronger the steroids, the greater the risk of both cataracts and glaucoma. These side effects are most common with dexamethasone, and least common with hydrocortisone. Rimexolone, clobetasone and fluoromethalone are all topical steroid preparations that are thought to be less likely to raise the intraocular pressure. They may be useful for patients who need long-term topical steroid treatment but who tend to get raised intraocular pressure from the steroids.

Topical steroid preparations are more misused than any other eye treatment. Almost all patients with a red inflamed eye will get relief of symptoms by using topical steroids, as the inflammation will subside. Unfortunately, the result can be disastrous if the inflammation results from herpetic or bacterial corneal infections. Before giving topical steroid treatment every patient should have the cornea carefully inspected with fluorescein dye. In general, if a corneal ulcer is present topical steroid treatment should not be given, unless it is done very carefully and with regular review by someone with expertise in corneal ulcer management. If there is no corneal ulcer, it is usually safe to give a short course of topical steroids. It is both a common and a bad habit to treat an inflamed eye with a mixture of antibiotics and steroids, without trying to diagnose the cause. If the disease is caused by an infection, only antibiotics should be used; if it is caused by inflammation, without any infection, only steroids should be used.

Systemic steroids

Systemic steroids are used to treat inflammations of the choroid, and occasionally the optic nerve and orbit. Unfortunately, systemic steroid treatment, especially when it is prolonged, may cause numerous side effects throughout the body (**Table 4.3**).

Topical non-steroidal anti-inflammatory drugs, mast cell stabilisers and anti-histamines

There are several other groups of drugs that can be used to suppress various inflammatory responses of the eye. They are all weaker than steroids but they do not have the same serious side effects especially from long-term usage. The different groups of drugs have different pharmacological actions and are therefore used for different eye conditions.

Antihistamines

Antazoline, azelastine, levocabastine and emedastine are all topical antihistamines. They are very useful for allergic conjunctivitis. Sometimes, they are combined with a vasoconstricting drug.

Mast cell stabilisers

Cromoglycate, nedocromil and olopatidine prevent histamine release and are also used in allergic conjunctivitis, especially vernal conjunctivitis.

Prostaglandin inhibitors (topical non-steroidal anti-inflammatory drugs)

Diclofenac, ketorolac and flurbiprofen have an anti-inflammatory action. They have a specific use in suppressing pain after injury or surgery, and they keep the pupil dilated during intraocular surgery. They are also used for treating cystoid macular oedema, which can occur after cataract surgery (see page 302).

Systemic 'steroid-sparing' immunosuppressive drugs

These drugs are sometimes used systemically to treat severe sight-threatening inflammatory disease in the eye, such as uveitis or choroiditis. Cyclophosphamide, cyclosporine, methotrexate and azathioprine are the most commonly used of these drugs. They must be given with very great care, monitored carefully with regular blood tests and preferably prescribed and monitored by an experienced clinician because they can have serious and even fatal side effects.

Table 4.3 Possible complications from systemic steroid treatment
Fluid and electrolytes: sodium and water retention, therefore increased blood pressure
Endocrine and metabolic: weight gain and swollen (Cushingoid) appearance to face and abdomen
Growth suppression: children
Dermatological: thin skin bruising, acne, striae, mild hirsutism
Haematological: increased bleeding, increased white cell count
Musculoskeletal: bone thinning (osteoporosis), fractures, osteonecrosis (bone death, most commonly of the head of the femur)
Behavioural: agitation, mood swings, poor sleep
Increased infection risk, especially tuberculosis
Gastrointestinal: stomach ulcer, pancreatitis, Candidiasis
Drug interactions: many, but particularly important: HIV treatments, rifampicin (for TB), diabetic treatments, epilepsy treatments
Eye: cataract, glaucoma

Mydriatics

Mydriatics are substances that dilate the pupil. There are two ways in which they act:

1. *Blocking the parasympathetic nervous system:* this makes the pupil sphincter muscle relax and relaxes the ciliary muscle. This prevents the eye from accommodating causing blurring of near vision. This is called 'cycloplegia'. Therefore this group of mydriatics are called cycloplegics. There are cycloplegics that dilate the pupil for a short time (a few hours), e.g. homatropine, cyclopentolate and tropicamide. There are also 'long-acting' cycloplegics, such as atropine (normal dose one drop of a 1% solution once a day) which may dilate the pupil for up to 2 weeks. Excessive use of atropine can cause systemic side effects: drying of the mouth, loss of sweating and tachycardia. Old patients may become confused even with normal doses.

2. *Stimulation of the sympathetic nervous system:* this stimulates the pupil dilator muscle. Phenylephrine 2.5–10% is the most effective drop for this. This does not cause cycloplegia, but can cause a rise in blood pressure, particularly the 10% concentration and must be used very cautiously in people who are known to already have high blood pressure.

The uses of mydriatics

Mydriatics have several very important uses in ophthalmology:

- Examination: dilating the pupil allows examination of the fundus. It is possible to use any of the short-acting mydriatics, but the best dilatation is achieved by using both types of agent, e.g. cyclopentolate 1% and phenylephrine 2.5%.
- Intraocular surgery: the pupil is dilated for cataract surgery and intraocular retinal surgery (see Chapters 12 and 13).
- Treatment: cycloplegics relax the smooth muscle in the iris and ciliary body, and are therefore used in the treatment of inflammatory eye disease. This has two benefits. Firstly, it stops the iris sticking to the lens (synechiae) and secondly can reduce the pain slightly as some of the pain comes from spasm of the iris.

Drugs used in the treatment of glaucoma

Miotics

Substances that constrict the pupil are called 'miotics'. They act by stimulating the parasympathetic system, which makes the iris sphincter muscle constrict.

Miotics are mainly used to treat glaucoma. Constricting the pupil opens up the angle of the anterior chamber (see page 390), which helps to relieve angle closure glaucoma. Miotics also increase the flow of aqueous through the trabecular meshwork, which lowers the intraocular pressure in open angle glaucoma as well. The most commonly used miotic is pilocarpine (1–4% drops), and its effect lasts for about 8 hours. Eserine and carbachol have similar actions. The cholinesterase inhibitors are another group of powerful and long-acting miotics. However, they are not often used because of their possible side effects.

Pilocarpine and drugs like it have several side effects:

- They produce some contraction of the ciliary muscle, which makes the eye accommodate involuntarily. This causes some blurring of distance vision, especially in young people.
- They can cause a headache in some patients, which is often described as an 'ice-cream' headache, i.e. the same pain as when you eat very cold food too quickly.

Beta sympathetic blocking drugs (beta-blockers)

Beta-blockers lower the intraocular pressure by decreasing the production of aqueous fluid. Several drops are available, e.g. timolol (also called timoptol) (0.25–0.5%), levobunalol (0.5%), carteolol (1–2%) and betaxolol (0.5%). They are all used twice daily and have very few side effects in the eye. However, they are absorbed into the circulation and may cause serious side effects in the body.

- Asthma is the most common, and these drops should not be given to anyone with any history of bronchospasm. Betaxolol has less risk of causing asthma than the others.
- Slowing of the heart rate in susceptible patients. They may cause heart failure and must not be given to anyone who is known to already have a slow heart rate.
- Lack of energy. Some patients are aware of this when taking beta-blockers.
- Impotence. This is occasionally described by patients.

Adrenaline (1% drops)

Adrenaline stimulates the sympathetic nerve endings, and lowers the intraocular pressure. The exact mechanism is uncertain, but it probably increases drainage of aqueous fluid from the eye. Sometimes, adrenaline causes eyebrow pain and vasodilatation of the conjunctiva. *Dipivefrin* and *brimonidine* are similar to adrenaline in their pharmacological action and more effective. This group of drugs does not have any obvious systemic side effects. However, they often have local complications, causing irritation, redness and chronic inflammation and are therefore not widely used anymore for treating glaucoma.

Carbonic anhydrase inhibitors

Carbonic anhydrase is an enzyme that is important for the production of aqueous fluid. Therefore, carbonic anhydrase inhibitors will lower the intraocular pressure. *Acetazolamide* is the most common drug of this type. It is taken as 250 mg tablets, once every 6 hours (or slow release formulation every 12 hours), and is more effective for short term treatment than long term treatment because it has numerous side effects. These include tingling in the fingers, gastrointestinal discomfort and occasionally, after prolonged use, kidney stones.

Topical carbonic anhydrase inhibitors, such as dorzolamide and brinzolamide, have less pressure lowering effect than acetazolamide but have fewer and less serious side effects.

Latanoprost and other prostaglandin analogues

This group of drugs are used topically and are thought to lower the pressure by causing increased drainage of aqueous through the trabecular meshwork. They only need to be used once daily (at night). There are no systemic side effects but they can cause some eye irritation, increased pigmentation around the eye and eyelash growth. Latanoprost has recently become much cheaper as the original patent has expired, and so its use is increasing.

Osmotic agents

These draw fluid out of the extracellular spaces throughout the body. This lowers the intraocular pressure. They are only used in emergencies to prepare a patient with very high intraocular pressure for surgery. Unfortunately, osmotic agents also produce a rapid flow of urine, and often cause headaches. Therefore, they are only used as a single dose in urgent and acute cases. The most convenient osmotic agent is *glycerol*, which can be given orally (1 g per kg body weight). Glycerol is usually diluted with fruit juice to make it taste better. Various osmotic agents can be given by intravenous injection, such as *mannitol, urea, sucrose,* or mixtures of these compounds.

Tear substitutes (artificial tears)

Tear substitutes are viscous substances that help to maintain a thin film of fluid over the corneal surface. Tear substitutes are used in the following situations:

- Dry eyes: if the patient has a lack of natural tears, tear substitutes can be used to keep the eye comfortable and protect the eye.
- Incomplete eyelid closure: tear substitutes should be used to protect the eye, as the eyelids will not spread the tears across the whole cornea. In this situation it is often necessary to use a very thick tear substitute, such as paraffin gel.
- Eye drop preparation: tear substitutes are also added to some eye drops to make them more viscous. This makes them stay in the conjunctival sac for longer.

Many preparations are sold as tear substitutes. The active substance is usually *methylcellulose* (up to 1% solution), but other celluloses, polyvinyl alcohol or dextran may also be used.

Local anaesthetics

Local anaesthetic drops are used to anaesthetise the cornea or conjunctiva. They are used in the following situations:

- Removing foreign bodies from the cornea or conjunctiva.
- For surgery: some surgeons use just topical anaesthetics for cataract surgery. Even if injected anaesthetic is going to be used (e.g. peribulbar or sub-Tenon's, see Chapter 12), topical anaesthetic should be used first to reduce the pain of these injections. Topical anaesthetic also stops the sterilising fluid that must be used for all eye surgery from stinging.
- For any examination that requires touching the cornea. e.g. tonometry (see Chapter 3)

Amethocaine is the most commonly used local anaesthetic but others are available, such as proxymetacaine, tetracaine and benoxinate. Cocaine is another very powerful local anaesthetic that also constricts the blood vessels and dilates the pupils. Because of the risk of addiction it is hard to obtain in most countries.

Topical anaesthetics are very safe. However, there are two situations in which great care must be taken:

1. They must not be used for the treatment of a painful eye. They prevent healing and stop the patient being aware that the eye is getting worse.
2. If a long-acting topical anaesthetic (such as amethocaine) has been used to examine or treat a patient, it is sensible to put a patch over the eye when they leave the eye clinic, as they will not be aware of foreign bodies such as dirt and dust, entering the eye on their way home.

Other medications used for the eyes

Most, effective medicines belong to one of the above groups. However, other types of eye medicine are often very popular. Most of these are not very effective, but fortunately have no or minimal side effects. The following are examples:

- Vasoconstrictor or astringent drops constrict the blood vessels, which makes a red eye look white. They usually contain zinc sulphate and dilute solutions of adrenaline (or other vasoconstrictors). Unfortunately, they do not treat the cause of the vasodilatation, and their effect wears off after frequent use.
- Antiseptic agents like mercuric oxide or boric acid are often used in minor eye infections.
- Several preparations containing mixtures of amino acids and vitamins claim to prevent the onset of cataract, and other degenerative changes in the eye. They are probably useless.

Problems with medications

Unfortunately, all medication can have complications. *Iatrogenic disease* means disease that is caused by doctors or the treatments that they give. In some cultures there is great enthusiasm for taking medicines even for minor complaints and often the doctor feels that he has to prescribe medicine even though it may not be necessary. Sometimes the public think that the more medicines a doctor gives the better he or she is. This leads to a higher risk of complications and side effects. You must check the possible side-effects and risks of each medicine that you use to treat patients, but below are some important general issues to consider when you are prescribing medicines:

Drug resistance

After some time bacteria often become resistant to new antibiotics. This happens even in the best of circumstances but there are two common mistakes that make it happen much more quickly:

- Inadequate treatment. In many countries patients cannot afford a full course of treatment, e.g. for tuberculosis. They have treatment for a few weeks only and not a full course. This does not kill the bacteria and only makes them resistant to the antibiotics.

- Inappropriate treatment. Sometimes powerful antibiotics are given for minor infections or for viral infections, which do not need antibiotics at all. This encourages resistance and it means that very useful and effective drugs very soon become ineffective. One example is chloramphenicol which was a very effective treatment for conjunctivitis but is much less effective now in many places because of resistance caused by overprescribing.

Compliance

Compliance refers to whether the patient takes the medicine as instructed. Most studies have shown that compliance even with educated patients may be very bad. Detailed advice and encouragement helps patients to comply with instructions. Community health workers are very valuable for reminding patients of the importance of good compliance. There are some schemes where the patient has to take the medicine under direct supervision, and these have given greatly improved compliance and the results of treatment, but these schemes are very time-consuming and expensive to run.

Counterfeit medicine

Most eye medicines are manufactured and distributed by good pharmaceutical companies and are reliable. Unfortunately, there are some unscrupulous dealers who market counterfeit or badly prepared medications in poor countries. This is a very sad and a difficult problem because poor people may try to save money by buying cheaper medicines and end up being deceived. Many medicines, especially newer ones, which are protected by manufacturers' patents, are much too expensive for the average person. However, many drops and ointments can be prepared in a small hospital pharmacy. This is very much cheaper and may be more reliable than drugs bought in the market. Fortunately, there are also many useful treatments available on the market which are not costly, such as chloramphenicol drops and steroid drops.

Time expired medicines

Reliable drugs may be donated or sold cheaply to poor countries when they have almost reached their so called 'expiry date.' It provokes a lot of resentment and government health officials often ban these medicines completely. Although some medicines may deteriorate with time the majority do not, especially if they have been stored in the recommended way. Often manufacturers are obliged by law to put an expiry date on their products even though they may be effective for much longer. Whether to use such medicine depends on what else is available but most medicines retain their effectiveness long after their 'expiry date.'

Eye complications from systemic drugs

Some drugs that are taken systemically for general diseases can cause complications in the eye. The problem is especially common when people take drugs excessively without proper supervision. Numerous non-ophthalmo-logical systemic drugs can cause ophthalmic complications, but three that are particular important are:

- Chloroquine, which is used against malaria, can damage the retina causing severe central visual loss.
- Ethambutol, which is used against tuberculosis, can damage the optic nerve, causing central or just off-centre visual loss.
- Parasympathetic blocking drugs, which are used for a variety of conditions, including, intestinal disorders, Parkinson's disease and depression, can occasionally cause acute glaucoma (see Chapter 15).

Principles of ophthalmic surgery

Surgical skills are learned not from a textbook, but from an apprenticeship training. The purpose of this section is therefore only to outline the basic principles of eye surgery. In particular, everybody seeing eye patients and not just surgeons themselves should know something about post-operative complications and how to recognise and treat common problems. It is convenient to divide the techniques of eye surgery into two groups: extraocular surgery and intraocular surgery. We will also discuss another surgical technique: the treatment of painful blind eyes.

Extraocular surgery

This is surgery outside the eyeball, i.e. the eyelids, extraocular muscles, lacrimal passages and orbit. The principles of extraocular surgery are the same as most other types of surgery. Many of the frequently performed surgical procedures, such as those for trachomatous trichiasis (see Chapter 8) are relatively straightforward. This is because most of the extraocular tissues are easily accessible and have a good blood supply. There is good healing with a low risk of infection. In most cases the tissues can be anaesthetised with local anaesthetic and dilute adrenaline (lignocaine 1% with adrenaline 1.200,000 is the usual preparation).

Intraocular surgery

This is surgery inside the eye. All over the world intraocular surgery has changed rapidly in the last few decades because of modern technology. The surgical instruments are delicate, intricate and most intraocular surgery is done with a microscope. The costs are high, but have reduced dramatically in recent years, particularly for cataract surgery, which is the most important intraocular surgical procedure throughout the world. The results are very good, and most surgery is now done without the patient spending a night in hospital. Intraocular cataract and its complications are discussed in Chapter 12, but below are some general principles to consider.

Anaesthetising an eye for intraocular surgery

The eye can readily be anaesthetised and paralysed with local anaesthetic blocks. The method is as follows:

- Instil local anaesthetic drops in to the conjunctival sac. Although cataract surgery can be done with just topical anaesthetic, this requires great co-operation from the patient so that they do not move their eyes or squeeze their lids shut during the surgery. Therefore, it is better to inject local anaesthetic around the eye. This is usually done with one of two methods:

1. Peribulbar/retrobulbar anaesthetic (**Figure 4.5**): Inject 3–5 mL of local anaesthetic (e.g. 2% lignocaine) in to the space behind the eye. This will paralyse the eye muscles and block the sensory nerve supply to the eye. It will also block the optic nerve, so that the light of the operating lamp cannot dazzle the patient. The injection may contain hyaluronidase to help the anaesthetic spread. It is usual to give the injection through the outer part of the lower lid. For a retrobulbar injection, the needle is directed backwards for 15 mm, then slightly upwards and inwards for 10 mm so that the tip penetrates 25 mm altogether. A peribulbar injection uses a shorter needle (approx. 20 mm), which reduces the risk of accidental penetration of the eye, but the anaesthetic may take longer to be effective.

2. Sub-Tenon anaesthetic: for this injection a small incision is made in the conjunctiva, usually in the inferomedial area. This is lifted up and a blunt cannula is passed into the sub-Tenon space around the eye ball. This anaesthetic has almost no risk of perforating the eyeball, but can cause the conjunctiva of the eye to puff up with local anaesthetic.

Prevention of intraocular infection

This is a critical part of intraocular surgery. Bacteria will multiply very easily and quickly in the aqueous and vitreous fluid inside the eye. Post-operative infection elsewhere in the body is a serious problem, but in the eye it is a

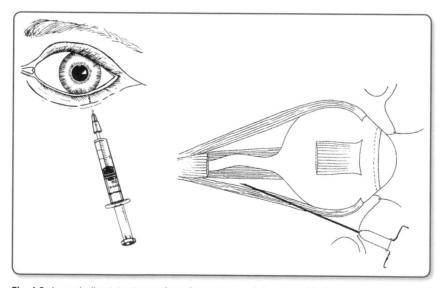

Fig. 4.5 A retrobulbar injection to show the position and direction of the injection.

disaster which if untreated will cause total destruction of the eye. Even with the most vigorous treatment the eye is often lost. It is therefore essential to sterilise the eye thoroughly to minimise the chance of infected material or bacteria entering the eye. The usual recommendation is to clean the eyelids and the conjunctival sac with 5–10% povidone iodine. Obviously, all the instruments should be scrupulously sterilised, and the surgeon and assistant should use a good 'no touch' surgical technique (i.e. only the sterile instruments touch the patient's eye)

Prevention of physical or chemical damage inside the eye

The delicate intraocular tissues are very susceptible to physical or chemical damage. Therefore, it is extremely important not to touch the inside of the eye any more than necessary in any intraocular manoeuvre. The endothelial cells lining the inner surface of the cornea are especially at risk. Even just touching these cells may cause permanent corneal oedema, which causes pain and loss of vision. The lens is also extremely sensitive to surgical trauma, and just touching it may cause lens opacity. It is also important not to introduce any fluids into the eye, apart from pure sterile isotonic saline or Ringer's or Hartmann's solution free from any added preservatives. Fluids that are not designed for use in the eye can cause severe and even permanent damage to the corneal endothelium.

Careful wound closure

Intraocular incisions must be made and closed carefully and correctly. This reduces the risk of complications. There are three normal places that the incision can be made: scleral, limbal and corneal. They each have advantages and disadvantages, but whichever you use, you must be sure that it is well sealed at the end of the operation. If the incision is made under a flap of conjunctiva, this will help to protect the wound. Some corneal incisions do not require suturing – they are referred to as self-sealing. However, they must be very carefully constructed and if there is any doubt about them being fully closed, sutures must be used. Very fine suture material is needed to close a surgical incision in the eye securely. These fine sutures inevitably act as foreign bodies, but if placed correctly they will cause very little discomfort or irritation. There are a number of different suture materials. The most popular suture materials are either 8/0 gauge virgin silk used as interrupted sutures, 10/0 monofilament nylon and 10-0 polyglactin (Vicryl), all of which should not irritate the eye if they are placed carefully across the wound.

Some years ago it was usual to advise patients to have long periods of bed rest after intraocular surgery. However, with better wound closure, there is now no need for this. Almost all eye surgery can now be done on an outpatient basis.

Padding/shielding the eye

Padding an eye increases the bacterial content of the conjunctival sac. However, padding is often recommended for 1–2 days after intraocular surgery. This will protect the eye from contamination, injury or irritation. Alternatively a clear shield can be worn; this allows the patient to see, but still protects the eye.

The treatment of painful blind eyes

Unfortunately blind, painful eyes are commonly seen in poor countries. They can be caused by numerous diseases, but they are more common in countries where eye trauma is more common and eye treatment less accessible. There are three different ways of treating blind, painful eyes:

1. Topical medication: frequent steroid drops and mydriatics once daily often relieves the pain as a temporary measure. If the eye is already blind, you do not need to worry about the possible complications of topical steroid treatment.
2. A retrobulbar injection to destroy the fine nerve fibres that transmit the sensation of pain. Usually, the function of the other nerves in the orbit is not affected, and this prevents the patient having to have the eye removed. Three different substances can be used (and if necessary repeated after a few days or if the pain returns some time after).
   a. Phenol is both a weak local anaesthetic and permanently destroys the fine nerve fibres which transmit pain. 2–3 mL of 5% phenol should be slowly injected into the retrobulbar space
   b. Alcohol 50% can be used if phenol is not obtainable. The injection first causes pain before relieving it and so a local anaesthetic injection should be given first
   c. Chlorpromazine is a phenothiazine medication that is used for treating psychosis. It is not exactly clear how it causes pain relief, but the high concentration (1–2 mL of 25 mg/mL) damages the nerves.

      Retrobulbar injection of toxic substances may be extremely painful and therefore it is much kinder to the patient to inject some retrobulbar anaesthetic first.
3. If these fail or if the eye is also disfigured and ugly, then removal either by evisceration or enucleation may be best (Figure 9.33). Artificial eyes are quite cheap and easy to insert.

Surgery in poor countries

In many areas, people have no access to even the most basic surgical treatment, and the community cannot afford expensive equipment and time-consuming operations. However, it is still very important that surgery in these situations should produce good results and be as free from complications as possible.

In many areas, but especially in parts of Africa, there are far too few eye surgeons. The only way of meeting the present needs of the community is to train other medical workers to perform certain operations. There is a great range of possible eye operations, but three are particularly important in preventing or curing blindness:

- *Cataract extraction.* This is by far the most important treatable cause of blindness.
- *The correction of inturning eyelashes* (trichiasis), following trachoma. If left untreated, these patients will develop corneal ulcers, scars and blindness.
- *Glaucoma surgery.* This can prevent blindness in patients with early glaucoma.

Ophthalmic optics and the correction of refractive errors

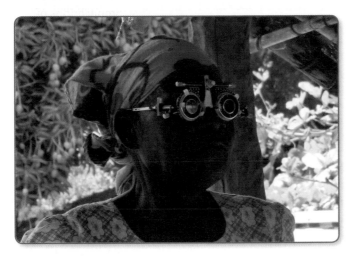

In much of the world people are still visually impaired simply because they do not have glasses.

Optics is the study of light. Ophthalmic optics is the study of the eye as an optical instrument and how it focuses the light. The eye can be compared to a camera. A camera captures an image of the outside world and records it on film or digitally. The retina of the eye captures an image of the outside world and transmits it to the visual centres of the brain where it is interpreted. However, the healthy eye is much more advanced than any camera because:

- The eye captures much greater detail than any camera.
- The eye can almost instantly change between focussing on both near and distant objects. Therefore, when you look ahead of you, it seems that everything from just in front of you to the far distance is in focus.
- The eye functions well in very bright light and in near total darkness.
- The eye continually records motion and changes. Even the best cameras can struggle to function well when objects are moving fast.
- The use of two eyes allows the image that reaches the brain to be in three-dimensions.

Basic ophthalmic optics

Light travels in straight lines. If the light ray strikes a surface like a mirror, it bounces back just like a ball bounces back from a wall. This is called *reflection*. If the light ray passes through a lens, the light ray will continue to pass forward, but the direction of the ray will be altered. This is called *refraction*. Different lenses will refract light in different ways.

Rays of light from a light source or an object far away are considered to be running parallel to each other. A *convex lens* will refract these rays of light towards each other, causing them to converge together at a point called the focal point (**Figure 5.1**). The focal length of the lens is the distance from the lens to the focal point when parallel rays of light enter the lens. Therefore, a very strong lens has a very short focal length and a weak lens a long focal length.

The power of a lens is not usually measured by its focal length, but by a unit called a '*dioptre*'. A lens with a power of 1.0 dioptre will focus parallel rays of light to a point one metre from the lens. A lens with a power of 2.0 dioptres is twice as strong and will focus parallel rays of light to a point half a metre from the lens, and a lens with a power of 10.0 dioptres is extremely strong and will focus parallel rays of light to a point one-tenth of a metre (10 cm) from the lens. In mathematical terms, this means that the power of a lens in dioptres is the reciprocal of its focal length. Dioptres are a much easier way of measuring the power of a lens than by recording its focal length.

A *concave lens* has the opposite effect of a convex lens (**Figure 5.2**). Parallel rays of light striking a concave lens will refract the rays away from each other so they never to come to a focal point. It can be imagined that they come from a focal point in front of the lens (see the dotted rays in **Figure 5.2**). Therefore, the focal length is a negative focal length, and the power of the lens is a minus number of dioptres.

Most simple lenses are *spherical lenses*. Their surface is part of a sphere. Therefore, wherever a ray of light hits the lens the focussing will be exactly the same. *Cylindrical lenses* are more complicated. A cylindrical lens is like part of the surface of a cylinder and the light rays are focused in one plane but not in the other (**Figure 5.3**). Therefore, the light rays are focussed to a line and not a point. Cylindrical lenses may be convex or concave and can be combined with a spherical lens.

The last common type of lens used in optics is a *prism*. Prisms alter the direction of light without focusing it (**Figure 5.4**). Prisms are used in ophthalmic instruments like the slit lamp and binoculars. Occasionally, prismatic lenses are used in spectacles to help patients who experience double vision because

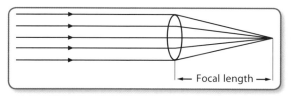

Figure 5.1 A convex lens. After passing through the lens, the rays of light converge to a point focus.

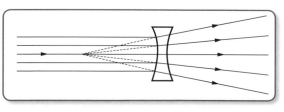

Figure 5.2 A concave lens. The rays of light diverge after passing through the lens and the focus is an imaginary point in front of the lens.

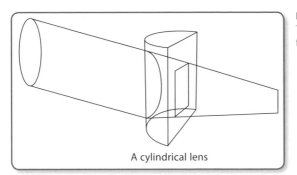

Figure 5.3 A cylindrical lens. The rays of light are only focused in one axis.

A cylindrical lens

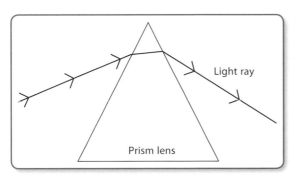

Figure 5.4 A prismatic lens. The direction of the light rays is changed without their being focused.

Light ray

Prism lens

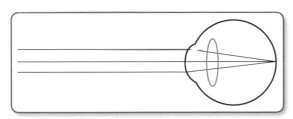

Figure 5.5 Focussing light rays from a distant object onto the retina.

their eyes are pointing in slightly different directions. Strong spectacle lenses can create a prismatic effect if the centre of the lens is not aligned correctly with the centre of the eye. Therefore, some patients feel discomfort or experience double vision from wearing spectacles that have strong lenses and are not centred correctly in the spectacle frame.

The optics of the eye

The cornea and the lens of the eye work as a very powerful convex lens and the normal healthy eye at rest will focus parallel light rays coming from a distant object on to the retina (**Figure 5.5**). For a sight test, the patient is usually seated 6 m from the test chart, and this is optically the same as an object in the far distance. The length of the eye from front to back is just over 2 cm, or one-fiftieth of a metre. Therefore, the total refractive power of the eye is about 50 dioptres. About 40 dioptres of this refractive power come from the curved surface of the cornea, and about 10 dioptres from the lens.

Accommodation

Rays of light from an object close to the eye (e.g. a page of a book) will be diverging when they reach the eye (**Figure 5.6**). Therefore, these light rays are focused behind the retina causing the image to be blurred. The focusing power of the eye must therefore increase in order to see near objects clearly (see the red dotted rays in **Figure 5.6**). To do this, the lens changes its shape, becoming more spherical and therefore a stronger lens. This is called 'accommodation', and the mechanism is as follows:

- The ciliary body forms a ring of smooth muscle around the lens, and it is attached to the lens by many tiny elastic fibres, called the 'suspensory ligament.'
- These fibres constantly pull on the equator of the lens, causing it to flatten slightly. When the ciliary body contracts, the muscle ring becomes smaller, causing the fibres of the suspensory ligament to become looser.
- The lens then relaxes into a more spherical shape, and becomes a stronger lens.

Refractive errors

In a normal healthy eye, the light rays that enter the eye are focused (or refracted) onto the retina. This is called *emmetropia* (**Figure 5.5**). If the eye is unable to focus the light rays correctly, this is known as a refractive error. Nearly all refractive errors can be corrected by spectacles. In the past, blindness prevention programmes have concentrated on eye diseases and refractive errors have often been neglected. Most older (and even many current) surveys of visual impairment have assessed the 'best *corrected* vision', and it was sometimes forgotten that the people who were being surveyed did not in fact always have the glasses to give them the best corrected vision. The correction of refractive errors has been identified in the '*VISION 2020 – The Right to Sight* programme as one of the main causes of avoidable loss of vision. There are several reasons for this.

- Refractive errors are very common. Many are not serious and will only cause inconvenience to the patient. However serious refractive errors, if not corrected with spectacles, can be quite disabling. An uncorrected refractive error of about 4.0 dioptres would leave the patient visually impaired, and an uncorrected refractive error of about 10.0 dioptres is bad enough for the patient to be classified as 'blind'.
- Most refractive errors develop in childhood. This is very likely to affect the education and therefore entire future life of the patient.

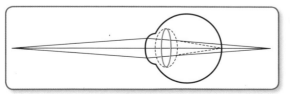

Figure 5.6 Accommodation. The change in shape of the lens makes it more powerful, so light rays from a near object can be focused on the retina.

- Almost all refractive errors can be fairly easily corrected with spectacles. Simple spectacles that would make an enormous difference to the patient's life can be prescribed by any health worker after a short-training course.

In an eye that has refractive error, the rays of light cannot come to a focus on the retina, and so the object appears blurred. In **Figure 5.7** the rays of light are focused behind the retina, and the image on the retina is blurred and out of focus. By narrowing the beam of light entering the eye, the blurred area on the retina becomes smaller, and the object appears clearer (**Figure 5.8**). This is called the 'pinhole effect'. The *pinhole test* is a simple way to detect refractive errors (see Figure 3.3). If the patient has better vision through a pinhole, it indicates a refractive error. People with refractive errors often see better in bright light when the pupil constricts, and sometimes screw up their eyelids to see better because both of these create a pinhole effect.

Correcting refractive error with spectacles

Most refractive errors can be corrected with spectacles. The purpose of the spectacle lens is to help focus the light rays on to the retina. The basic refractive errors are as follows:

1. **Myopia (or short-sightedness)**

   Myopia means that parallel rays of light are focused in front of the retina, and not on the retina itself (**Figure 5.9**). Therefore, distant objects appear blurred. A negative (or concave) spectacle lens will help to focus parallel rays of light onto the retina, and correct the myopia (see the red dotted rays in **Figure 5.9**). However, myopic people can see near objects clearly without the eye having to focus. The greater the

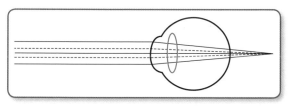

Figure 5.7 An eye with a refractive error. The rays of light are not focused on the retina.

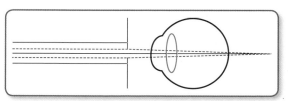

Figure 5.8 The pinhole effect. Only the narrow beam of dotted rays passes through the pinhole, so the blurred area on the retina is much smaller.

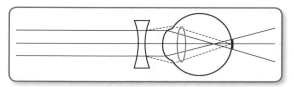

Figure 5.9 Myopia. With the eye by itself, the light rays (black) are focused in front of the retina. The concave lens causes the light rays to diverge (red) so that distant objects are then focused on the retina.

degree of myopia, the closer the patient has to hold things to see them clearly without any spectacles. One advantage for a myopic person is that they can read simply by taking off their glasses.

There are two possible causes of myopia:

- *Axial (length) myopia.* If the eyeball is too big, the rays of light will be focused in front of the retina. Patients with axial myopia have large eyes. Axial myopia usually starts between the ages of 5 and 15 years and progresses until about 20–25 years. This is the most common cause of myopia. There is a lot of research being carried out at present as to why people develop axial myopia. There is a definite genetic link and certain races and communities are much more likely to be myopic, but the other reasons for the development of myopia are unknown.

- *Index myopia.* If the refractive power of the eyeball is too strong, light rays will be focussed in front of the retina. This can occur for two reasons:
  - Increased curvature of the cornea. This can occur progressively in a disease called keratoconus (see page 217) in which the cornea becomes abnormally and excessively curved.
  - Increased refractive power of the lens. The refractive power of the lens often increases with the development of a nuclear sclerotic cataract (see page 278).

2. **Hypermetropia, (hyperopia or long-sightedness)**

Hypermetropia is the opposite of myopia. Parallel rays of light are focused behind the retina (**Figure 5.10**). A convex spectacle lens will add to the refractive power of the eye and focus the rays of light on to the retina, which corrects the hypermetropia (see the red dotted rays in **Figure 5.10**). However, young children can increase the power of their own lens by the process of accommodation, and so overcome hypermetropia by themselves. With age, the lens becomes harder and less able to accommodate (**Figure 5.11**). Therefore, as hypermetropic people get older, they have an increasing need for spectacles.

In the same way as myopia there are two possible causes of hypermetropia:

- *Axial hypermetropia.* If the eyeball is too small, the rays of light will be focussed behind the retina. Patients with axial hypermetropia have small eyes. This is the most common cause of hypermetropia. Axial hypermetropia usually starts at birth. However, some hypermetropia is normal in childhood (which is overcome by accommodating). Most young babies have short eyes and are

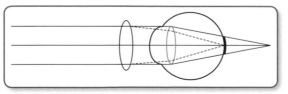

Figure 5.10 Hypermetropia. The light rays (black) are focused behind the retina. The convex lens causes the light rays (red) to converge so that distant objects are then focused on the retina.

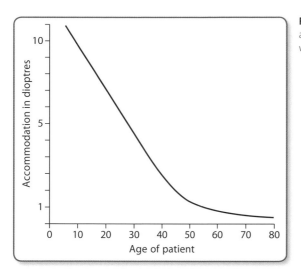

Figure 5.11 Presbyopia: accommodation decreases with age.

hypermetropic, but as the eyeball grows the hypermetropia gradually lessens.

- *Index hypermetropia*. If the refractive power of the eyeball is too weak, light rays will be focussed behind the retina. This can occur for two reasons:
  - Decreased curvature (flattening) of the cornea.
  - Decreased refractive power of the lens.

Hypermetropia often decreases with age and the growth of the eye, but hardly ever increases unless there is a significant problem with the eye such as something in the orbit compressing the eyeball. However, hypermetropia that is already present becomes more of a problem with increasing age, because the lens becomes progressively more rigid, and therefore cannot change its shape by accommodation to compensate for hypermetropia.

3. **Aphakia**

   Aphakia means that the patient's own lens has been removed (almost always by cataract extraction). Therefore, the eye is extremely hypermetropic. The patient needs a strong spectacle lens of about +10 dioptres to compensate for the loss of the lens. Nowadays, most patients have a plastic lens implant inserted into the eye instead when a cataract is removed, and they are called *pseudophakic.*

4. **Astigmatism**

   Astigmatism means that the eye has a different focus in different planes. For example, vertical rays of light may be focused on the retina, while horizontal rays of light are focused behind or in front of the retina. Astigmatism is usually caused by the cornea not being a perfect sphere, and instead being more curved in one axis than another. Occasionally, it can be caused by tilting or displacement of the lens in the eye. A cylindrical lens with power in only one axis is used to correct astigmatism. Astigmatism often occurs combined with either myopia or hypermetropia.

5. **Presbyopia**

The lens in the eye becomes harder with increasing age, and is therefore less able to change its shape (**Figure 5.11**). Therefore, the power of accommodation decreases with age, until after the age of about 50–60 years there is virtually no accommodation at all. An eye that cannot accommodate can still see distant objects clearly (unless there is also refractive error), but cannot focus on near objects. This explains why old people need spectacles with a convex lens for close work or reading. Presbyopia occurs in everyone and is part of the natural ageing process in the lens.

Refractive errors are usually due to alterations in the natural size, shape and curvature of the eye, and are not usually thought of as diseases. However, there are certain diseases especially of the cornea and the lens, which can affect the refraction in unusual ways. These are listed in **Table 5.1** and most of them are described in more detail elsewhere in the book.

Sometimes just having a refractive error can predispose to certain eye diseases, and these are listed in **Table 5.2**.

An optometrist or optician normally does the assessing of refractive error and fitting of spectacles. However, a simple assessment of the refraction should be part of a basic eye examination. Therefore, everyone who is responsible for seeing patients with eye disease should know something about refractive errors and how to prescribe spectacles to correct them. This is a particular need in places where there are not enough optometrists, like the rural areas of poor countries.

As well as prescribing spectacles, optometrists also need to know about eye disease. Often, patients think they need a pair of glasses when in fact their vision is reduced because of eye disease. Diseases such as glaucoma or diabetic retinopathy, which are very common, may be detected by an optometrist before the patient experiences any symptoms.

Table 5.1 Eye diseases causing refractive errors	
Refractive error	**Diseases that cause the refractive error**
Myopia	Nuclear sclerotic cataract of the lens Keratoconus (also causes astigmatism) Subluxed lens (also causes astigmatism)
Hypermetropia	Aphakia Masses in the orbit behind the eyeball, e.g. tumours, orbital inflammatory diseases
Astigmatism	Corneal scarring (causes irregular astigmatism) Eyelid masses, pressing on the eye, e.g. Meibomian cyst

Table 5.2 Refractive errors causing eye diseases	
Refractive error	**Associated eye diseases**
Myopia	Retinal tears and retinal detachment Glaucoma
Hypermetropia	Squint and amblyopia

Refracting a patient

When a patient is refracted, the aim is to measure the refractive error in each eye and to prescribe spectacles to correct this. There are two parts to refraction: objective refraction and subjective refraction.

Objective refraction

Objective refraction measures the refractive power of the eye with an instrument. This can be done in two ways, either by using a retinoscope or an auto refractor. A *retinoscope* (**Figure 5.12**) shines a light into the patient's eye. The person testing the refraction looks through the retinoscope along the path of these light rays and observes their reflection from the retina. By placing corrective lenses in a trial frame in front of the patient's eye, the refraction of the eye can be measured. *Auto refractors* are special machines that can measure the patient's refraction.

Subjective refraction

The purpose of a subjective refraction is to put different lenses in front of the patient's eye until the patient says that his vision is as clear as it can be, i.e. the patient himself is deciding which lens he thinks gives the clearest vision.

In ideal circumstances, a patient's objective refraction is measured first and using this as a starting point a subjective refraction is then performed. Slightly stronger or weaker lenses are used until the patient feels they have

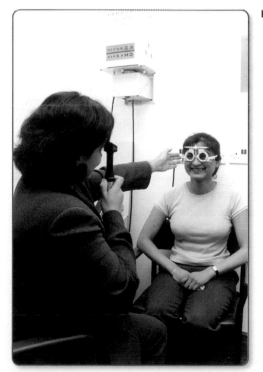

Figure 5.12 Performing a retinoscopy.

got the clearest possible vision. If the right equipment is not available to do an objective refraction, the entire refraction can be done subjectively. This is a skill that can be taught quite easily and is very useful for basic eye care workers who are seeing patients where optometrists are not available. The equipment required is listed in **Box 5.1**.

One disadvantage of only performing a subjective refraction is that it is difficult to correct astigmatism. Therefore, cylindrical lenses are not really needed for a subjective refraction alone. Spectacles which contain a cylindrical correction to treat astigmatism are also much more expensive, as well as harder to prescribe and fit. Therefore in general it is best for those working in rural areas using just subjective refraction to prescribe spherical lenses only. This is satisfactory for nearly all cases of refractive error, and it is not necessary to correct small amounts of astigmatism. The very few patients who have bad astigmatism and require special glasses can be referred to the nearest optometrist.

Steps of subjective refraction

1. Sit the patient 6 m from a Snellen chart, or 3 m from the chart if using a mirror (although **always** check that you are using a 6 m chart). Measure the distance visual acuity in each eye separately. Encourage the patient to read the smallest letters possible. If the visual acuity is 6/9 or better, there is no significant refractive error and the patient does not need glasses (the only possible exception is a young child with hypermetropia – see below).
2. If the visual acuity is 6/12 or worse, then check if it improves using the pinhole. If it does, there is almost certainly a refractive error. The level of visual acuity will give a rough idea of the size of the refractive error (**Table 5.3**). Start with a lens of approximately the right power according to the visual acuity (i.e. if 6/36, try 3.0 dioptres) and see if the patient prefers a minus lens or a plus lens.

Subjective refraction for myopia

If the patient prefers minus lenses, then they are myopic. Try giving weaker or stronger minus lenses until the patient sees 6/6. Always prescribe the weakest lens possible because it is very easy to overcorrect myopic patients,

---

Box 5.1 The equipment required for basic subjective refraction
- Snellen chart.
- Reading chart for near vision.
- Trial frame.
- Set of simple spherical lenses, both convex (plus) and concave (minus).
- Pinhole.
- Occluder to cover one eye at a time, so that each eye can be tested individually.

Table 5.3 Approximate visual acuities with different refractive errors	
Visual acuity	**Approximate refractive error**
6/12	1.0 dioptres
6/18	2.0 dioptres
6/36	3.0 dioptres
6/60	4.0 dioptres
Worse than 6/60	5.0 dioptres or more

especially young myopic patients. This is because young myopic patients, like all young patients, have active accommodation and the eye can focus easily. Therefore if the myopia is overcorrected, this will make the eye hypermetropic, and a young patient will automatically and subconsciously accommodate to bring the letters on the test chart into focus. It is very easy to prescribe a pair of glasses that are too strong, forcing the patient to accommodate all the time. This causes eyestrain, especially when reading, as the patient has to accommodate even more. There are two ways of avoiding the mistake of giving glasses that are too strong to myopic patients.

- Always give the **minimum** amount of **minus** lens that is needed for clear vision (**Box 5.2**).
- If the test chart has red and green letters also on it, this can confirm that the glasses are not too strong, using the optical principle called chromatic aberration. The test is called the duochrome test (see below).

Subjective refraction for hypermetropia

If the patient sees better with a plus lens, they are hypermetropic. Always prescribe the strongest lens possible to give the patient clear vision, i.e. the **maximum plus** lens. The reason is as follows: hypermetropic patients, especially if they are young, will subconsciously accommodate all the time in order to increase the focusing power of the eye and bring distant objects into focus. The aim of the spectacles is to allow the patient to relax their accommodation when looking in the distance and often they do not easily do this. Therefore, allow them to look through the lens for a few seconds to see if their vision will clear.

Chromatic aberration and the duochrome test

All eyes suffer from this minor optical defect. It means that different coloured lights, which have different wavelengths, are refracted in different ways (**Figure 5.13**). The red rays of light are refracted less than the green, so the green tends to be focused in front of the retina and the red behind the retina. If a myopic patient is slightly under corrected, the red letters will appear clearer than the green. If they are overcorrected, the green letters will

---

Box 5.2 The golden rule of subjective refraction

Remember the golden rule of all subjective refraction: prescribe the minimum amount of minus for myopia and the maximum amount of plus for hypermetropia. (For easy memory, minimum minus=myopia).

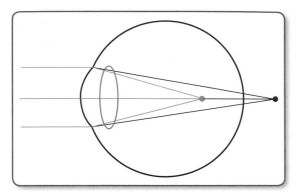

Figure 5.13 Chromatic aberration to show the optical principle of the duochrome test.

be clearer. The aim is to prescribe a lens through which the red letters appear slightly clearer, i.e. the myopia is slightly under corrected.

Subjective refraction for presbyopia

As the lens becomes harder with age, the patient's ability to accommodate becomes gradually less throughout life, but especially after the age of 40 years. Therefore, patients over 40 years usually need reading glasses for near vision. Usually:

- Patients between 40 and 50 years old will need +1.0 dioptre in addition to their distance correction.
- Patients between 50 and 60 years need +2.0 dioptres
- Patients over 60 years need +3.0 dioptres.

However, every patient is different and it is always best to prescribe the reading addition that is comfortable for the patient. This reading addition is, of course, added to the distance correction, i.e. patients who are emmetropic (normal sighted) only need the full reading correction; a hypermetrope of +3.0 dioptres would probably need 5.0 dioptres for reading when aged 50 years and a myope of –3.0 dioptres would not require any reading glasses. He would just have to take his glasses off to read.

Subjective refraction for aphakia

This is for aphakic patients who have had cataract surgery without an intraocular lens implant. These patients are very hypermetropic and require a lens of approximately +10.0 dioptres. Therefore, the subjective refraction should start with a lens of about +10.0. Very often these patients will not require extra reading glasses. The reason is that all plus lenses have increased power when they are positioned further from the eye. A strong lens like a +10.0 can increase its power at the surface of the eye to about +12.0 dioptres merely by sliding the spectacles down the nose and further from the eye.

More complex lenses

If the patient's vision improves with a pinhole but not with spherical lenses, then they should be referred to an optometrist or a specialist doctor. They probably have either astigmatism and need cylindrical lenses or they have a disease like an early cataract or keratoconus. These difficult cases need an objective refraction as well.

Interpupillary distance

The patient's interpupillary distance should be measured, especially if strong lenses have been prescribed. This is done with a ruler across the bridge of the nose and with the patient looking in the distance. The purpose is to make sure the optic axis of the lens corresponds to the centre of the eye, so the glasses will not have a prismatic effect and cause discomfort. This is only possible if the spectacles are being made up in an optical workshop.

Other ways of correcting refractive errors

There are two other ways of correcting refractive errors: with contact lenses or with refractive surgery.

Contact lenses

These are small lenses that rest on the surface of the cornea. As well as having the correct refractive power, they need to be the same shape as the surface of the cornea and must be fitted by an expert. Hard contact lenses are small and move over the surface of the cornea. Soft contact lenses are larger and do not move. Once the eye has become used to wearing a contact lens, most patients can wear them comfortably for several hours, or all day. However, serious and sight threatening complications can develop if contact lenses are not cleaned or looked after properly, or are badly fitted.

Refractive surgery

This is surgery to correct the refractive error. It is becoming increasingly popular in some areas of the world. A great variety of methods have been used in the past to try to achieve this, but the most effective and the only reliable way is to use a laser to shave off bits of the cornea, which changes its refractive power. There are two widely used procedures:

- *Photo refractive keratectomy (PRK):* The corneal epithelium is peeled off and a laser is used to alter the shape of the front surface of the cornea.
- *Laser intrastromal keratomileusis (LASIK):* This is a more complicated procedure. The eye is fixed in a suction clamp. A laser or sharp knife is used to slice off the front of the cornea, but leaving it attached by a small hinge. A laser is then used to excises a central part of the cornea and the surface flap of the cornea is replaced, which rapidly adheres spontaneously to the rest of the cornea.

The results of laser refractive surgery are very good when carried out by properly trained experts using the best equipment. However, there are limitations of the procedure:

- Myopia greater than 10 dioptres cannot safely be corrected and even between 5 and 10 dioptres has less predictable results.
- The results of treating hypermetropia are less predictable than myopia.
- The equipment required for refractive surgery is extremely expensive. If the procedure is done cheaply it is likely that the quality and safety are being compromised.
- Myopia may increase in early adult life. It is best to wait until it has stabilised before recommending laser treatment.

Minor complications occur commonly. These include dry eye and glare from lights at night. Serious complications happen occasionally including flap complications and infection, which can cause visual loss.

Aids for patients with low vision

Patients with low vision may be helped by visual aids, which magnify the image on the retina. There are many sorts of visual aids, some are very expensive, but cheap and simple visual aids can be helpful. The purpose of a visual aid is to enlarge the area of the retina on which the image is focused. The main disadvantage is that the field of vision (the area that is seen) is smaller.

The only type of visual aid for objects in the distance is to use telescopic spectacles. These may be for both eyes (binoculars), or for one eye only (monoculars). Unfortunately, they are expensive and they have the disadvantage of giving only a small field of vision.

It is much easier to provide visual aids for near vision, to help with activities such as reading. There are various possibilities.

- Spectacles with a very strong reading correction, e.g. plus 5 dioptres. With these, the print can be held at only 20 cm from the eye and will appear to be much larger.
- A simple convex lens can be placed in front of the print. This can either be held in the hand (a hand magnifier) or can be fixed on a stand (a stand magnifier).
- A good bright light also helps most people with poor vision to see better.
- The more expensive telescopic lenses can also be used for near vision.

Self-adjusting spectacles

Spectacles are now available in which the lenses have an adjustable focus. The patient puts them on and twists a small screw at the side of the frame which adjusts the power of the lens until he or she can see clearly through the lens. They are called 'Alvarez' lenses, named after their designer, and they are both cheap and reasonably good quality. They are a good way of providing spectacles to poor communities who have no other optical services. However, we consider that training eye care workers according to the methods described in this chapter is a more effective way to reach people in need. Complications with self-adjusting spectacles arise when patients over-correct myopia or adjust them unnecessarily. One possible solution would be to distribute these spectacles only through trained eye care workers, to ensure that they are used appropriately and effectively.

The eyelids and the lacrimal apparatus

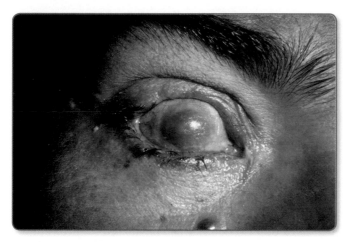

The most important function of the eyelid is to protect the cornea. This young patient has blinding, corneal scarring because of the loss of part of her upper eyelid.

The eyelid is very accessible and therefore most eyelid disorders are fairly easy to recognise with careful examination. Unlike other parts of the eye, examination of the eyelid does not require specialist equipment.

Eyelid disorders can be divided into three main groups:
1. Inflammations and infections.
2. Abnormalities of the function and position of the eyelids.
3. Tumours.

Inflammations and infections of the eyelids

The eyelids are exposed to the outside world and contain numerous glands. Infection and inflammation of these different glands is common. Fortunately, the eyelids have a very good blood supply, and so most of these infections either heal or remain localised. Because the eyelid skin is thin and loose, oedema and swelling of the eyelids may develop very easily in any inflammation. Sometimes inflammation in another site, such as the nose, scalp or orbit, causes oedema of the eyelids (see Figures 16.13 and 19.14 for examples).

Styes

A stye (also called a hordoleum) is an infection either of an eyelash follicle, or of a sebaceous gland (gland of Zeiss) near the eyelash roots. They are common and are usually caused by staphylococcal infection. They cause swelling, pain (mainly from pressure on the skin caused by swelling) and redness. They usually discharge and then heal without intervention or with simple hot compresses (pressing with a warm, clean cloth) and massage. Some people also use an antibiotic ointment. Occasionally it is helpful to incise them and they certainly should be incised on the extremely rare occasions when the infection spreads to cause significant skin cellulitis.

Inflammation or infection of the meibomian glands

Each eyelid has approximately 40 meibomian glands. Their openings are lined up along the eyelid margin and release the oil, one of the critical components of the tear film (**Figure 6.1**). Quite often, the mouths of one of these glands become blocked, causing a build-up of oil and an inflammatory reaction around the oil. This is a lipogranuloma and is called a Meibomian cyst or chalazion (**Figure 6.2**). For the first few days they can be tender and the surrounding skin can be red because of the rapid expansion and pressure, but the pain soon settles leaving a painless lump. These cysts are common, especially in adolescence. Sometimes there may be more than one of them, and they may recur. When they are large they can press on the eyeball causing astigmatism which causes the patient to have blurred vision. They are treated with hot compresses and massage (see above) and they often shrink away over a few months. If they do not they can be incised surgically in the following way:

1. Instil local anaesthetic drops in the conjunctiva and inject local anaesthetic with adrenaline into the eyelid.
2. Evert the eyelid with a small eyelid clamp.
3. Incise in a vertical direction through the conjunctiva into the tarsal plate over the cyst.
4. Curette out the contents of the cyst and apply antibiotic ointment.

Occasionally, an acute bacterial infection develops in a meibomian gland, causing an abscess (**Figure 6.3**). These infections can be quite severe, because the pus cannot drain away easily. There may be some general malaise and fever and the preauricular lymph node just in front of the ear may become enlarged and tender. Occasionally, the inflammation may spread to the orbit, causing orbital cellulitis. Eventually, the abscess either bursts through the skin

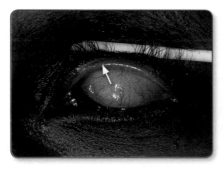

Figure 6.1 Normal meibomian gland openings on the lid margin (arrow).

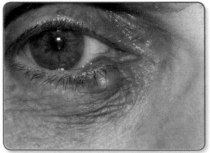

Figure 6.2 A meibomian cyst. Often the meibomian cyst is easier to see from the conjunctival surface of the eyelid.

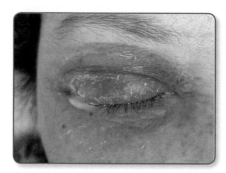

Figure 6.3 An acute infection of a meibomian gland. The gland is full of pus and the surrounding tissues are inflamed.

or conjunctiva, or settles down to leave a meibomian cyst. The abscess should be treated with systemic antibiotics and incised and drained surgically.

Inflammatory and allergic swelling of the eyelids

The eyelids frequently swell in response to allergens, irritants, bites and stings (**Figure 7.22**). Often the specific cause cannot be found, but the symptoms usually settle down quickly without treatment. Occasionally, recurrent swelling of the eyelids indicates a significant systemic autoimmune condition, which may require further investigation and systemic treatment.

Blepharitis

Blepharitis is the name for a more generalised and widespread inflammation of the eyelids. The usual cause is either a chronic infection with staphylococci or excess sebaceous secretion (called seborrhoea), or sometimes a combination of both of these causes. Blepharitis is often a minor, mildly irritating eyelid condition, which causes the patients some discomfort of the eyelids and irritation and redness of the conjunctiva. However, severe blepharitis may lead to permanent scarring at the eyelid margin, and the eyelashes may be absent, distorted, irregular or inturning (trichiasis).

Blepharitis is divided into two types: anterior and posterior. Anterior blepharitis is an inflammation of the skin, eyelash roots and sebaceous glands along the eyelid margin. It causes small scaly deposits to develop around the base of the eyelashes (**Figure 6.4**). Posterior blepharitis is an inflammation of the tarsal plate and the meibomian glands. It causes the meibomian gland openings to be blocked and capped with thick, oily secretions (**Figure 6.5**). This is also called meibomian gland dysfunction. In some patients both anterior and posterior blepharitis are present.

Blepharitis is often found with two skin conditions: seborrhoea and acne rosacea. In seborrhoea, the skin elsewhere is flaky and these patients also have dandruff of the scalp and eyebrows and external ears. *Seborrhoeic blepharitis* is a more severe form of anterior blepharitis. The crusts and scales irritate the eye and may cause secondary chronic staphylococcal infections of the eyelid margin. After some time scarring of the lid margin, and loss or misdirection of the eyelashes may occur. Acne rosacea is an inflammatory disorder in which spots and redness of the skin develops with blocked glands and more oily secretions. These patients are likely to have severe posterior blepharitis. It is important to recognise the associated

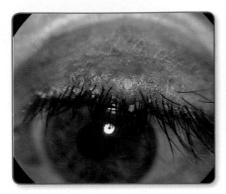 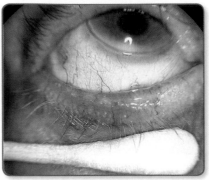

Figure 6.4 Seborrhoeic blepharitis. Note the scales from sebaceous material sticking to the lid margin and the eyelashes.

Figure 6.5 Posterior blepharitis. Note the occluded meibomian gland openings and the rounding and small vessels on the lid margin (telangiectasia).

skin condition as treating the blepharitis alone, often does not give a significant improvement of symptoms, or the blepharitis relapses as soon as the treatment is stopped.

Treatment

There are various different treatments that may help to keep blepharitis under control.

Eyelid hygiene and hot compresses: The crusts of sebaceous secretions irritate the eye, and their presence encourages chronic infection. The crusts and secretions should be gently removed with warm saline or very dilute detergent. Warm water and eyelid massage helps to melt the sebaceous secretions and to express the viscous secretions out of the meibomian glands.

Topical steroids and antibiotics: Steroid cream or drops applied to the lid margin, preferably after removing all the crusts, prevent the inflammation and minimise the scarring. Sometimes topical antibiotics are given in combination with the steroids. They usually give excellent and immediate symptomatic relief but they should not be used long-term.

Broad spectrum systemic antibiotics: The tetracycline antibiotic group (e.g. tetracycline, doxycycline and minocycline), appear to reduce the sebum production perhaps through anti-matrix metalloproteinase (MMP) activity combined with killing bacteria at the lid margin. However, they need to be given for several months and can have side-effects, such as increased likelihood of sunburn, and gastric reflux. These antibiotics should be reserved for cases that do not resolve with topical treatment and must not be given to children or pregnant or nursing mothers.

Ophthalmic herpes zoster (ophthalmic shingles)

This is caused by the herpes zoster (HZV)/varicella virus, which also causes chicken pox. Chicken pox is the result of the primary infection with HZV and is therefore more common in children. Shingles is the reactivation of the virus that has remained dormant in the nerve endings. It usually only involves one sensory nerve root area and is much more common in adults. The ophthalmic branch of the fifth nerve is the most common site: herpes zoster ophthalmicus (HZO).

The disease often starts with malaise and fever, and then pain over the area supplied by the affected nerve (the forehead, scalp and eye in ophthalmic herpes zoster). After a few days, the rash appears on the forehead, scalp and eyebrow (**Figure 6.6**). Sometimes the side of the nose is also involved, this signifies that the nasociliary branch of the ophthalmic nerve has been affected, and means that eye complications are more likely. Herpes zoster infections usually occur in the elderly or in patients whose cellular immunity is depressed. If it occurs in children (**Figure 6.6b**) or young adults it is often a sign that the patient is immunocompromised, most likely with HIV.

Treatment

In the early stages of the disease (within 48 hours of the rash appearing), systemic antiviral drugs (acyclovir or famcyclovir) taken by mouth, will reduce the disease severity. There is probably no point starting these drugs later on when they only produce limited improvement and they are expensive. Analgesics are helpful to control the pain. Sometimes secondary bacterial infection can occur in the rash and may require topical or systemic antibiotics.

Acute complications

Intraocular inflammation and infection: HZO can cause infective and inflammatory changes in the eye, although it is rare for it to cause serious ocular problems. During the acute HZO episode, conjunctivitis is common and infective keratitis occurs occasionally. These usually settle as the episode settles. However, they are sometimes accompanied or followed by inflammatory changes in the cornea (stromal keratitis) and in the anterior segment (anterior uveitis) of the eye. These inflammatory changes are treated with topical steroids and mydriatics. HZO can infect the retina (viral retinitis, see Chapter 13). Although this is extremely rare, it carries a very high likelihood

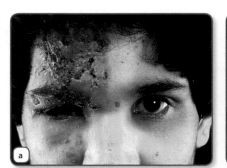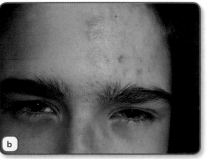

Figure 6.6 Ophthalmic herpes zoster. (a) An adult with HZO with a rash only affecting one side of the forehead; the side of the nose is spared. If the side of the nose is also involved this means the nasociliary branch of the ophthalmic nerve is affected and the eye is more likely to be affected also. (b) A child with HZO – this case is milder than in part a, but if you see a child with HZO, they are almost certainly immunocompromised. In this case, he was having chemotherapy for cancer.

of visual loss. Immunocompromised and elderly patients are more likely to develop viral retinitis than healthy patients with HZO.

Ocular muscle palsies: Very rarely, herpes zoster virus affects the extraocular muscles, causing squints and double vision.

Long-term complications

Postherpetic neuralgia: This is persistent pain in the area that had the shingles long after the rash has settled. It is quite common, can be very severe and may persist for years. Simple analgesics may help. The antidepressant amitriptyline and the antiepileptic drugs (carbamazepine and gabapentin) are often helpful.

Skin changes: More severe attacks of shingles can cause scarring, contracture and depigmentation of the skin.

Loss of corneal sensation: The herpetic viruses frequently impair corneal sensation. This can make the eye more at risk of other corneal disease, such as erosions, ulcers and damage from foreign bodies.

Intraocular long-term complications: Herpetic anterior uveitis can cause iris atrophy (see **Figure 11.10**) and chronic glaucoma.

Molluscum contagiosum

This is a viral wart, which appears especially on the margins of the eyelids (**Figure 6.7**). It is easily diagnosed, but frequently missed, particularly when it is a cause of chronic conjunctivitis). It is discussed in more detail in Chapter 7 (conjunctiva).

Infections of the eyelids caused by 'tropical' diseases

The eyelids are exposed, and are therefore prone to various infections, which occur only, or mainly, in the tropics. This occurs because of the prevalence of insect vectors combined with poor hygiene and malnutrition that occurs with hot climates and poverty. It is sometimes possible to make the correct diagnosis from a careful examination and a good knowledge of common local diseases. However, it may be necessary to ask for laboratory investigations, such as a bacterial culture or a histological examination.

Cutaneous leishmaniasis

This is common in many desert areas of the world. It is caused by a protozoan parasite, which is spread by the bite of certain sandflies. The disease usually occurs in young children or in people who have recently arrived in

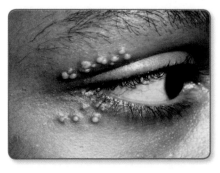

Figure 6.7 Molluscum contagiosum.

a tropical area. A granulomatous nodule develops first and later a localized chronic necrotic ulcer occurs where the sandfly has bitten (**Figure 6.8**). The lesion may be on any exposed tissue but is most common on the face. A histological examination at the base of the ulcer will show macrophages containing large numbers of parasites. Secondary infection with bacteria is very frequent, and probably causes some of the scarring and contracture, which occurs when the ulcer eventually heals. If the contracture occurs on or near the eyelids it can cause ectropion and ptosis (see below) (**Figure 6.9**).

Treatment: The majority of cutaneous leishmaniasis lesions heal without intervention. However, it is important to prevent or treat secondary infection by applying antiseptic or antibiotic dressings. Multiple other treatments have been tried with variable reports of success, including: scraping away the necrotic granulation tissue under local anaesthetic, oral fluconazole, oral metronidazole, oral allopurinol (usually used for gout) injections of amphotericin B and sodium stibogluconate, either given into the base of the ulcer, or given as a course of intravenous injections. In the long term, oculoplastic surgery may be required for the contractures and lid complications.

Cancrum (noma)

This is a poorly understood condition, which occurs in malnourished young children, usually following a severe generalised infection. In cancrum, there is rapidly progressive, severe inflammation of the tissues, which leads to gangrene and tissue destruction, especially around the lips and cheeks, and

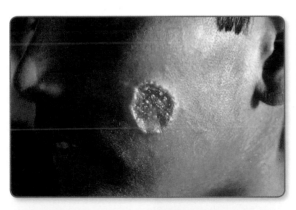

Figure 6.8 Active cutaneous leishmaniasis of the face. This ulcer has been cured of secondary infection but there is often pus and necrotic tissue on the surface.

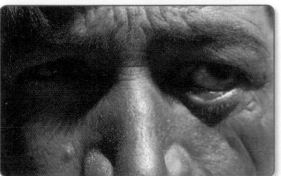

Figure 6.9 Contraction and ectropion of the left lower eyelid following cutaneous leishmaniasis.

sometimes on the eyelids (**Figures 6.10** and **6.11**). These children are desperately ill. The exact cause is uncertain but measles, herpes simplex and bacterial infection or a combination of these are all likely. The immediate treatment is improved nutrition, multivitamins and intravenous antibiotics and acyclovir. In the later stages complex plastic surgical reconstruction may be possible.

Leprosy

Leprosy is an important cause of eyelid abnormalities. It is discussed in Chapter 17.

Other tropical infections

Various other bacterial, fungal and parasitic infections may involve the eyelid and cause problems including: chronic inflammation, granulomas, ulcers, scars and lid position abnormalities. The most important of these infections are:

- *Chronic bacterial infections*, such as actinomycosis, tuberculosis and yaws.
- *Anthrax*: this is a bacterial infection spread by spores usually found on animal skins. Anthrax of the face is found among people who handle the skins of animals, or people who sleep on infected sheepskins. The disease presents acutely with one or more small raised spots on the surface of the skin, and severe oedema and tissue reaction. It can then progress rapidly to gangrene and generalised illness. It is treated with penicillin in large doses.

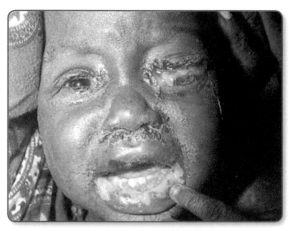

Figure 6.10 Early cancrum ulcers in the mouth, the eyelid and the base of the nose. Severe necrotic ulcers have developed in a malnourished child recovering from measles. Herpes simplex may be a cause of these ulcers.

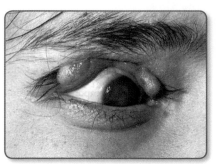

Figure 6.11 Old cancrum which has destroyed most of the upper eyelid. Note the secondary scarring in the exposed cornea.

- *Eyelash lice*: the lice are usually found embedded near the roots of the lashes, and their eggs (called nits) are stuck to the lashes.
- *Fly larvae*: flies may lay their eggs under the surface of the eyelids of young or debilitated patients. As the larvae develop, they cause a chronic infection and inflammation.
- *Onchocerciasis and loiasis* are both caused by parasitic worms, and may involve the eyelids (see Chapter 16).

Abnormalities of the function and position of the eyelids

Facial palsy

The facial nerve (cranial nerve VII) supplies the orbicularis oculi muscle. Therefore, paralysis of the facial nerve prevents the eyelid from closing properly (**Figure 6.12**). The paralysis is usually on one side only. In dense (complete) palsies, the diagnosis is obvious because the whole face appears lop-sided and droops on the side of the palsy. However, if the facial palsy is incomplete or bilateral, the diagnosis is often missed, as the defect is much less obvious or completely symmetrical. Patients with facial palsy often complain of a watering eye. This is because the loss of the blink reflex and the sagging, ectropic, lower eyelid prevents the tears from draining properly.

When the eyelids cannot close properly (lagophthalmos) or the blink reflex is reduced, the cornea is at risk from damage from exposure and infection. The majority of people do fortunately have a natural reflex which makes the eye roll upwards when they blink or attempt to blink: the Bell's reflex. This must be checked for in patients with a facial nerve palsy. If it is present, it is likely to give some protection to the cornea, but if it is absent the cornea is even more at risk.

Lagophthalmos is treated with various measures to protect the cornea. These include lubricant drops, taping the eyelid shut at night and surgery to

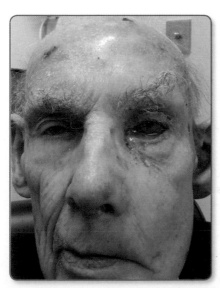

Figure 6.12 Facial nerve palsy. The left side of the face has drooped. Fluorescein dye drips out of the eye because of the ectropion and paralysis of the eyelid muscles, which should squeeze the tears towards the puncta. There is also lagophthalmos (inability to completely close the eye).

either help eyelid closure or reduce the size of the eyelid aperture. This is discussed in more detail in Chapter 17.

The anatomy of the facial nerve

The facial nerve passes from the brain stem into the temporal bone. Inside the bone it passes near the middle ear in a bony canal, and emerges at the base of the skull. It then breaks up into branches running across the face. It can be damaged at all of these different sites and there are therefore numerous possible causes of facial nerve palsies. Any patient with facial palsy should be carefully examined to exclude possible serious disease. It is particularly helpful to test for hearing loss and other cranial nerve abnormalities, to ask the patient if they had any facial or neurosurgery and to look for signs of leprosy. The most important causes of facial nerve palsy are:

- *Intracranial damage*, e.g. from a tumour pressing on the nerve. These patients are usually deaf in the same ear. The most common tumour to cause this is an acoustic neuroma (vestibular schwannoma).
- *Middle ear disease*, damaging the nerve in the facial canal. These patients will probably have chronically infected ears and hearing loss.
- *Leprosy* is a common cause of a unilateral facial palsy and practically the only cause of acquired bilateral facial palsy. The damage occurs in the superficial branches of the nerve and there may be some inflammation in the facial canal. If detected early it can be treated with steroids. It is discussed in detail in Chapter 17.
- *Surgery*: surgery anywhere along the path of the facial nerve can cut or damage its branches. It is particularly at risk during parotid gland surgery (e.g. for a parotid tumour) and acoustic neuroma surgery (see above).
- *Herpes zoster infection (Ramsey Hunt syndrome)*: these patients present with sudden facial nerve palsy similar to a Bell's palsy (see below). However, they also have pain and shingles vesicles in and around the ear and sometimes have decreased taste sensation, a dry mouth and dizziness. The infection can also affect other cranial nerves.
- *Bell's palsy*: this is the name given to a sudden facial palsy in which the cause is not known. It is a diagnosis of exclusion, i.e. the other causes of facial nerve palsy must be excluded before making a diagnosis of Bell's palsy. It often follows a mild upper respiratory infection. There is often partial or complete recovery of function some months later. Bell's palsy probably should be treated with a course of oral steroids, as this seems to reduce the length and severity of the episode.

Ptosis

Ptosis is drooping of the upper eyelid (**Figure 6.13**). Mild cases are only a cosmetic problem, but in severe cases the lid may obstruct the vision. There are many causes of ptosis. Most ptoses are caused by disorders of the muscle (or its nerve supply) that open the eyelid, called the levator palpebrae superioris muscle. It is supplied by the third (oculomotor) cranial nerve, and therefore ptosis may be a sign of serious neurological disease. Occasionally, ptosis is caused by other problems such as lid scarring, thickening or

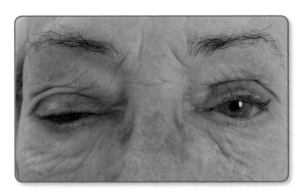

Figure 6.13 Right ptosis. The normal position of the pupil margin is between the pupil margin and the upper limbus. On the affected side, the eyelid covers most of the pupil. Patients with ptosis often raise their eyebrows subconsciously to lift the eyelid a little bit with their forehead muscles.

disorders of the nerve supply to a small sympathetic system controlled eyelid muscle called *Müller's* muscle. We will discuss the more common causes of ptosis and we have also put a danger flag next to causes, that although rare may be very serious and even life-threatening.

Ptosis caused by disorders of the muscle

Senile (involutional) ptosis: This is the commonest cause of ptosis. The levator muscle still works normally, but the aponeurosis that joins it to the tarsal plate has become thin and stretched allowing the lid to drop. This problem is repaired surgically, by identifying the aponeurosis and re-attaching it to the eyelid.

Congenital ptosis: This is quite common and may be unilateral or bilateral. There is usually a failure of the levator muscle to develop normally and therefore the function is greatly reduced, unlike a senile ptosis. If the drooping eyelid completely covers the pupil, the eye may develop amblyopia (see page 438). Congenital ptosis must be treated quickly if the lid is causing amblyopia, but can otherwise be left until the child is a bit older. The treatment is surgical, but the choice of surgery depends on the amount of function of the levator and therefore should be conducted by a specialist. There are some more rare causes of congenital ptosis such as blepharophimosis syndrome where the entire palpebral fissure is small.

Ocular myopathy: In ocular myopathy all the extraocular muscles are weak, but ptosis is often the first sign of this weakness. There are different types of ocular myopathy, they are mostly inherited disorders and are quite rare. Many of them are also associated with weakness of muscles elsewhere in the body. Myotonic dystrophy is the commonest one and causes widespread muscular weakness, and is associated with cataract.

Ptosis caused by problems with the nerve supply to the muscle

Third cranial (or oculomotor) nerve palsy: Complete 3rd nerve palsy will cause a total ptosis, a dilated pupil and limitation of all eye movements except abduction (from the lateral rectus muscle and a small amount of downwards movement from the superior oblique muscle) (see page 444). The eye is often described as being 'down and out'. If the palsy is only partial, some of these signs may be absent. A third nerve palsy can have various causes. However, the most serious is an expanding cerebral aneurysm.

This is an emergency and must be referred to a neurosurgeon urgently if at all possible.

Cervical sympathetic nerve palsy: The sympathetic nervous system supplies *Müller's* muscle in the eye, which has a small role in lifting the eyelid. Therefore, damage or interruption of this system causes a mild ptosis, as well as causing the pupil to constrict (because pupil dilatation, which is controlled by the sympathetic nervous system is paralysed), and reduce sweating on the affected side of the face. This condition is called 'Horner's syndrome'. The cervical sympathetic fibres may be affected anywhere from the thoracic spinal cord to the eye. Most causes of Horner's syndrome are not serious, but there are some life-threatening causes of a Horner's syndrome including a tumour at the top of the lung (Pancoast tumour) and an aneurysm of the internal carotid artery.

Myasthenia gravis (MG): MG is a complex disorder, which affects the neuromuscular junction between the motor nerve and the muscle. It is sometimes associated with tumours of the thymus gland. One of the first signs of MG is ptosis, which is usually bilateral. The ptosis is very variable, but is worse when the patient is tired. It is often associated with weakness of other muscles, causing double vision or difficulty in swallowing. The condition rapidly improves with a small dose of a drug, such as neostigmine, which strengthens neuromuscular transmission.

Ptosis caused by excess weight, volume or thickening of the upper lid

Extra volume, thickness or weight in the upper lid can cause ptosis, e.g. in trachoma, or an eyelid tumour. The eyelid is simply weighed down or held down by the extra weight or scarring.

Management of ptosis

The most important part of managing a ptosis is to diagnose the cause as this will guide the treatment. Surgical treatment is the final stage after medical conditions have been treated.

Eyelid retraction

Eyelid retraction is the opposite of ptosis. It is caused by overaction of the levator muscle and the smooth muscle fibres in both the upper and lower eyelid. It is usually associated with thyroid eye disease (see page 464 and **Figure 19.16**). It may also occur after trauma or excessive surgical correction of trachomatous entropion or ptosis.

Ectropion

Ectropion is out-turning of the eyelid, exposing some of the tarsal conjunctiva. The four main types are:

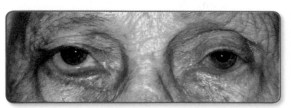

Figure 6.14 Atonic ectropion of the lower eyelids, especially on the right. The exposed conjunctiva has become inflamed and hypertrophic.

1. *Atonic (involutional) ectropion* (**Figure 6.14**): the lower lid loses it tension and is too loose to rest against the eyeball. It is caused by senile stretching of the tissues. The exposed conjunctiva is likely to become chronically inflamed, thickened and swollen. This in turn will cause further eversion.
2. *Paralytic ectropion:* this is caused by a facial palsy (see above)
3. *Cicatricial ectropion* (a cicatrix is an old-fashioned word for a scar): scarring and contracture of the eyelid skin, causes the eyelid to turn outwards (**Figures 6.15** and **6.16**). This usually occurs from extensive sunlight exposure, skin tumours that tether the skin, chronic skin infections and trauma/burns.
4. *Mechanical ectropion:* the weight of a large lid tumour can cause ectropion.

The treatment of ectropion is surgical. For atonic ectropion, the lid needs to be tightened, which is often done by removing a section of the lid ('wedge excision') or by tightening the lid laterally ('lateral tarsal strip'). It may help to give a short course of topical antibiotic and steroid ointment before surgery to suppress the inflammation in the exposed conjunctiva. Paralytic ectropion also requires lower lid tightening, but sometimes more complex surgery to minimise the lagophthalmos is also required. For cicatricial ectropion, a skin graft (often taken from in front or behind the ear) is often required in order to increase the skin volume. Mechanical ectropion obviously requires removal of the tumour or mass that is weighing down the lid.

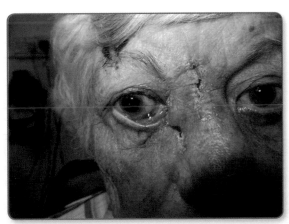

Figure 6.15 Cicatricial ectropion from trauma. This eyelid had a laceration from a fall. Although the wound was stitched up, the scarring has caused cicatricial ectropion.

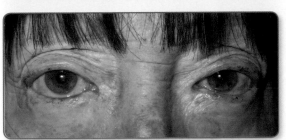

Figure 6.16 This lady has had long term sun exposure causing early cicatricial ectropion, symmetrically on both sides.

Entropion

Entropion is the inturning of the eyelid. This can cause the eyelashes to touch the cornea (trichiasis) causing irritation and damage. If this is not treated it can cause keratitis and corneal ulcers and produce scarring of the cornea and eventually blindness. Upper lid trichiasis is more damaging than lower lid trichiasis because the lashes are in greater contact with the central cornea. There are two main types of entropion:

1. *Cicatricial entropion:* This is caused by scarring and contracture of the tarsal conjunctiva and tarsal plate, causing the eyelid to turn in. This may occur after any chronic conjunctival infection or inflammation, but by far the most common cause is chronic trachoma (**Figure 6.17**), which is discussed in more detail in Chapter 8. Trachomatous cicatricial entropion is much more common in the upper lid. The treatment is surgical and must be done as soon as possible to avoid damage to the cornea.

2. *Atonic (involutional) entropion* occurs only in the lower lid in older patients. The tarsal plate becomes weak and floppy, and the connective tissue in the eyelid stretches. This allows the eyelid to roll inwards when the orbicularis oculi muscle contracts to close the eyelid (**Figure 6.18**). It is possible to restore the lower lid to its normal position by gently pulling it down. However, closing the eyes will invert it again. A good test for atonic entropion is to put in an eye drop that stings a little, e.g. topical anaesthetic. The patient will squeeze their eyes shut and this will bring out an intermittent entropion. The problem can be temporarily corrected by holding down the lower lid with tape or by putting in everting sutures (**Figure 6.19**). The long term treatment is surgical, and as with atonic ectropion, most of the surgical procedures involve tightening the eyelid.

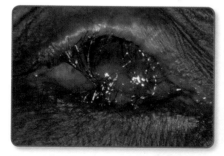

Figure 6.17 The upper and lower lids have a cicatricial entropion from trachoma and the lashes are rubbing against the cornea.

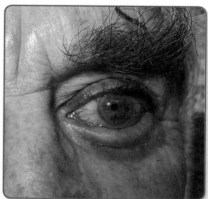

Figure 6.18 The lower lid has a senile (or atonic) entropion. The lower lashes and lid margin have turned in completely. This can easily be corrected just by pulling down the lower lid skin, but it will turn in again on closing the eyelids tightly.

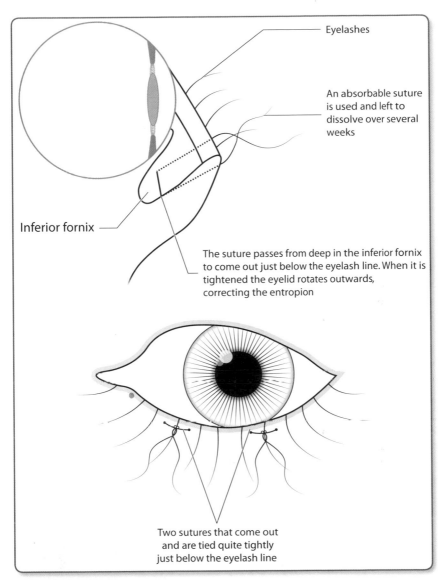

Eyelashes

An absorbable suture is used and left to dissolve over several weeks

Inferior fornix

The suture passes from deep in the inferior fornix to come out just below the eyelash line. When it is tightened the eyelid rotates outwards, correcting the entropion

Two sutures that come out and are tied quite tightly just below the eyelash line

Figure 6.19 Everting sutures.

Tumours

Eyelid tumours are quite common. The eyelids have a fairly complex structure, with lots of different parts, which can form tumours. It can be difficult to distinguish clinically between a tumour and some chronic inflammatory conditions in the eyelid. The most important distinction is whether a tumour is benign or malignant.

Benign tumours and cysts of the eyelid

Sebaceous cysts and cysts of other eyelid glands are the most common causes of lumps in the eyelid (see above) and may look like tumours (**Figure 6.7**).

Benign tumours are also common. They may originate in the skin or the connective tissue. A papilloma is a common benign tumour of the skin, which is usually found near the eyelid (**Figure 6.20**) margin. Occasionally, several papillomas may be present. Connective tissue tumours like haemangiomas or neurofibromas may also occur in the eyelids.

Malignant tumours of the eyelid

Basal cell carcinomas (BCC) (rodent cell ulcers)

These are the most common malignant tumours of the eyelids. They are found especially in fair-skinned people who have been exposed to excessive sunlight (**Figure 6.21a** and **6.22, 6.23**). They are therefore common in rural communities in the desert areas of the Middle East and central Asia and Southeast Asia. They are much less common in dark-skinned people and virtually unknown in blacks.

BCCs may occur anywhere on the eyelids and skin, but are most common on the lower lid. The typical appearance is a raised nodule with a rolled edge, a central ulcerated area and blood vessels (telangiectasia) running into and around it. When they are on the lid margin, there is likely to be loss of eyelashes (madarosis). Sometimes, the tumour may look like a cyst, or there may be inflammatory changes without any ulceration. The

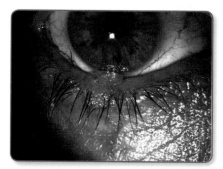

Figure 6.20 A squamous papilloma of the eyelid; a very common benign eyelid lesion.

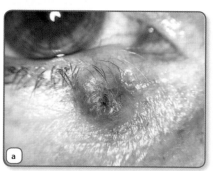
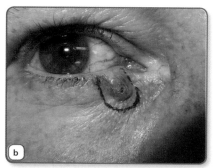

Figure 6.21 A small basal cell carcinoma (BCC). (a) An early small basal cell carcinoma of the lower lid. It has the characteristic features of a shiny ('pearly') rolled edge, small blood vessels (telangiectasia) and central ulceration. (b) The same BCC has been marked pre-operatively with a 3 mm border. As this BCC is close to the punctum, the patient must be warned that this may be damaged during surgery, which might cause a permanently watery eye.

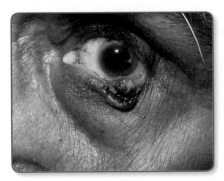

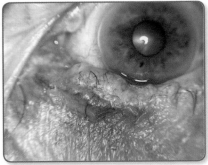

Figure 6.22 A large nodular basal cell carcinoma involving approximately half of the lower lid. This tumour presents in an Asian patient; although these tumours are less common in more pigmented skin, they still can occur.

Figure 6.23 A large ulcerating (morpheic or infiltrating) basal cell carcinoma. These can be more difficult to detect, as they do not form a lump. This one already involves over half the eyelid.

tumour is only locally invasive, and does not spread to other parts of the body. However, it continues to grow and spread locally on the face, and if left without treatment can be very invasive (growing into the orbit), disfiguring, and eventually fatal. One must be suspicious that any chronic ulcer or inflammation of the eyelid skin in a patient over the age of forty could be a BCC, especially if the patient is fair-skinned and has been exposed to excessive sunlight.

Other malignant tumours of the eyelids
The tumours described below are less common than BCCs, but are more dangerous and some of them can be fatal.
Squamous cell carcinomas (SCC): These are also associated with over-exposure to sunlight. They can grow quickly causing great local destruction and may spread through the local lymph nodes to other parts of the body.
Sebaceous gland carcinomas: These tumours are rare in Western countries and Africa but are more common in South and South East Asia, where they are as common as SCC. They are frequently mistakenly diagnosed as blepharitis or meibomian cysts. They can be fatal if not treated early.
Malignant melanomas of the eyelids: These are highly malignant, but fortunately very rare.
Kaposi sarcoma: Prior to the AIDS epidemic this was an extremely rare tumour. It has become much more common in recent years and is described in more detail in Chapter 20.

The treatment of eyelid tumours

Most eyelid tumours can be treated surgically by local excision (**Box 6.1**). The eyelids heal well and there is usually plenty of spare tissue that can be pulled in to fill the defect. It is possible to excise at least a quarter of the eyelid margin as a V-shaped wedge, and to close the wound edges with direct sutures. If a more extensive excision is necessary, various plastic surgical procedures can be used to reconstruct the eyelid (**Figure 6.24**). Skin grafts sometimes

> ### Box 6.1 Important considerations when doing lid tumour excisions
>
> - If there is a risk of the tumour being malignant, a margin of healthy skin 3 mm or more, depending on how invasive the tumour is) should be excised as well as the tumour (Figure 6.21b). It is better to leave the patient with a noticeable scar than to leave tumour in the tissues.
> - It is sometimes unclear from a clinical examination whether the eyelid tumour is benign or malignant, or even some type of chronic inflammation. If histology services are available then a small biopsy (incisional biopsy) will help make the diagnosis in doubtful cases. Knowing the exact nature of the tumour makes the planning of the surgery much easier.
> - If histological assessment is locally available, all tumour excision specimens should be sent for examination. This will confirm the diagnosis and inform the surgeon if the whole tumour has been removed and may even be able tell you exactly where residual tumour should be re-excised from.
> - Patients who have had skin tumours removed should be followed up for recurrence. The length of time depends on how malignant the tumour is and whether there was complete or incomplete excision initially.

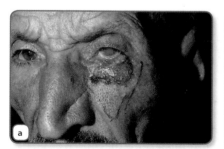

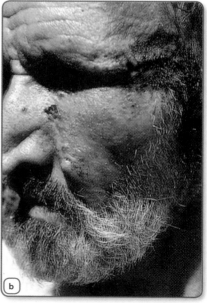

Figure 6.24 (a) This very large basal cell carcinoma has infiltrated the whole of the eyelid and part of the cheek. It must be excised with a healthy margin of tissue which is marked out with a pen. (b) After rotating a large flap of tissue from the lateral part of the cheek and angle of the jaw it was possible to close this large defect.

need to be used to fill in big defects, but these take very well on the eyelids because of their good blood supply. Other treatments such as cryotherapy and radiotherapy have been used to remove eyelid tumours, but these are not recommended as they can leave more scar tissue than conventional surgery and it can be very difficult to see recurrence in the residual scarred tissue.

Eyelid trauma

Eyelid trauma is common because the eyelids are very exposed. They are therefore frequently damaged when people are assaulted, in falls, road traffic accident and dog bite injuries (**Figure 6.25a** and **b**). They usually should be repaired surgically and it is important to ensure good alignment of the eyelid margin. Eyelid trauma that cuts through the canaliculus needs more complicated surgery (see below). Defects in the upper lid need urgent repair because of the risks of the exposed cornea becoming damaged.

Problems with the lacrimal apparatus

Tears are produced by the lacrimal gland superolaterally and drain down and medially across the eye to the upper and lower puncta and into the nasolacrimal drainage system (Figure 2.7). Problems can develop in any part of this system.

The lacrimal gland and lacrimal accessory glands

Diseases of the lacrimal gland are not common. Occasionally, however, the lacrimal gland is the site of inflammation, infection or of a benign or malignant tumour. As the lacrimal gland lies in the orbit, swelling of the gland will behave like an orbital mass, and cause forward displacement of the eye (proptosis) (**Figure 6.26**). The lacrimal gland can also swell with some infections, such as mumps.

Numerous inflammatory and autoimmune conditions cause scarring of the lacrimal gland and lacrimal accessory glands, e.g. Sjögren's syndrome, trachoma and mucous membrane pemphigoid. This will reduce the production of the watery component of tears, causing dry eye. The dry eye can be very severe and cause corneal damage and visual loss (see Chapter 8).

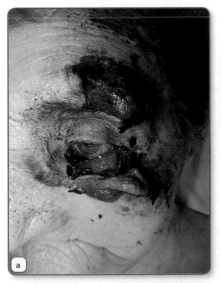

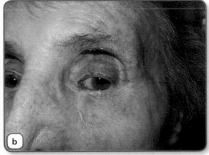

Figure 6.25 Eyelid trauma and repair. (a) This injury occurred when an elderly patient fell. (b) The wounds were surgically repaired. Eyelid and facial skin is very vascular, which greatly assists the recovery.

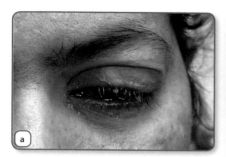

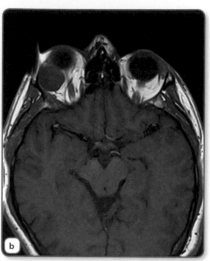

Figure 6.26 Diseases of the lacrimal gland. (a) Inflammation and swelling of the lacrimal gland (dacryoadenititis). This has caused the outer eyelid to be pushed forwards (proptosis) and downwards. (b) An MRI scan showing a left lacrimal gland tumour which is pushing the eye forwards and down.

The nasolacrimal passages

Disorders of the nasolacrimal passages are common, and usually produce excessive watering of the eye (epiphora). A watering eye can be caused either by poor drainage of the fluid because of an obstruction, or over-production of tears because something is irritating the eye or causing inflammation. There are two ways to find out if the nasolacrimal passages are obstructed:

1. A simple and very effective method is to instil a drop of fluorescein dye into the conjunctival sac of both eyes. After 1 or 2 minutes, look at the patient and see if there is still any fluorescein dye in the conjunctival sac. If one side still has fluorescein dye and the other side has no dye, the side with the dye has obstruction of the nasolacrimal passages. Further confirmation that the duct is patent can be obtained by asking the patient to blow their nose vigorously. Any dye on the handkerchief indicates that the tears are passing from the conjunctival sac into the nose.
2. The nasolacrimal passages can be syringed to see if any fluid passes down into the nose. This will also help to discover the exact site of the obstruction.

There are three common sites where the nasolacrimal passages may become blocked: the punctum, the common canaliculus and the nasolacrimal duct (see Figure 2.7).

1. **The punctum**
   Most of the tears pass through the lower punctum and the lower canaliculus. The upper punctum and canaliculus are less important. The punctum may become narrowed, occluded or everted, so that it no longer rests against the eye. A careful examination will detect defects of the punctum. An occluded or everted punctum can be corrected with a simple surgical procedure, such as widening the punctum with scissors.
2. **The upper and lower and common canaliculus**
   This is one of the narrowest parts of the nasolacrimal passages. Obstruction anywhere here or at the punctum usually causes epiphora without any conjunctivitis or discharge. If only the lower canaliculus

is blocked the symptoms are less marked and if only the upper one is blocked it usually does not cause any symptoms. The obstruction may occur following conjunctivitis which then causes scarring, but sometimes the common canaliculus becomes obstructed in old age. The canaliculus can become chronically infected and blocked with pus and debris, in which case slitting it open may allow this to drain and cure the problem. The site and extent of the blockage can usually be determined by passing a lacrimal syringe into each canaliculus after applying topical anaesthetic drops to the conjunctiva. Obstruction caused by scarring is very difficult to treat as the DCR operation (see below) is only possible if the canaliculus is normal. It is possible to insert a plastic, glass or silicone tube (Jones tube) through the medial caruncle and straight into the nose, but the tubes often become blocked or fall out.

3. **The nasolacrimal duct**

   This is the commonest site of obstruction. There are two ages at which this is usually seen: in infants, i.e. congenital nasolacrimal duct obstruction, and in older people, i.e. acquired obstruction. These two different situations behave and are managed very differently.

Congenital obstruction: The nasolacrimal duct only opens close to the time of birth and it sometimes hasn't opened when the baby is born. In most infants it will open naturally soon after birth, or in the first year. Approximately 90% of congenital obstructions will clear without intervention by the time the baby is 1 year old. Although the baby has continuous watering and some crustiness from dried tears, it rarely gets infected and does not trouble the baby (although it may trouble the parents and they should be reassured). It is advisable not to intervene with syringing and probing in the first year as this risks unnecessary damage to the tear drainage system. The occasional episode of infection can be treated with topical antibiotic drops. After the first year, it may become necessary to syringe and probe the nasolacrimal system under general anaesthetic in order to rupture the thin membrane that usually blocks the duct. However surgery is not obligatory as some obstructions will still clear independently in the second year of life.

Acquired obstruction: In acquired nasolacrimal duct blockage, the lacrimal sac usually fills up with stagnant tears and frequently becomes infected; this is called 'dacryocystitis' (**Figure 6.27**). The infection usually spreads to the conjunctiva, so that there is a chronic mucopurulent conjunctivitis as well as epiphora. The enlarged lacrimal sac can be seen or felt between the eye and the nose. Gentle pressure over the lacrimal sac may cause mucopurulent

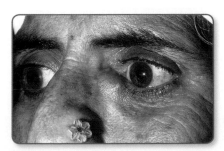

Figure 6.27 An enlarged lacrimal sac in a patient with dacryocystitis.

material to be squeezed back through the system and expelled from the punctum (**Figure 6.28**). It is helpful to teach the patient or the parents to massage the lacrimal sac. This helps keep it empty and reduce the risk of infection while they are waiting for permanent surgical treatment. Topical antibiotic drops are also helpful during episodes of infection. They should be applied after this massage so that they get right into the infected lacrimal sac.

Sometimes, an acute infection develops in the lacrimal sac with pain, redness and inflammation over the sac (**Figure 6.29**). In this case, the patient should be given systemic antibiotics. However, if the abscess bursts through the skin, this may leave a permanent fistula, so that tears pass out of the fistula and run down the cheek.

In adults, nasolacrimal duct obstruction cannot usually be treated successfully just by probing. There are two main treatment options.

1. *Lacrimal sac excision* (dacryocystectomy). This is the simplest treatment and can easily be done under local anaesthetic. It will cure the infection but the patient will be left with a watering eye.

2. *Dacryocystorhinostomy (DCR):* This is a more complex operation, which makes a new passage between the lacrimal sac and the nose. The bone between the lacrimal sac and the nasal mucous membrane is excised and the lacrimal sac mucosa joined to the nasal mucosa. This brings about a complete cure. The operation can be done under local anaesthetic but general anaesthesia is easier and often preferable for both the patient and surgeon. In some centres DCR is now being done from the nasal side using endoscopic instruments. This avoids the scar but the results are very dependent on the skill and experience of the surgeon.

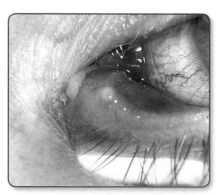

Figure 6.28 The obstructed, stagnant tears become purulent and infected. Pressure on the nasolacrimal sac with a cotton bud causes the pus to come out from the punctum. of the punctum.

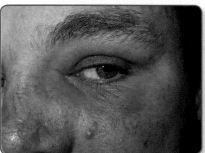

Figure 6.29 The blocked nasolacrimal system has become infected causing a lacrimal sac abscess. These abscesses can sometimes burst leaving a permanent fistula.

Diseases of the conjunctiva, episclera and sclera

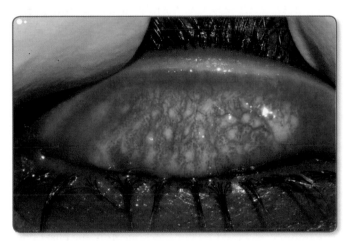

Conjunctival diseases are often not very serious, but they can give vital clues to the diagnosis of more serious disease. These conjunctival follicles are caused by active trachoma infection.

Conjunctivitis

Conjunctivitis is the general word for any infection or inflammation of the conjunctiva. The conjunctiva is the most exposed mucous membrane in the body, because the eyes are normally open during the day. Therefore it is vulnerable to infection and inflammation.

Conjunctivitis is the most common eye disease. It is more common and more serious in hot climates for the following reasons:

- Warm and humid climates are ideal for micro-organisms to survive and multiply.
- Dust, indoor wood fires and possible solar radiation are constant or repeated causes of ocular surface irritation.
- Insect vectors, such as flies, are common in hot and poor countries.
- Overcrowding, poor ventilation and poor hygiene all promote the spread of micro-organisms from person-to-person.

The symptoms of conjunctivitis

Discomfort

Conjunctivitis is usually uncomfortable but not very painful, because there are comparatively few sensory nerve endings in the conjunctiva. Irritation, itching or a foreign body sensation can all occur. Some causes of conjunctivitis, particularly viral, also affect the corneal epithelium. In these cases, there may be more pain and/or photophobia. If the pain is very severe then one should be suspicious that the diagnosis of conjunctivitis is not correct and there is pathology affecting the cornea or sclera.

Vision

The vision should be normal in conjunctivitis unless the corneal epithelium is also affected (see above). It may be intermittently blurred by excess secretions that form a film across the cornea. This usually improves when the patient blinks. If there is any visual loss, you should suspect that conjunctivitis is not the correct diagnosis.

Time course

The time-course depends on the cause of the inflammation, but viral and bacterial conjunctivitis is usually a self-limiting condition lasting a few days (except trachomatous conjunctivitis), while the length of symptoms of allergic conjunctivitis will depend on the season or exposure to allergens.

The signs of conjunctivitis

The signs vary according to the cause of the conjunctivitis. However some of the features below will be seen. A magnifying lens or loupes helps one to see these signs, although most of them can be seen with the naked eye. Examination of the conjunctiva should include everting the upper lid to see the upper tarsal conjunctiva. The normal everted upper lid can be seen in **Figure 7.1**.

1. **Vasodilatation**
    Dilatation of the superficial blood vessels is part of an inflammatory response. It causes the eye to go red and therefore conjunctivitis is sometimes called 'pink eye'. The redness is either spread all over the conjunctiva (**Figure 7.11**), or is most obvious towards the fornices. Conjunctival vasodilatation that is only found or is much more marked around the limbus it strongly suggestive of corneal or intraocular disease. In certain acute infections, petechial conjunctival haemorrhages may also be visible (**Figure 7.5**). In chronic conjunctivitis, the vasodilatation may be much less noticeable and confined to certain areas, such as the inner canthus or the upper fornix.

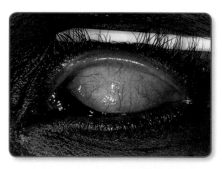

Figure 7.1 A normal everted upper lid showing the tarsal conjunctival surface. There is no inflammation and the blood vessels are clearly seen.

2. **Increased secretions**

   Increased secretions are a feature of most types of conjunctivitis. There are two reasons for this; firstly, irritation of the inflamed conjunctiva provokes a reflex increase in tear production; secondly, inflammation causes protein exudate and inflammatory cells to leak from the blood vessels. The character of these secretions often helps to diagnose the cause of the conjunctivitis:

   - Purulent or mucopurulent yellowy-green secretions are suggestive of acute bacterial infections (**Figures 7.2, 7.7 and 7.8**).
   - Watery (serous) secretions are more typical of viral infections (**Figure 7.11**).
   - Long, thick, 'stringy' white discharge is usually a sign of chronic allergic conjunctivitis (**Figures 7.15–7.18**).

   At night, when the eyelids are closed, the secretions become dry and 'crusted'. It can be difficult to open the eye(s) in the morning and the symptoms of conjunctivitis are also sometimes worse at this time. This may be because the temperature behind the closed eyelid increases, allowing micro-organisms to multiply.

3. **Oedema**

   Oedema of the conjunctiva (chemosis) and occasionally the eyelids may be visible in more severe cases. However, it does not usually indicate any specific cause (**Figure 7.8**).

4. **Follicles**

   Follicles are nodules of lymphoid tissue **beneath the surface** of the conjunctival epithelium, which guard against infection. These lymphoid follicles enlarge, especially in viral and chlamydial infections (**Figures 7.3**). Clinically, they must be looked for, particularly to help diagnose trachoma. They appear as small, slightly pale nodules just visible to the naked eye under the conjunctival surface. They are usually most numerous in the fornices, and may also appear on the inside of the upper eyelid. The upper fornix is difficult to examine, and so it is

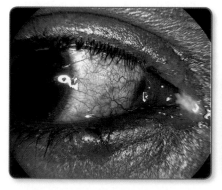

Figure 7.2 Bacterial conjunctivitis. The blood vessels are dilated, getting more dilated further away from the cornea. There is obvious purulent discharge in the inner corner of the eye.

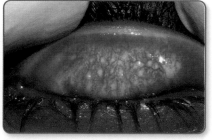

Figure 7.3 Follicles on the upper tarsal conjunctival surface appear as small, pale, glistening lumps. This patient has trachoma.

easier to identify follicles in the lower fornix. The lymphatic drainage from the conjunctiva passes to the preauricular node, which is just between the temporomandibular joint and the front of the ear. This preauricular node is sometimes enlarged and tender in conjunctivitis.

5. **Papillae**

   Papillae are raised areas **on the surface** of the epithelium in the conjunctiva lining the tarsal plates especially the upper tarsal plate (**Figure 7.4**) and occasionally near the corneal limbus (**Figure 7.16**). At these two places the conjunctiva is firmly adherent to the underlying tissues. Papillae are formed in response to any chronic inflammation and are composed of blood vessels and inflammatory cells growing in the subconjunctival tissues. To the naked eye, the papillae make the conjunctival surface appear rough, red and velvety rather than smooth and glistening. The conjunctiva also loses its normal transparency, so that it is difficult to see the underlying blood vessels very clearly. The individual papillae are not usually visible to the naked eye. However, with a slit lamp, and especially in green light, it is possible to see each papilla with its small central blood vessel. Occasionally, the individual papillae are very large and can be seen with the naked eye (**Figure 7.15**). This is called 'cobble- stone' hypertrophy, and is a characteristic feature of vernal conjunctivitis.

   It can be difficult to distinguish between follicles and papillae without a slit lamp. They are both features of chronic conjunctivitis, and are often present together, especially in trachoma. However, it helps to remember that follicles are found beneath the conjunctival surface and are most numerous in the fornices. Follicles usually enlarge in response to an infection. Papillae are found on the conjunctival surface, and especially in the upper tarsal conjunctiva and have a central blood vessel. They are an inflammatory response either to an allergy or an infection.

6. **Keratinisation (Figures 7.20 and 10.7)**

   Keratin is a hard protein, which skin cells produce to resist wetting. In certain diseases, the conjunctival epithelium produces keratin, making it hard and unwettable. The most important of these diseases is vitamin A deficiency (see Chapter 10). However, keratinization is also a feature of various rare types of inflammatory conjunctivitis (see page 155).

7. **Membrane formation**

   A membrane is a skin or plaque composed of organised fibrinous and inflammatory material, which covers and sticks to the conjunctiva

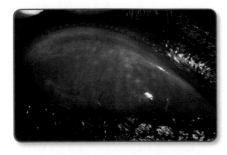

Figure 7.4 Upper tarsal papillae. These slightly obscure the view of the underlying conjunctival blood vessels. There are also a few follicles which are little white spots.

(**Figure 7.5**). The membrane can usually be peeled off the conjunctiva. They are uncommon, but may occur more frequently in streptococcal, diphtheria and some strains of adenoviral infection.

8. **Scarring**

   Scarring (fibrosis) is the end result of any inflammatory process in the conjunctiva. It is especially common in trachoma (see **Figure 8.4**). White, fibrous scar lines are seen on the tarsal conjunctiva and as the scarring worsens these converge into white plaques of scar tissue that can distort the eyelid, reduce the forniceal depth and obliterate and obscure the underlying blood vessels of the eyelid. Sometimes the tarsal conjunctiva eyelid adheres to conjunctiva of the globe. This is called 'symblepharon' (**Figure 7.19**). If the scars are severe, the conjunctiva will be unable to lubricate and protect the cornea properly and secondary corneal damage may occur.

9. **Increased pigmentation**

   Chronic conjunctivitis can cause increased pigmentation, particularly in more dark skinned people and especially in children. The pigment is most noticeable around the limbus and in the exposed conjunctiva between the eyelids (**Figures 7.6** and **7.16**). These pigmentary changes are characteristically diffuse and do not have well-defined margins. It is important not to confuse them with quite normal pigmentation which is often found around the limbus but is in irregular patches and has well-defined margins. The two most common conditions to cause increased pigmentation are vernal conjunctivitis and vitamin A deficiency xerophthalmia.

Causes of conjunctivitis

Numerous conditions can cause inflammation of the conjunctiva. In fact almost any infective or inflammatory skin condition can cause conjunctival inflammation, as the conjunctiva is a mucous membrane that extends

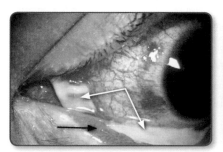

Figure 7.5 Acute haemorrhagic conjunctivitis with pseudomembrane formation from adenovirus infection. A greyish membrane at the inner canthus and lower fornix has developed (white arrow) and scattered haemorrhages are present under the conjunctiva and papillary hypertrophy of the lower tarsal conjunctiva (black arrow).

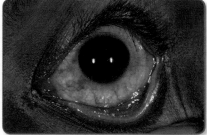

Figure 7.6 Pigmentation around the limbus. This patient is a 13-year-old girl who has had chronic trachoma. She also has upper lid entropion and trichiasis.

from the skin onto the globe. **Table 7.1** shows a list of causes. This list is not exhaustive, but does provide a system for helping you to make a diagnosis and decide on treatment.

Diagnosis of conjunctivitis

The list in the table of possible causes of conjunctivitis is very long. However, do not be dismayed by this, as most cases of conjunctivitis have one of four

Table 7.1 The main causes of conjunctivitis	
Infective	
Bacterial	Acute bacterial conjunctivitis†
	Blepharitis associated conjunctivitis (chronic) †
Chlamydial	Trachoma (*Chlamydia* A, B, C)†‡
	Adult inclusion body conjunctivitis (*Chlamydia* D-K)
Ophthalmia neonatorum	Gonococcus‡
	Chlamydia*‡
Viral	Adenovirus†
	Herpes virus (simplex and zoster)
	Molluscum contagiosum
	Measles‡
Rare infective causes	Syphilis, tuberculosis, actinomycosis, lymphogranuloma venereum, parasitic worms, myiasis
Immunological	
Type 1 hypersensitivity reactions	Seasonal and perennial allergic conjunctivitis (hay fever) †
	Vernal keratoconjunctivitis†
	Atopic keratoconjunctivitis†
	Giant papillary conjunctivitis
Type 2 hypersensitivity reactions	Mucus membrane pemphigoid‡
Type 3 hypersensitivity reactions	Sjögren syndrome
Type 4 (delayed) hypersensitivity reactions	Contact conjunctivitis: some irritants, chemicals and eye drops produce a true delayed hypersensitivity reaction, i.e. it takes around 2 days to develop
	Phlyctenular conjunctivitis
	Erythema multiforme/Stevens–Johnson syndrome/toxic epidermidis necrolysis‡
	Superior limbal keratoconjunctivitis
Others	
Chemical: e.g. cleaning products, chilli peppers, some traditional medicines, snake venom†, smoke†	
Traumatic/irritant: foreign body, e.g. dust, sand, eyelashes†, conjunctivitis artefact (self-induced)	
Poor tear film /primary dry eyes†	
Vitamin A deficiency†‡	
Exposure, e.g. facial nerve palsy†	

*Neonatal chlamydial conjunctivitis is unlikely to be blinding, but is often present with chlamydial pneumonia which can be fatal.
† More common causes in tropical and poor countries.
‡ Potentially blinding causes.

basic causes: bacterial infection, viral infection, trachoma and allergic/vernal (**Table 7.2**). Below are some questions to think about and ask the patient when you are faced with a patient with conjunctivitis.

Is the history acute or chronic/recurrent?

Acute conjunctivitis is usually caused by a bacterial or viral infection. Mucopurulent secretions indicate a bacterial cause. Watery secretions and follicles indicate a viral cause.

Chronic conjunctivitis can be caused by an abnormality of the eyelids, conjunctiva or lacrimal apparatus and all of these must be examined carefully. The commonest lid causes are blepharitis and inturning eyelashes. The commonest conjunctival causes are allergy (which can cause recurrent or chronic conjunctivitis), dry eyes and foreign bodies. The commonest lacrimal cause is nasolacrimal obstruction with lacrimal sac infection. Therefore, always look at the punctum for signs of discharge (see Figure 6.28) and the skin overlying the lacrimal sac for evidence of a lump or tenderness (see Chapter 6).

Is it unilateral or bilateral?

One very useful rule is that conjunctivitis is nearly always in both eyes. Infective causes often start in one eye but frequently become bilateral before long. If only one eye is affected, one must look for a predisposing cause, such as a foreign body or nasolacrimal obstruction. Alternatively, you should look for other causes of a red eye such as anterior uveitis.

What age is the patient?

Almost all the causes of conjunctivitis can affect children. However, allergic disease, trachoma and xerophthalmia are particularly common.

Where is the patient from?

The cause of conjunctivitis depends greatly on the location. For example, trachoma and xerophthalmia, which are both blinding diseases are only seen in poverty, while allergic disease is more common and often more serious in hot climates.

What symptoms does the patient have?

The symptoms can guide the diagnosis. For example, itchiness is more suggestive of allergic disease, the type of discharge can point towards bacterial (purulent), viral (watery) or allergic disease (white, stringy) and pain and photophobia indicate corneal involvement as well. Xerophthalmia, despite being potentially blinding, causes very few symptoms in the early stages.

What conjunctival changes does the patient have?

There is a lot of overlap in conjunctival signs, and inflammatory papillae occur in almost all types of conjunctivitis. However follicles are more suggestive of trachoma or viral infection, and giant 'cobblestone' papillae are strongly suggestive of allergic disease.

What other ocular signs does the patient have?

Examination of the limbus and cornea can be very informative: vernal keratoconjunctivitis (VKC), xerophthalmia and trachoma all cause limbal changes. In the cornea, xerophthalmia is associated with destructive corneal ulcers, trachoma causes superficial keratitis and VKC can cause 'shield ulcers'.

Table 7.2 A summary of the common causes of conjunctivitis

Cause of conjunctivitis	Age and background	Secretions	Duration of illness	Typical clinical picture	Cytology of conjunctival cells	Treatment
Bacterial	Any	Mucopurulent	1–2 weeks	Conjunctival vasodilatation, sticky eyes, eyelid oedema (if chronic or recurrent, look for eyelid or lacrimal disease)	Neutrophils	Topical antibiotics
Viral	Any	Watery	1–8 weeks	Follicles, papillae, superficial punctate keratitis, pseudomembrane if severe	Lymphocytes and monocytes	Symptomatic only
Trachoma	Mainly young children, poverty and crowded living conditions	Slightly mucopurulent	1 month to long term chronic symptoms	Follicles, papillae, corneal pannus	Mixed neutrophils and lymphocytes, inclusion bodies seen	Azithromycin orally or tetracycline ointment
Vernal/allergic	Children and adolescents, particularly in hot countries	White, stringy mucus	Chronic intermittent	Itchiness, papillae (sometimes cobblestone), limbal infiltrate and pigmentation, keratitis and corneal ulcers if severe	Eosinophils	Topical corticosteroids and mast cell stabilisers
Xerophthalmia	Infants and young children, poverty and malnutrition	Watery and foamy	Chronic	Bitot's spots, non-wetting of conjunctiva and cornea, corneal ulcers if severe, limbal pigmentation	Mixed	Vitamin A orally or injection

Acute bacterial conjunctivitis

Bacterial conjunctivitis (**Figures 7.2** and **7.8**) is common. The bacteria may invade a normal, healthy conjunctiva to produce a primary bacterial conjunctivitis. The inflammation is typically acute, severe (marked redness and discharge) and bilateral. The disease lasts for 1–2 weeks, and then resolves spontaneously, usually without any significant scarring. In some cases, the bacterial invasion is secondary to weakened defences, for example:

- Eyelid abnormalities, e.g. ectropion, entropion, trichiasis, facial palsy, chronic blepharitis.
- Lacrimal abnormalities, e.g. dacryocystitis, xerophthalmia/ keratoconjunctivitis sicca (dry eyes).
- Blepharitis: this extremely common condition is not fully understood, but is probably a combination of an abnormally oily tear film and chronic bacterial lid infection.

Secondary bacterial conjunctivitis usually has a more chronic course. It is important to look carefully for other abnormalities in cases of chronic conjunctivitis and particularly if it is unilateral when there may be a predisposing abnormality that requires treatment.

Numerous different bacteria can cause conjunctivitis and if swabs are taken it can often be difficult to determine if any bacteria that are cultured are pathogenic or are normal lid commensals. A few specific organisms that have particular characteristics are:

- *Staphylococcus:* can cause an acute primary conjunctivitis, and is a very common cause of secondary conjunctivitis.
- *Haemophilus influenzae:* often responsible for seasonal epidemics of conjunctivitis in hot, dusty climates.
- Gonococcus: usually comes from contact with genital discharges, and can causes a very severe conjunctivitis, particularly in neonates (see below).
- *Moraxella lacunata:* causes a more mild conjunctivitis and is sometimes called 'angular conjunctivitis' because the inflammation is in the inner and outer canthus.

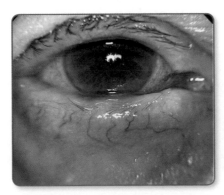

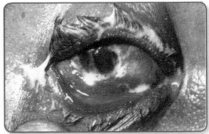

Figure 7.7 Mild bacterial conjunctivitis. There is a small amount of purulent discharge on the eyelashes and the conjunctiva is injected.

Figure 7.8 Severe bacterial conjunctivitis. The eyelashes, conjunctiva and lid margin are covered in purulent discharge and the conjunctiva is grossly swollen (chemotic) and injected.

The clinical appearance of bacterial conjunctivitis will depend on how severe it is. However, a characteristic feature is mucopurulent discharge (**Figure 7.8**). In more severe cases, there is the continual production of yellowy-green pus, but in milder cases the patient may simply report that the eyelids are stuck together on waking. There is always vasodilatation of the conjunctival vessels causing a red or pink eye. In severe cases there may be chemosis of the conjunctiva, oedema of the eyelids and general malaise.

It is not possible to identify particular bacteria by clinical examination. To identify the causative organism of any bacterial conjunctivitis requires a Gram stain of a conjunctival smear, or a culture. However, even where such facilities are available, it is only necessary to do this if the condition does not respond to first line antibiotics. Most cases are responsive to broad-spectrum topical antibiotics or resolve without treatment, and without any complications. The eye should not be padded, as this impedes cleaning and allows discharge, debris and micro-organisms to accumulate.

Treatment protocols vary, but one might consider a broad-spectrum antibiotic drop or cream four times a day, or two hourly in more severe infections.

Chlamydial infection

Trachoma

In many poor communities, chlamydia sub-types A, B and C is the commonest cause of conjunctivitis and unlike most other causes, trachoma is potentially blinding. It is discussed in detail in Chapter 8.

Adult inclusion body conjunctivitis

This rather clumsy phrase refers to adult chlamydial conjunctivitis. In adults the primary source of infection is the genital tract. It is more common in women than men. The eye infection is unlikely to heal properly until the genital tract infection is identified and treated. Untreated genital *Chlamydia* is an important cause of infertility.

Ophthalmia neonatorum (neonatal conjunctivitis)

Newborn babies are at risk of severe conjunctivitis within the first couple of weeks of birth. Their eye is especially susceptible to conjunctivitis, and the disease is more serious, for several reasons:
- The immune response and the protective tear film are poorly developed. Therefore, the neonate is less able to fight any infection.
- The neonate is exposed to potentially virulent infections in the vaginal tract, particularly gonococcus and chlamydia.
- The infant cornea is comparatively soft and vulnerable to invasion. An attack of conjunctivitis is more likely to infect and damage the cornea.

Gonococcus

This bacterium can be devastating to the eye. Vaginally transmitted infection causes acute and purulent conjunctivitis within the first 2 weeks of life. The infection can cause suppurative keratitis, corneal perforation and blindness (**Figure 7.9**).

Chlamydia

Vaginally transmitted *Chlamydia* usually produces a less severe conjunctivitis than gonorrhoea and usually occurs a few days later (perhaps between about day 5 and day 14) (**Figure 7.10**). However, the eye infection is an indicator that the patient is at risk of chlamydial pneumonia, which can be fatal and must be treated with systemic antibiotics.

Others infections

Neonates are of course at risk of other causes of infective conjunctivitis. However, initially one should treat the infant as if they have gonococcus or chlamydia because of the potentially devastating consequences of these infections.

Treatment

Neonatal conjunctivitis must be treated very quickly and vigorously because of the risk of permanent corneal damage or even death. If laboratory services are available a Gram stain of the conjunctival discharge will help to diagnose the precise cause, e.g. Gram-negative cocci will be seen in gonococcal infection. A culture is also helpful but treatment should be started immediately and the results simply used to support or guide treatment. Where laboratory services are not available, any severe neonatal conjunctivitis should be treated for both infections. Antibiotics should be given topically and systemically. If possible the child should be admitted to hospital as frequent topical and systemic antibiotics should be used and careful observation is essential.

Initial topical treatment should include very frequent tetracycline/erythromycin/azithromycin when the infection is severe and then less frequently as it improves. These are all effective against gonococcus and *Chlamydia*. Initial systemic treatment depends on availability and local guidelines, but

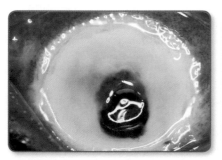

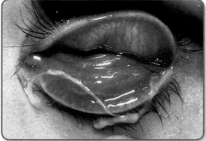

Figure 7.9 Acute and severe ophthalmia neonatorum. This baby had gonococcal conjunctivitis which caused ulceration and total destruction of the cornea. It is unusual to see a case as severe as this, but the neonatal cornea will ulcerate much more rapidly than in an adult.

Figure 7.10 Ophthalmia neonatorum from a chlamydial infection causing redness and swelling of the eyelids and mucopurulent discharge.

might include intravenous or intramuscular third (or later) generation ceph-alosporin (e.g. cefotaxime 100 mg/kg body weight) for gonococcus and/or erythromycin (50 mg/kg/day divided q.d.s.) or azithromycin (10 mg/kg for 3 days) for chlamydia. Gonococcus used to be treated with penicillin but resistance is now very common.

Mild neonatal conjunctivitis may only require topical treatment but still re-quires careful monitoring. Don't forget that the mother and her partner will also need assessment and treatment for genital infections.

Prevention

For many years Credé's treatment was performed to prevent neonatal con-junctivitis. The eyelids were cleaned with saline swabs as soon as the head was born and before the infant's eyes opened and then 1% silver nitrate drops were applied. However, silver nitrate may evaporate or decompose and thus cause burns to the eye. Therefore, tetracycline 1% ointment or erythromycin 0.5% or 2.5–5% povidone-iodine is now used. One of these preventative measures should be used routinely wherever there is a risk that the mother may be infected with gonococcus or chlamydia.

Viral conjunctivitis

Numerous different viruses can cause conjunctivitis, with a wide variety of clinical pictures. The disease may be so mild that it is impossible to recog-nise it clinically. At the other extreme, viral conjunctivitis may be a severe and disabling condition. There is no treatment for the majority of viruses that cause conjunctivitis, but fortunately it is usually a self-limiting condi-tion without long-term complications.

The typical symptoms and signs of a viral conjunctivitis are:
- Gritty foreign body sensation.
- Serous (watery) discharge.
- Dilated conjunctival vessels, causing red/'pink' eye (**Figure 7.11**).
- Lymphoid follicles and/or papillary hypertrophy.
- Mild to moderate photophobia. This is quite common because some viral infections also involve corneal epithelium.(**Figure 7.12**).
- Associated mild coryzal symptoms, e.g. sore throat, cough, runny nose.

Adenovirus conjunctivitis

Adenovirus conjunctivitis is the most common viral infection of the con-junctiva. There are many different strains of adenovirus. They are highly contagious; the infection is easily spread from person-to-person by direct contact. Therefore, the disease is particularly common where people live close together in unhygienic conditions, and often occurs in epidemics. Interestingly, epidemics also occur in eye clinics, as the infection is spread by eye workers, or contaminated equipment, such as slit lamps or tonom-eter tips. The old-fashioned name for adenovirus conjunctivitis was 'ship-yard conjunctivitis', after an epidemic in an American shipyard; workers fre-quently went to an eye clinic for removal of foreign bodies and treatment of

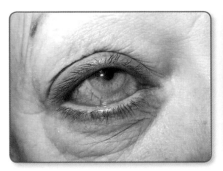

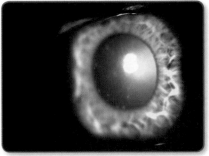

Figure 7.11 Acute viral conjunctivitis causing dilated blood vessels, which are most prominent towards the fornix and away from the limbus. There is increased watery tear secretion.

Figure 7.12 Adenovirus keratoconjunctivitis. There are white punctate opacities in the cornea.

welding injuries, but unfortunately they would catch epidemic adenovirus whilst they were there.

Adenovirus conjunctivitis is usually bilateral but often affects one eye first and more severely than the other. There are two specific signs to look for that are suggestive that adenovirus is the cause:

1. Numerous fine punctate areas of inflammation in and under the epithelium of the cornea. These opacities are only visible with good magnification and are more easily seen with focal illumination from a slit lamp (**Figure 7.12**).
2. A membranous layer of fibrin may form anywhere on the conjunctival epithelium, but most commonly on the upper tarsal surface (the eyelid must be everted to see it). This is sometimes called a pseudomembrane (**Figure 7.5**), as it not a layer of cells, just debris. They can be difficult to peel off.

The acute disease usually lasts for about 1–3 weeks. However, the small superficial opacities in the cornea may persist for many months, and cause discomfort, photophobia and slight blurring of the vision.

Some strains of adenovirus and sometimes other viruses like enterovirus can produce a very severe and contagious infection with conjunctival haemorrhages. This is called epidemic haemorrhagic conjunctivitis (**Figure 7.5**). There was a widespread epidemic in West Africa at the time of the 'Apollo' space missions and it is sometimes called Apollo disease in West Africa. In severe cases there may be residual corneal and conjunctival scarring.

Treatment

There is no specific treatment for the virus, so any treatment is essentially symptomatic, e.g. cold compresses and artificial tear drops if available. Antibiotic drops or ointment may help to prevent secondary infection. In severe cases, topical steroid drops 3 or 4 times a day may help the inflammation subside more quickly and can be a useful treatment for the inflammatory opacities that remain in the corneal epithelium after the infection has resolved. Steroid drops must always be used carefully and under supervision.

Measles

Measles is a generalised viral infection, which also invades the conjunctival and corneal epithelium. For this reason all children with measles have some conjunctivitis and superficial keratitis. Normally, these eye changes are quite mild compared to the other symptoms of the disease. However, measles in malnourished children is often very severe. It can cause serious corneal ulceration, blindness and even death. It is described in detail in Chapter 10.

Molluscum contagiosum

Molluscum contagiosum is a viral infection, which causes small dome shaped lesions with a central depression to develop in the skin, commonly on the face and trunk. Sometimes the lesions are very obvious (**Figure 7.13**) but often they are very small and easily missed particularly when they are on the eyelid margin. The lesions themselves are not a concern, but they shed virus, and when they are near the eye this causes a persistent follicular conjunctivitis. They are a frequently missed cause of chronic secondary conjunctivitis, which will not resolve until the lesion is removed. The lesions can be removed by scraping them off, or by using a sterile needle to open the centre out and cause them to bleed a little. If the child is very resistant to having them removed in this way, some people report that painting clear nail varnish on them clears them relatively quickly. This virus has become much more common with the HIV epidemic.

Herpes simplex virus

The herpes simplex virus may cause conjunctivitis, particularly when there are herpetic lid vesicles (herpes simplex blepharitis). It does not usually require treatment, but ocular acyclovir cream can be used (five times/day) if the lid lesions are painful, or if the patient is at risk of developing herpetic corneal ulcers (see page 191).

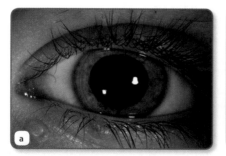
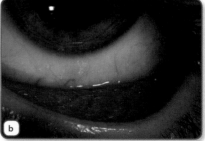

Figure 7.13 Molluscum contagiosum. (a) Two molluscum vesicles can be seen on the lower lid. These look quite harmless and could easily be missed. However, if the lower lid is everted (b) a chronic inflammatory conjunctivitis can be seen. This is frequently either missed (despitethe patient complaining of eye irritation) or misdiagnosed as allergic conjunctivitis. The inflammation is unlikely to resolve until the lesion disappears or is removed.

Granulomatous conjunctivitis (Parinaud's oculoglandular conjunctivitis)

Granulomatous conjunctivitis is the name for a follicular conjunctivitis with a local inflammatory granuloma and sometimes ulceration in the conjunctiva (**Figure 7.14**). It is nearly always unilateral and is often associated with visible swelling of the lymph glands on the same side (typically preauricular and submandibular). Sometimes fever and malaise are present. Granulomatous conjunctivitis is also known as 'Parinaud's oculoglandular conjunctivitis/syndrome'. Numerous, often rare, different infective agents can cause this clinical picture. Cat-scratch disease, tuberculosis and syphilis are probably the commonest causes, but others are given in **Table 7.3**. Parasitic worms, fly larvae and embedded foreign bodies can provoke a similar conjunctival granulomatous appearance, but without the systemic signs. A biopsy and culture are usually necessary to identify the causative organism, and the correct treatment can then be given.

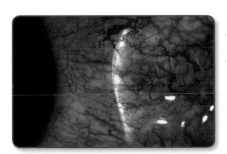

Figure 7.14 Granulomatous conjunctivitis. The conjunctiva is very inflamed and the slit lamp beam is used to show a raised area from the granuloma.

Table 7.3 Causes of granulomatous conjunctivitis

Disease	Infective agent	Type of infection
Cat-scratch disease	Bartonella henselae	Extracellular bacteria
Syphilis	Treponema pallidum	
Tularaemia	Francisella tularensis	
Yersinia infection ('plague')	Yersinia pseudotuberculosis	
Actinomycosis	Actinomyces israelii	
Tuberculosis	Mycobacterium tuberculosis	Intracellular bacteria
LGV *	Chlamydial LGV	
Rickettsiosis (Mediterranean spotted fever)	Rickettsia conorii	
Blastomycosis	Blastomycosis israelii	Fungal
Sporotrichosis	Sporothrix schenckii	
Coccidioidomycosis Paracoccidioidomycosis	Coccidioides immitis Paracoccidioidomycosis	
Infectious mononucleosis	Epstein–Barr virus	Viral
Mumps	Paramyxovirus	
* LGV, Lymphogranuloma venereum		

Immune response (inflammatory) conjunctivitis

The normal immune system should first react to and then eliminate an invasion or provocation and then should die down. However, sometimes the immune response is exaggerated or inappropriate; this is hypersensitivity. Hypersensitivity causes inflammation, which can cause tissue damage. There are four major types of hypersensitivity reactions: types 1, 2, 3, and 4.

Conjunctivitis from type 1 (allergic) hypersensitivity reactions

Type 1 (immediate) hypersensitivity occurs when histamine and other inflammatory mediators are released by mast cells and basophils. These cells have already been sensitised by immunoglobulin E to a specific antigen and when they encounter that antigen again, they hypersensitivity reaction occurs. This is atopic disease and typically happens in the skin, nose and eyes in children aged from 3–16 years, although occasionally, a younger child or a young adult may be affected. Type 1 conjunctivitis is very common and can sometimes cause serious and debilitating disease. There are three main types of type 1 hypersensitivity in the eye:

Vernal keratoconjunctivitis (VKC)

VKC (**Figures 7.15–7.17**) is a chronic allergic conjunctivitis, which is particularly common in children. In temperate climates, these children usually suffer from other atopic diseases such as asthma and eczema. However, in hot climates where vernal conjunctivitis is much more common and severe, many patients have no associated atopic diseases. VKC was originally called 'spring catarrh', but it often occurs throughout the year and particularly in countries where there is no spring. Furthermore the damaging consequences of the disease are conjunctival and corneal, while 'catarrh' (secretions) is a less significant symptom of the disease. Also, 'vernal' is also not accurate, as this is simply the Latin for spring. Therefore, some people refer to the

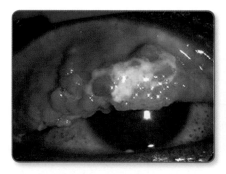

Figure 7.15 Vernal conjunctivitis. The upper eyelid has been everted to show the 'cobblestone' papillae on the upper tarsal conjunctiva and typically allergic, white 'stringy' discharge. Dark pigmented spots are also visible at the limbus.

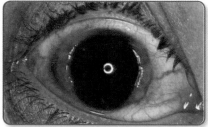

Figure 7.16 Limbal hypertrophy in vernal keratoconjunctivitis. There is fleshy papillary hypertrophy of the conjunctiva and increased pigmentation at the limbus.

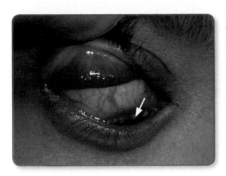

Figure 7.17 Severe vernal keratoconjunctivitis. This causes very marked papillary inflammation of the upper tarsal conjunctiva and Trantas spot (arrow). Courtesy of Dr N Rogers.

disease as VKC when it is seasonal and atopic keratoconjunctivitis (AKC) when it is not. Other people use the term VKC when it is in children and AKC when it is in adults.

The symptoms and signs of VKC

VKC is a bilateral disease, usually with similar severity in the two eyes. Severe and persistent itching and irritation in both eyes is the characteristic symptom. There is often a sticky, white discharge which forms long 'ropey' strands (**Figure 7.15**), caused by increased secretion of viscous mucus in the tears; the patients often complain of 'string' or 'worms' in their eye. Thickening of the tarsal conjunctiva with the formation of papillae is a characteristic feature of vernal conjunctivitis. This can give the conjunctiva a 'velvety' appearance and obscures the underlying blood vessels. Sometimes the papillae are huge, when they are referred to as 'cobblestone papillae' (**Figure 7.15**). The spaces between the papillae are filled with mucus, and it is possible to demonstrate this mucus with special stains like Alcian blue. Often the symptoms and signs do not match: some patients have cobblestone papillae, but mild symptoms, whilst others have severe itching, but minimal conjunctival changes.

Inflammation also occurs at the limbus (**Figure 7.16**). The limbal conjunctiva appears thick and swollen and the underlying blood vessels may be dilated. Limbal vasodilatation is unusual for a conjunctival disease, as it is usually a sign suggestive of corneal or intraocular disease. Small pin-point white fluorescein staining spots may appear on the corneal epithelium at the limbus; they are called Trantas spots (**Figure 7.17**). They represent spots of necrosis of the epithelium. The changes at the limbus are more common in younger children. Increased pigmentation also occurs at the limbus in dark-skinned races (Figure 7.17). It often spreads to affect the entire exposed conjunctiva between the eyelids. These pigmentary changes are fine and diffuse, and often very obvious.

Occasionally, the cornea is affected in VKC. This is probably because the limbal inflammation spreads to the peripheral cornea, but also the thick mucus sticks to the corneal epithelial cells and the tarsal papillae rub against the cornea. The first sign of any complication in the cornea is a superficial punctate keratitis (see page 215). Occasionally, the epithelial cells are stripped away to form a shallow oval ulcer, usually just above the centre of the cornea (**Figure 7.18**). These ulcers are sometimes called 'shield' ulcers, because of their shape. They are sometimes bilateral. They have a lot of mucus in their base, which can form a thick sticky plaque which adheres

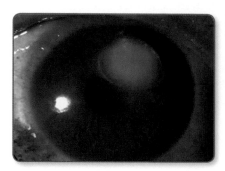

Figure 7.18 A shield ulcer in severe vernal keratoconjunctivitis.

firmly to the cornea, and prevents the ulcer from healing by stopping the corneal epithelial cells growing over the ulcer. If the ulcer will not heal, one can scrape away the mucous plaque with a scalpel under local anaesthetic. Eventually, the ulcer will heal to become a vascularised scar.

VKC appears to die out in adult life. There is only a risk of permanent damage to the eye if corneal ulcers have developed. Limbal changes fade away quickly, and the inflammation and hypertrophy of the conjunctiva gradually subsides usually leaving little or no scarring. There is an association between VKC and keratoconus (see page 217), but the reason for this is uncertain.

The treatment of vernal conjunctivitis

Topical steroid drops is the main treatment. In a typical case, prednisolone or dexamethasone drops about 4 times a day for 1–2 weeks will relieve most of the symptoms. After that, drops perhaps twice daily will maintain the relief. However, they should not be used long-term and should be reserved for short periods when the disease is very bad. Unfortunately, many patients or their parents obtain further supplies from local chemists and continue treatment for months or years. They risk causing cataracts, glaucoma and infective ulcers. Patients and parents should be warned of these dangers. Sometimes a subconjunctival injection of steroid, under the upper tarsal conjunctiva, may have a better effect than drops, especially if there is marked inflammation and hypertrophy of the upper tarsal conjunctiva. Mast cell stabilisers such as sodium cromoglycate, nedocromil, lodoxamide or olopatadine can support steroid treatment. These prevent the release of histamine and other toxins from the mast cells. They should be commenced at the same time as steroids and can be continued longer term to maintain the response to the steroid, but must be used regularly (two to four times daily depending on preparation). They have few side effects, although they are more expensive than steroids. Oral antihistamines are also useful, but many of them cause unwanted drowsiness. In severe cases that do not respond to topical steroids, topical cyclosporine can be used. However, this is a very expensive treatment at present. In some chronic cases the response to medical treatment is disappointing, or it cannot be given because of side effects.

In the past various surgical treatments have been used to destroy the papillae on the upper tarsal conjunctiva. They are rarely used nowadays because of the risk of permanent damage to the conjunctiva, but there is possibly still a place for them in intractable cases or if the side effects of medical treatments are prohibitive. Treatments that have been used in the past include tarsal conjunctival cryotherapy and diathermy/cautery/beta radiation destruction of the papillae. In desperate cases people sometimes try occlusive goggles to prevent allergens reaching the eye or they have been advised to emigrate to a cooler country if they can afford it!

Seasonal and perennial allergic conjunctivitis (hay fever)

Hay fever conjunctivitis is an acute allergic reaction to airborne allergens such as pollen, moulds, dust and animal particles (dander). These allergens react with IgE immunoglobulins bound to mast cells to provoke the release of histamine and other inflammatory mediators. It is often not possible to identify the specific allergen. It is usually associated with acute rhinitis. There are none of the structural changes which vernal conjunctivitis causes in the conjunctiva. The symptoms of hay fever conjunctivitis usually subside with a short course of antihistamines given topically or systemically. Mast cell stabilisers, and in severe cases topical corticosteroids, may also be helpful.

Numerous substances in the environment can provoke an immediate hypersensitivity response. Common ones, worth considering if a patient has chronic and itchy conjunctivitis, are animal hairs or dander and house dust mite. If facilities allow, these can be tested for with skin prick testing.

Giant papillary conjunctivitis (GPC)

GPC is a type I hypersensitivity occurring locally in response to contact with a foreign material, for example, a contact lens (particularly a soft lens if there are deposits on the lens) or an artificial eye. Giant papillae that look similar to those in VKC form on the upper tarsal conjunctiva. The symptoms are typical of allergic conjunctivitis, with itching and stringy discharge. The treatment is to identify and remove or clean the provoking material and then treat the inflammation with mast cell stabilisers. Topical steroids are rarely required, except in patients with ocular prostheses, when there are fewer concerns about side-effects.

Conjunctivitis from type 2 hypersensitivity reactions

Type 2 (antibody-dependent cytotoxic) hypersensitivity occurs when antibodies bind either to the patient's own tissues or to foreign antigens that are attached to the patient's cells surfaces. This provokes an immune attack on these tissues.

Mucous membrane pemphigoid

In this condition, there is gradual shrinkage and fibrosis of the conjunctiva. The disease is often referred to as ocular cicatricial pemphigoid, but in fact the scarring changes occur in mucous membranes other than the eye, including the inside of the mouth (buccal mucosa) from where biopsies can be very helpful for diagnosing this condition. It is a rare, but potentially blinding condition, which is frequently missed. The earliest sign of the disease is the reduction in depth of the fornices and the development of adhesions between the tarsal and bulbar conjunctiva called 'symblepharon'

(**Figure 7.19**). In more severe cases there is keratinization of the conjunctival epithelium, which may spread to produce severe scarring of the cornea (**Figure 7.20**). The treatment of MMP is very difficult and often not very effective unless a wide range of lubricants, anti-inflammatories and immune-suppressants are used as well as surgery to correct lid deformities.

Conjunctivitis from type 3 hypersensitivity reactions

Type 3 (immune complex mediated) hypersensitivity occurs when excess quantities of antigen-antibody immune complexes form and cannot be cleared by the immune system.

Sjögren syndrome

Sjögren syndrome is an immune condition, which results in dry eyes [also known as keratoconjunctivitis sicca (KCS)]. Sjögren syndrome can be primary, when dry eyes and dry mouth are the only symptoms, or secondary when these features are found together with an autoimmune condition such as rheumatoid arthritis. Primary Sjögren syndrome is quite common especially in old people. Secondary Sjögren syndrome is less common overall, but does occur very frequently among patients with several different auto-immune conditions. The lacrimal gland and accessory conjunctival glands become inflamed and then scarred, making them less able to produce tears. The eyes feel sore and gritty and the conjunctiva becomes inflamed. These patients are also more prone to developing other forms of conjunctivitis, such as bacterial and herpetic as the eyes' tear film defence is weaker. The epithelial cells in the exposed conjunctiva and cornea become degenerate and dehydrated, producing a superficial punctate keratoconjunctivitis,

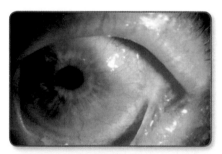

Figure 7.19 Mild mucous membrane pemphigoid. There is adherence between the tarsal conjunctiva and the bulbar conjunctiva.

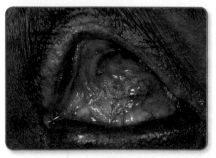

Figure 7.20 Severe mucous membrane pemphigoid. The conjunctiva and cornea have become completely keratinised and the fornices obliterated. The only hope for useful treatment for an eye like this, where both the conjunctiva and the cornea are severely diseased, is a very complex and difficult operation to insert an artificial cornea called keratoprosthesis (see Figure 9.31 page 224).

particularly in the lower more exposed parts of the cornea. This can be detected in the usual way with magnification and fluorescein dye (**Figure 9.18**).

To diagnose keratoconjunctivitis sicca, it is necessary to demonstrate the lack of tears. This is done with a small strip of filter paper, the end of which is left in the lower fornix (Schirmer test) (**Figure 7.21**). Typically the test is done for 5 minutes and the length of wetting along the filter paper is measured; less than 10 mm is abnormal. The test is not always reliable, although will usually pick up very dry eyes. It can give different results with and without prior instillation of topical anaesthetic, because anaesthetic eliminates reflex tearing. A careful slit lamp examination of the tear film and the speed at which it breaks up will also show that the tear film is deficient.

KCS is treated with frequent instillation of tear substitutes such as methylcellulose. Antibiotic drops and ointment will help to prevent or treat secondary conjunctivitis, and acetylcysteine drops (5%) will help to dissolve the excess mucus, although they can sting and can be difficult to obtain. In severe cases, it may help to close the lacrimal puncta. This can be done with cautery under local anaesthetic. This is easy and cheap to do; under local anaesthetic the tip of a cautery is placed in the punctum and the cautery turned on for a few seconds. However, it is irreversible. In some places punctum plugs may be available. These have the advantage of being easily removed, but they also often fall out or can accidentally be pushed too far in, where they may cause chronic irritation or infection.

Conjunctivitis from type 4 hypersensitivity reactions

Type 4 (delayed) hypersensitivity occurs when a group of immune cells called the T cells are initially sensitised by an antigen and then encounter this antigen again, causing a vigorous inflammatory response. Unlike type 1 reactions, type 4 reactions do not provoke eosinophil release.

Contact (irritant) conjunctivitis

Almost any substance can provoke an irritant reaction in the conjunctiva and usually the eyelids as well, which become red and swollen (skin dermatitis). Sometimes this is a delayed response (i.e. a true type 4 reaction) and sometimes an immediate reaction. Commonly encountered culprits

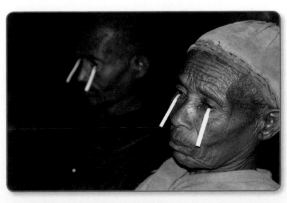

Figure 7.21 Schirmer test for dry eyes.

include: eye medication (e.g. neomycin, gentamicin, thimerosal, chloramphenicol) and preservatives or other 'vehicles' in eye medication (e.g. benzalkonium chloride), cosmetics and toiletries (**Figure 7.22**). A careful history and occasionally allergy testing may help identify the causative agent. Topical steroids will relieve the symptoms, but the long-term solution is to identify and avoid the particular medication or chemical that is provoking the conjunctivitis. An allergic response to topical medication is surprisingly common and often missed, with the inflammation being attributed to the underlying infection or disease process rather than the treatment. In some culture, over-prescribing of medicines is a major problem and the unfortunate patient is given yet more medicine, when the best treatment may be to stop all the treatment and re-assess the situation in a few days.

Phlyctenular conjunctivitis and keratoconjunctivitis

'Phlycten' is the Greek word for a blister and it describes the clinical appearance of this disease (**Figure 7.23**). Phlyctenular conjunctivitis is caused by a localised hypersensitivity reaction to bacterial proteins in the bloodstream. These bacterial proteins are often tubercular, and the highest incidence of the disease is in poor communities where tuberculosis is common and any patient with a phlycten is a tuberculosis suspect. However, other bacterial proteins, e.g. staphylococcal antigen or even fungal proteins, e.g. *Candida albicans*, can also provoke them. Even if the response is to a tubercular protein, it does not necessarily mean that there are living bacilli in the body. The phlyctenular reaction itself represents a high degree of antibody formation

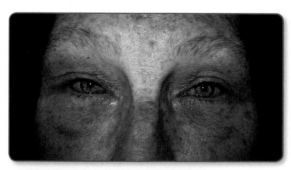

Figure 7.22 Allergic reaction to eye drops causing vasodilatation of the conjunctival blood vessels as well as redness and swelling of the eyelids and the cheek.

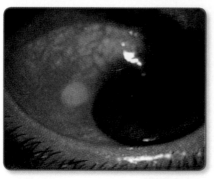

Figure 7.23 Phlyctenular conjunctivitis. The patient has a grey, raised lesion with intense inflammation around it.

and is suggestive of some resistance to the infection. However, a Mantoux test and chest X-ray should be done if possible.

Children and young adults are most at risk of developing phlyctens, probably because they have particularly reactive cell-mediated immunity. They may appear anywhere on the bulbar conjunctiva, but are especially common at or near the limbus. It is not known why they only occur here, and not in other parts of the body. A phlycten first appears as a raised pinkish nodule surrounded by an area of hyperaemia. It then develops a necrotic grey centre surrounded by reactive inflammation. Finally the necrotic centre sloughs out and the phlycten heals. Conjunctival phlyctens produce only mild symptoms and heal without obvious scarring. However, corneal phlyctens cause considerable photophobia, pain and discomfort, and may leave significant scars (Figure 9.13). The whole process normally takes about 2 weeks. Sometimes the disease process can be much more severe: limbal phlyctens can 'migrate' towards the centre of the cornea. The edge that is advancing upon the cornea shows superficial ulceration and inflammation. The limbal edge heals with vascularisation and scarring. If these ulcers are not treated, they may eventually reach the central area of the cornea. The final scar is characteristically superficial and forms a wedge pointing towards the centre of the cornea.

Phlyctens respond very well to topical corticosteroids. The inflammation will rapidly resolve and the amount of final scarring and visual loss will be far less. A few patients may need systemic treatment for tuberculosis.

Erythema multiforme, Stevens–Johnson syndrome (SJS) and toxic epidermal necrolysis (TEN)

These three conditions are thought to be the same pathological process, but with differing severity. An immune mediated cytotoxic reaction causes acute inflammation of skin and mucus membranes. It is often provoked by taking a new medication, particularly some antibiotics. In milder cases (erythema multiforme) 'target lesions' occur on the skin (**Figure 7.24a**), but resolve without intervention. However, in more severe cases (SJS and TEN), the disease can be associated with profound conjunctival inflammation and then scarring. All the mucous membranes can be affected, and the top layers of skin can peel away from the underlying layers (**Figure 7.24b**). TEN is frequently fatal, particularly if good intensive care facilities are not available. However, for patients who do survive, the damage is particularly devastating in the eyes and patients are frequently left with poor or no vision, from corneal scarring and severe dry eye (**Figure 7.24c**). Ocular treatment in the acute stage involves intensive lubricant use, topical steroid and antibiotic and frequent monitoring to assess for corneal complications.

Other causes of conjunctivitis

Rosacea

Rosacea is a chronic inflammatory disease of the skin. It particularly affects the central face and is associated with meibomian gland dysfunction of the eyelids, which can cause a chronic conjunctivitis. It is considered in more detail in Chapter 6.

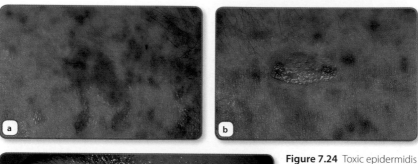

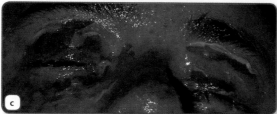

Figure 7.24 Toxic epidermidis necrolysis. (a) 'Target' lesions. (b) Skin peeling away. (c) Severe periocular disease in toxic epidermidis necrolysis.

Traumatic conjunctivitis (see Chapter 21)

Conjunctival foreign bodies are extremely common, and are easy to miss both in the history and the examination. They can cause a chronic conjunctivitis if they are not removed.

Chemical conjunctivitis

Ocular chemical injuries will inevitably cause conjunctival inflammation. One chemical injury that is almost exclusively seen in tropical countries is snake-bite venom, particularly from spitting cobras. Although this can cause vigorous conjunctivitis and corneal epithelial erosions, the vision should return to normal. Traditional medicines can also contain substances such as euphorbia sap, which may cause a vigorous immediate inflammatory reaction.

Psychological causes of conjunctivitis

Tension, anxiety or depression can produce symptoms all over the body. The exact pattern of these symptoms varies both with the cultural background and with the individual patient. It is very common for young students who have no significant refractive error or evidence of eye disease to complain of irritation and discomfort in their eyes and difficulty in reading. It is of course necessary to check thoroughly that there is no underlying organic disease, refractive error or extraocular muscle imbalance. Probably the best treatment then is to reassure the patient that nothing is wrong, but some of these patients are very resistant to reassurance. In these situations one might consider a topical lubricant which sooths the eye and probably works as a good placebo.

Very rarely, patients deliberately damage their own conjunctiva; this variant of Münchausen disease (a condition in which a person pretends to be ill or harms themselves) is called *conjunctivitis artefacta*.

Degenerative changes in the conjunctiva

Pinguecula (plural pingueculae)

A pinguecula is a fatty degenerative deposit which is found under the conjunctival epithelium in the exposed interpalpebral fissure (**Figure 7.28b**). Pingueculae are common in older patients who have been exposed to the sun and probably dust and other environmental insults for many years. They do not usually cause any symptoms unless they become raised and inflamed. If this occurs, localised inflammation is seen. They usually settle without intervention or just with artificial tears for comfort, although a mild topical steroid such as fluorometholone can be used if required.

Pterygium

A pterygium is a wedge of conjunctival tissue, which grows over the surface of the cornea (see Figures 9.24 and 9.25). It is discussed in detail in Chapter 9.

Concretions (Figure 7.25)

Concretions are tiny, hard, yellow or white granules, which are found on the inside of the eyelids. They are formed of the degenerative products of old epithelial cells and mucus, and may also contain calcium deposits. They often develop after infection like trachoma but may occur in otherwise healthy eyes. They usually do not cause any symptoms but they can erode to the surface, where they may scratch the cornea and give a gritty feeling to the eye. If they are causing symptoms they can be removed with the point of a needle using local anaesthetic drops.

Conjunctival tumours

Conjunctival tumours are quite common in tropical countries, and usually occur at or near the limbus. They have become much more common in recent years, probably because of the HIV/AIDS epidemic.

Conjunctival carcinoma

Conjunctival carcinoma appears to be brought on by excessive exposure to sunlight, and perhaps also irritation from dust, sand and smoke. Over the last few years there has been an epidemic of conjunctival carcinoma especially in Africa, and these patients have a high risk of being

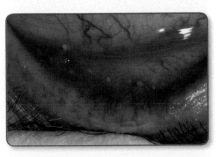

Figure 7.25 Conjunctival concretions in the lower tarsal conjunctiva.

HIV positive. It is thought that the HIV virus suppresses the immunity to another virus (possibly one of the human papilloma viruses) which multiplies and encourages tumour formation. Sunlight also seems to be needed to provoke the growth of the tumour because they only appear in the exposed part of the conjunctiva.

Conjunctival carcinoma starts in the epithelial cells. When the disease is confined to the epithelium it is called 'carcinoma in situ' and can easily be removed (**Figure 7.26**). It later spreads to the subconjunctival tissues and surrounding conjunctiva but can still be totally excised (**Figure 7.27**). After removing all the tumour cells as deeply as possible, the surface of the wound on the sclera should be treated to kill any remaining tumour cells. This can be done using cryotherapy, diathermy or cytotoxic drugs like mitomycin. Neglected conjunctival tumours can become large fungating masses filling the whole orbit, and may need radical surgery, or can even be fatal (see Figure 19.13).

Other conjunctival cysts and tumours

- *Congenital dermoid cysts* are found at the limbus. They occasionally have hair coming out of them. They can usually be easily excised.
- *Pigmented naevi* are common especially near the limbus, particularly in darker skinned races (**Figure 7.28**) and no treatment is usually necessary. However, if there is evidence of growth or inflammation, they should be removed by local excision and if possible they should be examined by a pathologist.
- *Melanomas* are very occasionally seen in the conjunctiva.

Scleritis and episcleritis

Episcleritis

Episcleritis is a common, localised inflammation of the episcleral layer of the eye (**Figure 7.29**). It causes a mild to moderate ache and no visual symptoms. One can confirm that only the episcleral vessels and not the deeper scleral vessels are inflamed by putting a drop of phenylephrine 2.5% in the eye. Episcleral vessel dilatation will temporarily disappear, while the larger scleral vessels will

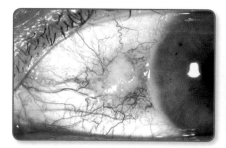

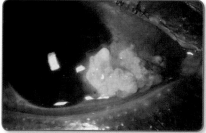

Figure 7.26 Early conjunctival carcinoma. There are some slight inflammatory changes around the lesion. This carcinoma can easily be excised.

Figure 7.27 A more advanced conjunctival carcinoma which has spread extensively over the conjunctiva, but can still be locally excised.

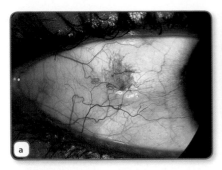
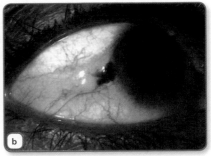

Figure 7.28 Conjunctival naevus. (a) A small naevus. This normal area of conjunctival pigmentation is very common in darker skinned people. There is no inflammation and this lesion is quiet and not progressive. (b) A more obvious pigmented naevus at the limbus. There is also some fatty degenerative tissue under the conjunctiva in the palpebral fissure which is called a pinguecula. Because this naevus is slightly vascularised and raised, it is safer to excise it.

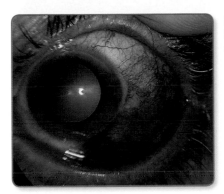

Figure 7.29 Episcleritis. The inflamed vessels look slightly bigger and deeper than in conjunctivitis.

be unaffected. Episcleritis is usually self-limiting, although a mild topical steroid (e.g. fluoromethalone) can be used for a short period if required.

Scleritis

Diseases of the sclera are not common, but are important because they are serious. Scleritis is the commonest and most important one to recognise (**Figures 7.30 and 7.31**). It can be blinding and also often an indication that significant, systemic autoimmune disease is present. Patients report severe pain in, around and behind the eye, which is worse on eye movements. The inflammation is usually unilateral but when associated with systemic auto-immune disease may be bilateral. The anterior and/or the posterior sclera can become inflamed. Posterior scleritis is particularly likely to be sight-threatening and as it does not cause much anterior inflammation it can be difficult to diagnose. Fundus examination may show inflammation of the choroid and retina, and fluid exudates under the choroid. In scleritis there may be patches where the sclera becomes necrotic. These often look like inflamed nodules (**Figure 7.31**) and can be very painful.

Scleritis should usually be treated with systemic steroids, and in very severe cases more powerful immunosuppressive drugs like cyclophosphamide may be needed. When the inflammation has subsided, the sclera may become thin, causing it to bulges from the intraocular pressure, and patches of it may become blue, because of scleral tissue destruction allow the uvea beneath to be seen (**Figure 7.32**). This is called scleromalacia.

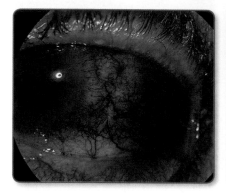

Figure 7.30 Scleritis. The dilated blood vessels on the surface of the sclera are underneath the conjunctiva.

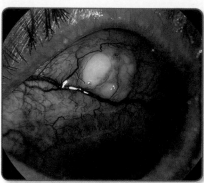

Figure 7.31 Nodular scleritis. In very severe cases of scleritis, inflammatory nodules can form.

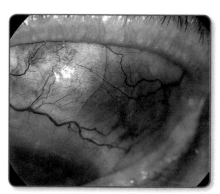

Figure 7.32 Scleromalacia. The sclera has been destroyed by scleritis allowing the uvea beneath to be seen.

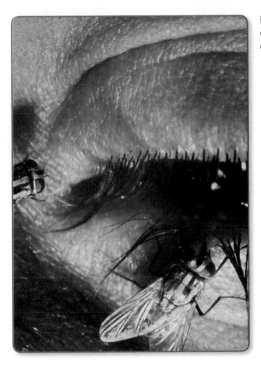

Poor water supplies, poor hygiene and eye seeking flies are some of the major enemies in trachoma prevention.

Trachoma is the commonest infectious cause of blindness worldwide. The disease starts with conjunctival infection in childhood and causes entropion (in-turning of the eyelid) and trichiasis (eyelashes turning in to rub on the eyeball). Approximately 40 million people worldwide have active trachoma infection, over 8 million have trichiasis and 1.2 million are blind from the disease. Trachoma is still found in 56 countries, but it has been described as 'a forgotten disease of forgotten people', because it is the rural poor who suffer from it, and they tend to get forgotten both economically and politically (**Figure 8.1**). However, non-governmental organisations and health ministries have scaled up efforts to control and treat the disease in recent years.

The earliest descriptions of the disease are in ancient Egyptian texts (approximately 1600 BC), but the word 'trachoma' comes from the Greek word for 'rough', which describes the surface appearance of the conjunctiva in chronic trachoma. The disease was widespread throughout the world and many of the large eye hospitals of rich countries were set up around 200 years ago to treat people, and particularly soldiers returning from war that had trachoma. However, it was about another 100 years before the characteristic inclusion organisms were demonstrated in 1907, and another 50 years before the organism – *Chlamydia trachomatis* – was first isolated in 1957.

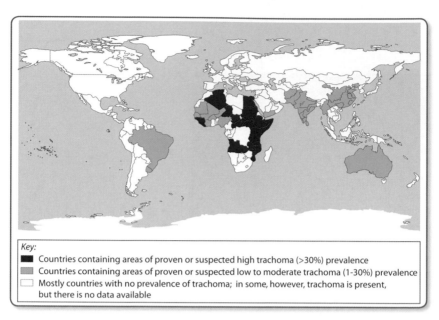

Key:
■ Countries containing areas of proven or suspected high trachoma (>30%) prevalence
■ Countries containing areas of proven or suspected low to moderate trachoma (1-30%) prevalence
☐ Mostly countries with no prevalence of trachoma; in some, however, trachoma is present, but there is no data available

Figure 8.1 Map showing the prevalence of active trachoma in different countries of the world. The Sahel belt across Sub-Saharan Africa is the worst affected. Although this simplified map suggests that the prevalence is uniform in a country, it does vary widely.

The clinical and laboratory research into trachoma in the last 25 years and the translation of this to 'the field' has been very important for the control of trachoma. We now know that the causative organism is sensitive to broad-spectrum antibiotics, and that a single dose of azithromycin can eliminate the disease for months if not longer. We now have mass treatment campaigns for treating whole communities with azithromycin. We also understand the importance of hygiene and facial cleanliness and programmes have been introduced to supply clean water and hygiene education to affected communities. We have also improved the surgical treatment of the later stages of the disease: we have developed simpler surgical procedures, which are taught to nurses and integrated eye-care workers who conduct almost all of the surgery for the disease. Despite all this, at present, the total eradication of trachoma remains a distant goal. However, the knowledge and technology are now available to control trachoma relatively cheaply, and so prevent blindness and many areas are making effective use of this, but Ministries of Health and the global health community must not ignore this disease of poor people.

Trachoma is most prevalent in a 'belt' that stretches across Northern Africa called the Sahel belt. In some countries, such as Southern Sudan and Ethiopia, over 40% of the children suffer from trachomatous conjunctivitis and children as young as 10 years old have entropion and trichiasis. Trachoma is still present in all the continents except Europe and North America. It is always associated with poverty.

The organism that causes trachoma is called *Chlamydia trachomatis*. Chlamydiae are bacteria, but behave differently to 'regular' bacteria. They spend most of their time living inside cells, but also have another form – called the elementary body – which lives outside cells and allows it to be spread from person-to-person. There are several different types (serovars) of *Chlamydia trachomatis*; serovars A, B, Ba and C survive and multiply most comfortably in conjunctival epithelium and are responsible for trachoma. Serovars D to K survive in genital epithelium and cause pelvic inflammatory disease and infertility, although they can also infect the eyes causing a follicular conjunctivitis which looks clinically similar to trachoma, either in sexually active individuals or in neonates who are infected from the mother's vaginal tract (see Chapters 7 and 22).

Symptoms and signs of trachoma

Trachoma is often a lifelong disease starting with the infective stage in childhood and continuing to the scarring stage with entropion and trichiasis in adulthood. The clinical picture varies enormously from a mild infective condition without any complications to a severe chronic infection resulting in complete entropion and corneal blindness in early adulthood.

Acute infective trachoma

Initially the symptoms of infective trachoma are the same as any infective conjunctivitis, with an irritable red eye and a mucopurulent discharge. It is nearly always bilateral although one eye may be more affected than the other. In severe cases, there may be eyelid oedema, or pain and photophobia because the cornea is involved.

There are some clinical signs that may help to distinguish trachoma from other causes of conjunctivitis. These include:
- tarsal conjunctival inflammatory follicles
- conjunctival papillary inflammation (see page 140) particularly on the conjunctival surface of the everted upper lid
- limbal inflammation
- scar lines on the tarsal conjunctiva from previous episodes of trachomatous infection and inflammation.

Follicles are enlarged nodules of lymphoid tissue under the conjunctival epithelium. (**Figure 8.2**) They are usually just visible to the naked eye. As the disease progresses, they become larger and develop pale, necrotic centres. They are most easily seen on the everted upper tarsal plate and in the lower fornix.

Papillae are found on the surface of the conjunctiva, especially on the inside of the upper eyelid (**Figure 8.3**). They cause the conjunctiva to look like red velvet to the naked eye, and obscure the underlying blood vessels.

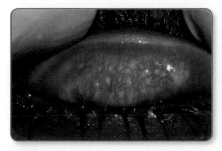

Figure 8.2 Active trachoma. Follicles on the tarsal conjunctival surface of the upper lid.

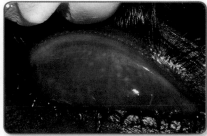

Figure 8.3 Active trachoma. Intense papillary inflammation of the tarsal conjunctiva of the upper lid.

However, if you look closely with loupes or a slit lamp, you can see the individual red dots, which are the papillae with their central blood vessel.

In mild cases, only a few follicles or papillae can be seen on the upper eyelid conjunctiva. In severe cases, the follicles and papillae will completely obscure the underlying tarsal conjunctival blood vessels. These severe cases are the ones that are more likely to develop blinding complications later.

Trachomatous infection and inflammation also affects the bulbar conjunctival and corneal epithelium, especially the upper part under the upper eyelid. This may be because the upper cornea is in close contact with the upper eyelid. Superficial punctate keratitis (Figure 9.18) is an early sign of corneal involvement, which is usually only visible with a slit lamp. However, fluorescein dye will stain the individual epithelial defects, so that a faint green haze may be visible to the naked eye. As the infection becomes more severe, the inflammation in the superficial cornea becomes more obvious. Blood vessels grow from the limbus into the cornea. These blood vessels and inflammatory changes are called a pannus (*pannus* is the Latin word for a sheet because it looks like a thin sheet of blood vessels and inflammatory tissue).

Scarring trachoma

In areas where infective trachoma is common, children may suffer from repeated acute infections and/or have a chronically red and inflamed eye. Over time this causes scar formation. Although scar tissue can form in other chronic inflammatory conditions, it is a very characteristic feature of trachoma. Scar tissue, sometimes called 'fibrous tissue', consists of collagen fibres. These collagen fibres are formed following any damage to the tissues. For unknown reasons, in trachoma, the scarring is more severe in the upper eyelid. At first, individual white scar lines (**Figure 8.4a**) can be seen on the everted upper lid, but as the scarring increases this becomes thick bands and areas of scar tissue (**Figure 8.4b**). This scarring can obliterate all the underlying blood vessels and cause distortion, thickening and vertical shortening of the upper lid. The scarring also causes damage to other ocular tissues, including the lacrimal gland and ductules, the meibomian glands and the mucin-secreting Goblet cells. This can cause a very dry eye and the normally wet conjunctival surface can become dry and keratinised (like skin), which may worsen the scarring process and corneal damage.

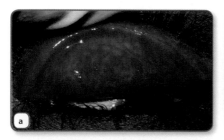
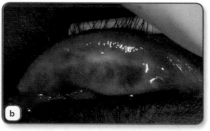

Figure 8.4 Tarsal scarring. (a) White bands of early tarsal scarring in amongst the intense papillary inflammation. (b) More advanced tarsal scarring. A large area of the tarsal surface of the upper lid is now scarred. There is still some inflammation between the scarred areas.

Trichiasis

The contraction of the inner surface of the upper lid caused by the scarring causes the eyelid to roll inwards. This 'in-rolling' of the eyelid is called entropion (**Figure 8.5**). Also, scarring changes around the eyelash follicles cause the eyelashes to emerge further back (closer to the eye) on the lid margin (metaplastic lashes) (**Figure 8.6**) or to point backwards towards the eyeball (misdirected lashes) (**Figure 8.7**). Entropion, metaplastic lashes and misdirected lashes are all present together in the eyelids of many patients with scarring trachoma (**Figure 8.8**). All three processes cause the eyelashes to rub against the eyeball, which is called trichiasis. They can rub anywhere, but lashes touching the cornea are the most damaging, and require treatment most urgently.

Corneal scarring

Trichiatic lashes cause corneal scarring by directly rubbing on and scratching the cornea, as well as encouraging corneal infections to develop. This is probably made worse by the cornea's defences, i.e. conjunctiva and tear production, also being damaged by trachomatous scarring. The scarring is often in the centre of the cornea and therefore greatly affects vision. The scars may correspond to specific trichiatic lashes (**Figure 8.8**). However, many individuals with trichiasis do not yet have corneal opacity and therefore if treatment is given quickly, visual loss can be avoided. Corneal scarring usually starts in adulthood but like trichiasis, can occur in children in areas with very high trachoma prevalence (**Figure 8.9**). Corneal opacification increases with age

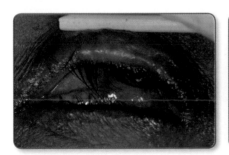

Figure 8.5 Trachomatous entropion.

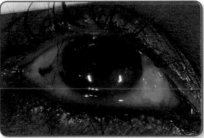

Figure 8.6 Metaplastic lashes. Three trichiatic eyelashes are coming from an abnormally posterior place on the eyelid.

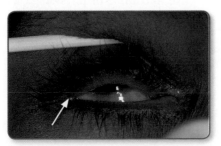

Figure 8.7 Misdirected lashes. The trichiatic eyelashes are coming from the normal line of eyelashes, but pointing towards the eye (arrow).

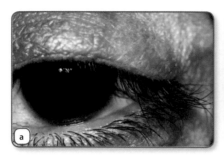
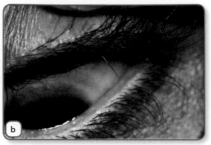

Figure 8.8 Trachomatous trichiasis can be difficult to see. In (a) the eyelid looks quite normal but in (b) the same eyelid has been slightly everted and trichiatic lashes are seen clearly.

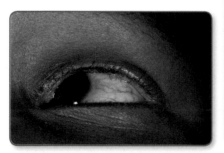
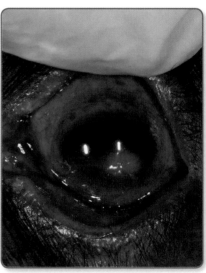

Figure 8.9 This girl is 12 years old and already has quite severe upper lid entropion trichiasis. Although the eyelashes have been cut short, it will not be long before they start damaging the cornea.

Figure 8.10 Superior corneal pannus and Herbert pits, which are small pigmented dimples at the superior limbus.

because as entropion worsens, the cornea is exposed to trichiatic lashes for longer and the protective tear film gets less and less. The disease is more common and severe in women, although it is not known if this is because of increased exposure to children with active trachoma, or physiological/ anatomical differences or because they have less access to healthcare than men and therefore only get treatment when the disease is more advanced.

The inflammatory changes in the superior cornea and limbus (see above) also result in scarring. The fibrovascular pannus leaves a dense white scar sometimes with persistent vascularisation usually in the upper third of the cornea. The limbal follicles become scarred and pigmented leaving small depressions, called Herbert's pits. (**Figure 8.10**). Herbert pits are a diagnostic sign that the patient has previously had active trachoma.

The rubbing of trichiatic eyelashes every time the patient blinks can be extremely painful and cause photophobia and eyelid spasm (blepharospasm). Affected individuals are often unable to work or look after their homes or families, which causes a huge economic and social burden on families and communities. Patients can be excluded from society and young women with severe trachomatous trichiasis often report that their chance of finding a husband is greatly reduced.

The classification of trachoma

Trachoma is a complicated disease affecting the conjunctiva, cornea, eyelids and eyelashes. Specialists have tried to classify the different features of the disease. Classification systems can help eyecare workers to make a diagnosis and can help scientists who are researching the disease. McCallan who worked in Egypt over 50 years ago was the first person to create a classification, but this is too complicated for routine use and assesses many very rare signs. Currently the most useful classification is the 'WHO simplified trachoma grading system' and the more detailed 'WHO follicles, papillae, cicatriciales grading system'. The simplified system helps to identify the major different clinical signs of the disease and is used for recording the numbers of patients with the major different stages of the disease during treatment campaigns and simple prevalence surveys (**Table 8.1** and **Figure 8.11**). The more detailed system is mainly used for research.

We will describe the WHO simplified system as this is the most widely used system 'in the field' and can be taught in a short-training course. This system is very helpful for classifying the major stages of the disease, but it does not describe the severity of each of these stages. Therefore, it cannot be used to assess if the disease is becoming worse e.g. it cannot be recorded if there is increased corneal scarring in a patient who was seen previously. It therefore has limited value for research studies.

Trachoma blindness in the community

Within trachoma endemic areas, the overall pattern of trachoma in the community varies enormously. For example, it is quite possible for most of the young children to have active trachoma in one village, but very few of them to have it in a neighbouring village. The prevalence of active infection and

Table 8.1 The WHO simplified system for the assessment of trachoma		
Grade		**Description**
Trachomatous inflammation – follicular	TF	The presence of five or more follicles (>0.5 mm) in the upper tarsal conjunctiva
Trachomatous inflammation – intense	TI	Pronounced inflammatory thickening of the tarsal conjunctiva that obscures more than half of the deep normal vessels
Trachomatous scarring	TS	The presence of scarring in the tarsal conjunctiva
Trachomatous trichiasis	TT	At least one lash rubs on the eyeball
Corneal opacity	CO	Easily visible corneal opacity over the pupil

TRACHOMA GRADING CARD

> – Each eye must be examined and assessed separately.
> – Use binocular loupes (× 2.5) and adequate lighting (either daylight or a torch).
> – Signs must be clearly seen in order to be considered present.

The eyelids and cornea are observed first for inturned eyelashes and any corneal opacity. The upper eyelid is then turned over (everted) to examine the conjunctiva over the stiffer part of the upper lid (tarsal conjunctiva).

The normal conjunctiva is pink, smooth, thin and transparent. Over the whole area of the tarsal conjunctiva there are normally large deep-lying blood vessels that run vertically.

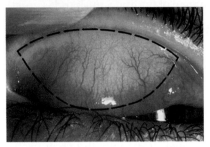

Normal tarsal conjunctiva (x 2 magnification). The dotted line shows the area to be examined.

TRACHOMATOUS INFLAMMATION – FOLLICULAR

(TF): the presence of five or more follicles in the upper tarsal conjunctiva.

Follicles are round swellings that are paler than the surrounding conjunctiva, appearing white, grey or yellow. Follicles must be at least 0.5 mm in diameter, i.e., at least as large as the dots shown below, to be considered.

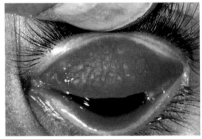

Trachomatous inflammation – follicular (TF).

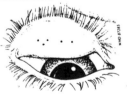

TRACHOMATOUS INFLAMMATION – INTENSE

(TI): pronounced inflammatory thickening of the tarsal conjunctiva that obscures more than half of the normal deep tarsal vessels.

The tarsal conjunctiva apperas red, rough and thickened. There are usually numerous follicles, which may be partially or totally covered by the thickened conjunctiva.

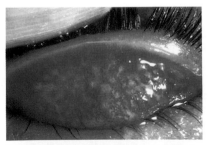

Trachomatous inflammation – follicular and intense (TF + TI)

TRACHOMATOUS SCARRING (TS): *the presence of scarring in the tarsal conjunctiva.*

Scars are easily visible as white lines, bands or sheets in the tarsal conjunctiva. They are glistening and fibrous in appearance. Scarring, especially diffuse fibrosis, may obscure the tarsal blood vessels.

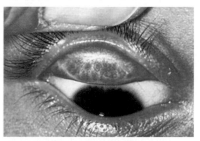

Trachomatous scarring (TS)

TRACHOMATOUS TRICHIASIS (TT): *at least one eyelash rubs on the eyeball.*

Evidence of recent removal of inturned eyelashes should also be graded as trichiasis.

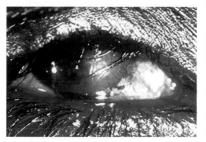

Trachomatous trichiasis (TT)

CORNEAL OPACITY (CO): *easily visible corneal opacity over the pupil.*

The pupil margin is blurred viewed through the opacity. Such corneal opacities cause significant visual impairment (less than 6/18 or 0.3 vision), and therefore visual acuity should be measured if possible.

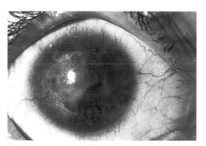

Corneal opacity (CO)

TF: – give topical treatment (e.g. tetracycline 1%).

TI: – give topical and consider systemic treatment.

TT: – refer for eyelid surgery.

 WORLD HEALTH ORGANIZATION PREVENTION OF BLINDNESS AND DEAFNESS

Support from the partners of the WHO Alliance for the Global Elimination of Trachoma is acknowledged.

Figure 8.11 The World Health Organization simplified system for the assessment of trachoma.

the length of infective episodes decreases as people get older. However, most adults who have had infective trachoma as a child will have some conjunctival scarring. In some adults this will be 'quiet scarring', i.e. the process is not active and the eyelid not inflamed. But in others, there will be continuous tarsal conjunctival papillary inflammation, even though follicles and *Chlamydia trachomatis* infection are rare in adults. It is not known why the inflammation continues in some adults even though they are probably not being reinfected with *Chlamydia*. However, it seems that frequent acute infections can cause chronic inflammation in some people that continues for many years or even decades. Trichiasis and entropion start to become a problem from about age 15 years and blindness from corneal scarring after the age of about 30 years. Both entropion/trichiasis and corneal scarring are likely to progress throughout life in hyperendemic areas. In the very worst areas up to 10% of the community may have some sight loss from trachoma.

In areas where the spread of the disease is less, either for climatic or hygienic reasons, many children may still have active trachoma. However, the scarring is less severe, and complications that can cause blindness, such as trichiasis and corneal scarring, are uncommon. As communities become richer, the prevalence of infection and subsequent eyelid complications decreases. However, even in communities where the infection has been eradicated, the older generation may continue to have potentially blinding entropion/trichiasis that requires treatment.

Risk factors for trachoma

Trachoma can vary from a mild to a very severe disease in different situations. It is possible to produce a mild form of trachoma by inoculating a volunteer (who has had no previous infection) with *Chlamydia trachomatis* infected discharge that comes from someone known to have the infection. The volunteer soon develops active trachoma with a typical follicular and papillary conjunctivitis. After a few weeks, however, the infection heals spontaneously with only very slight subconjunctival scarring and no significant damage to the eye. However in places with high trachoma prevalence, the disease is very different; children are persistently infected with *Chlamydia trachomatis* and most adults have conjunctival scarring from previous infection and many of these will have entropion/trichiasis.

Why does the same infection produce a mild disease in one situation, and a severe blinding disease in another situation? In general, poverty is responsible for trachoma. Whenever the standards of living improve the incidence and severity of trachoma falls. Trachoma was a significant problem in Europe in the last century, but almost completely disappeared when living conditions improved. This was long before the discovery of any antibiotics, or even before there was any understanding of how trachoma is transmitted. However, it is not known exactly which of the many factors associated with poverty (e.g. poor hygiene, poor healthcare, malnutrition, dirty and inadequate water supplies) are the most important in causing the disease. Some of the important risk factors for becoming infected and re-infected include:

1. **Factors that promote the spread of infection.**

Trachoma is thought to be mainly spread by the five 'F's:
- Flies: the *Musca sorbens* face seeking fly feeds on facial secretions (discharge from the eye and nose) and is thought to transmit the disease from person-to-person (**Figure 8.12**).
- Faeces: hyperendemic environments often have few if any latrines. The Musca sorbens fly lays its eggs in the human faeces, which are left in the open.
- Fingers: infection is easily transferred from the fingers of an infected child to the face of another child. This occurs more commonly in crowded living conditions where children often share beds.
- Faces: Infected children often have thick infected ocular and nasal discharges and rarely clean or wipe away these discharges.
- Fomites (materials and objects such as towels and clothing): these items are rarely washed and may be a reservoir of infected secretions.

All of these factors occur mainly in poor countries, which are frequently unhygienic and have poor water supplies and latrine facilities. As communities become wealthier, these factors improve and so trachoma becomes less severe and even disappears by itself.

2. **Weather conditions.**
   Trachoma can exist in all climatic conditions. However it is more prevalent and causes more blindness in hotter, drier, dustier areas. A comparison of two areas in West Africa shows how important climatic factors are. Near the coast, the climate is very humid. Trachoma is common, but is not a very significant cause of blindness. Further north towards the Sahara desert, however, the climate becomes much drier, and blinding trachoma becomes increasingly common. In all other ways the economic conditions and general way of life are almost identical. It is not clear which factors are responsible: lack of water, poor hygiene, irritation by dust exacerbating the inflammation and more flies could all be responsible.

3. **The presence of high levels of trachoma in a community.**
   Once an area has high levels of trachoma infection, then re-infection is much more likely. It becomes a vicious circle, i.e. the more people are infected, the more people will become re-infected and then even more people will have infection. In this way, over half of the children in some communities are infected. A mass treatment campaign can suddenly reduce the number of infected people and break the vicious circle.

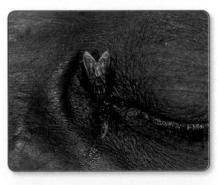

Figure 8.12 Musca sorbens. The eye seeking fly that spreads trachoma.

Differential diagnosis

Other eye infections and scarring diseases can look like trachoma. However, in areas where trachoma is common, patients with possible disease must be treated as if they have trachoma.

Differential diagnosis for active trachoma

The two diseases that are most often confused with trachoma are epidemic keratoconjunctivitis, caused by an adenovirus infection, and vernal conjunctivitis which is an allergic disease:

Adenovirus infection (see page 148) causes a more acute infection than trachoma. It produces superficial punctate keratitis over the whole cornea. By contrast, trachoma usually involves the upper cornea only. However, these fine corneal changes are very difficult to see with the naked eye.

Vernal conjunctivitis (see page 152) is a chronic disease, which is sometimes present as well as trachoma. Patients with vernal conjunctivitis usually complain of itching, and have characteristic changes on the upper tarsal conjunctiva and at the limbus.

Differential diagnosis for scarring trachoma

Scarring conjunctivitis can develop in a wide variety of conditions. In some of these conditions the scarring can be severe enough to distort the eyelids, leading to entropion and trichiasis. They include:

- Infections, e.g. adenovirus. Although acute infection is very common it rarely causes scarring.
- Autoimmune and inflammatory conditions, e.g. mucous membrane pemphigoid (see page 155), Stevens–Johnson syndrome, graft-versus-host disease and atopic keratoconjunctivitis. These are very rare but frequently cause conjunctival scarring.
- Ocular rosacea. This is a common condition, but rarely severe enough to cause significant scarring.
- Chemical injuries, some ocular medications (practolol, topical adrenaline) and some traditional eye medicines (particularly euphorbia sap based treatments).

Assessing a trachoma patient

Start by taking a brief history. It is helpful to know how long the patient has had symptoms and if they are pulling out their lashes (epilating). In some cultures epilation is done secretly and patients may be embarrassed to admit this to you. It can also be helpful and interesting to enquire about the symptoms of trichiasis (pain, photophobia and watering) and how these affect the activities of daily living. In some patients it is debilitating disease, but the symptoms are very variable.

Examination for the signs of trachoma can be done anywhere, including in the patient's village or home, with very little equipment (**Figure 8.13**). A torch and magnifying loupes are helpful but not essential; most signs can be seen with the naked eye (**Figure 8.14**).

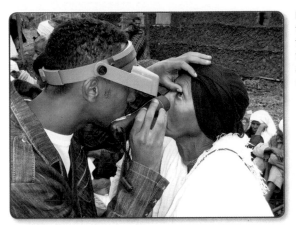

Figure 8.13 Examination for the signs of trachoma in the field. Loupes and a torch help to see trichiatic eyelashes, although they can often be seen even without these.

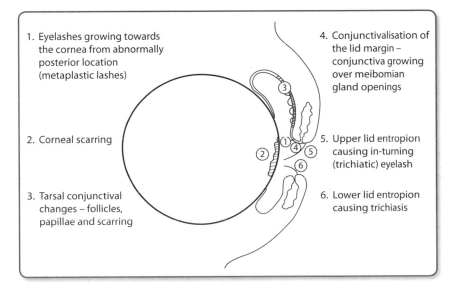

1. Eyelashes growing towards the cornea from abnormally posterior location (metaplastic lashes)

2. Corneal scarring

3. Tarsal conjunctival changes – follicles, papillae and scarring

4. Conjunctivalisation of the lid margin – conjunctiva growing over meibomian gland openings

5. Upper lid entropion causing in-turning (trichiatic) eyelash

6. Lower lid entropion causing trichiasis

Figure 8.14 Signs of trachoma.

1. Examine the eyelid position and eyelashes

The first signs of entropion are a rounding of the lid margin; its loses it usually square profile. If you look closely you may also see conjunctivalisation of the lid margin. This is where the meibomian gland openings, which are normally surrounded by skin, are instead surrounded by abnormal conjunctiva. Trichiatic eyelashes can be seen more easily with the patient looking upwards. Eyelashes touching the globe can be counted and can be divided into those that touch the cornea and those touching conjunctiva. Those touching the cornea are of greater risk to vision. Remember to look at the lower lid also, as in highly endemic areas approximately 10% of patients with trachomatous trichiasis will also have lower lid trichiasis (**Figure 8.7**).

2. Evert the upper eyelid (see Chapter 3, examination) (Figure 8.15)

This allows examination for follicles, papillary inflammation and conjunctival scarring. Look for the tarsal vessels (**Figure 8.16**). If these are clearly visible with their normal branching pattern, it is very likely that there is not significant inflammation or scarring, but if they are not visible, is it because the eyelid is red and inflamed or are they obliterated by scar tissue?

3. Examine the cornea for corneal scarring

This can be difficult without a slit lamp as some scars are very faint and there may be multiple reflections in the cornea. However, by adjusting the position of your torch and your viewing position you should be able to see even the smallest, faintest scars.

4. Examine the lower fornix and the plica semilunaris/caruncle area

Some patients develop forniceal shortening and symblepharon and many lose the plica/caruncle architecture. This shows that the scarring occurs throughout the mucous membrane surface of the eye (**Figure 8.17**).

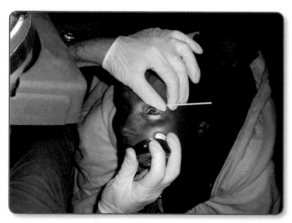

Figure 8.15 Upper lid eversion to look for tarsal scarring, follicles and inflammation.

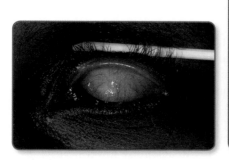

Figure 8.16 The normal tarsal plate.

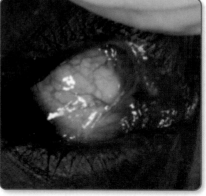

Figure 8.17 Symblepharon and loss of the plica from trachomatous scarring.

The laboratory diagnosis of active trachoma

The diagnosis of trachoma is almost always made from the clinical signs, and so you do not need to use laboratory tests to confirm it. Laboratory diagnosis is mainly used in research studies and at present there is no reliable and instant on the spot test for ocular *Chlamydia trachomatis.*

There is still not a 'gold standard' test, although there have been many advances in laboratory diagnosis in recent years. Some years ago cytological analysis was done using Giemsa staining of the chlamydial inclusion body, but this missed a considerable number of active cases. More recently, *C. Trachomatis* antigens were looked for using direct immunofluorescence with monoclonal antibodies. This increased the sensitivity of the test, and several commercially available kits were manufactured, but they required expensive and sophisticated laboratory equipment and expertise. Laboratory testing is now mainly done with polymerase chain reaction. Unfortunately, all these tests have their own problems, although they are very good at picking up all cases of chlamydia (high sensitivity and specificity):

1. They require great care with collecting and processing the specimens
2. They require expensive, high-tech laboratories and equipment
3. They are so sensitive that they may be detecting the presence of chlamydia that is not clinically meaningful.

Sensitivity and specificity are important concepts for evaluating a clinical or laboratory test. In a perfect world a test would correctly identify all the patients with the disease (and therefore also identify all the people who do not have the disease). In other words, the perfect test is always positive in people who have the disease and never positive in those who do not have the disease. However, the perfect test is very rare!

Sensitivity

This is the ability of the test to correctly identify those patients with the disease. A test with 100% sensitivity correctly identifies all patients with the disease. A test with 90% sensitivity will find 90% of people with the disease, but 10% of people who do have the disease, will be missed by the test. A highly sensitive test is important for diseases that are serious but treatable, and therefore missing the diagnosis may be disastrous, e.g. cancer. The sensitivity of a test does not tell us about whether a test is also finding lots of positives in people who actually do not have the disease. This is when specificity is important.

Specificity

This is the ability of the test to correctly identify people without the disease. A test with 100% specificity correctly identifies all patients without the disease. A test with 90% specificity correctly reports 90% of people who do not have the disease as being disease free, but is also incorrectly positive (i.e. reports the disease to be present) in 10% of people who actually do not have the disease.

Therefore a test with high sensitivity but low specificity will correctly find the people with the disease, but will incorrectly tell quite a lot of people that they have the disease, when in fact they don't have it. A test with high specificity and low sensitivity, will miss quite a lot of people who actually have the disease, but when it does identify someone with the disease, this is very likely to be the correct diagnosis.

The treatment of trachoma

Trachoma can be 'treated' at each of the stages of the disease process (**Figure 8.18**). Like most major public health diseases the best trachoma treatment is *prevention*. However, once a patient becomes infected with *C. trachomatis*, they can be treated with antibiotics, reinforced by good hygiene. Finally, once a patient has scarring of the eyelid, causing entropion/trichiasis, surgery to correct the lid position is the main treatment, but this can be supported with epilation.

The need to attack all stages of the disease was recognised by the WHO. In 1998 the WHO and international partners launched VISION2020, an initiative to eliminate avoidable visual loss by the year 2020 (see Chapter 1). Within VISION2020, a specific initiative was set up for trachoma, called the Global Elimination of Blinding Trachoma (GET2020). This promotes the **SAFE** strategy: **S**urgery to correct trichiasis, **A**ntibiotic distribution to treat chlamydial infection, **F**acial cleanliness and **E**nvironmental improvements to reduce transmission and re-emergence of the infection within treated communities. It should be noted that the sequence of treatment should be **EFAS**, but the acronym is less memorable!

Environmental improvements

The environmental risk factors for trachoma infection have been discussed above. Trachoma programmes are attempting to reduce these by improving and increasing clean water supplies, latrine building, insecticides to reduce the number of flies and education about hygienic living. Although it is not known exactly which of these measures is the most important or effective, they are probably all helpful. It is these changes that eliminated trachoma in richer countries, where the disease disappeared in the pre-antibiotic era.

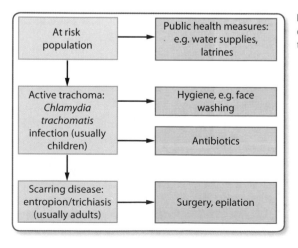

Figure 8.18 Treatment options at different stages of trachoma.

Face washing

Children with active trachoma often have purulent eye and nasal discharges, which are infected with *C. trachomatis*. Face washing probably reduces disease transmission and also encourages good hygiene in children and families.

Antibiotics

Chlamydia trachomatis is sensitive to certain classes of antibiotics: macrolides (e.g. azithromycin and erythromycin), tetracyclines (tetracycline, chlortetracycline, doxycycline and oxytetracycline) and the sulphonamides.

For several decades, trachoma infection was treated with several weeks of topical tetracycline cream. However, in the early 1990s a study found that a single oral dose of azithromycin (1 g for adults, 20 mg/kg for children) to be as effective as 2 weeks of topical tetracycline cream. This has significant advantages:

- Much higher compliance.
- Treatment can be directly observed.
- Chlamydial infection outside the eye, e.g. genital infection, is treated.
- Possible reduced mortality. The mortality rate is reduced in some groups of patients taking azithromycin, perhaps because respiratory and/or gastrointestinal infections are also treated.

Systemic treatment does have disadvantages:

- Some patients are reluctant to take an oral treatment for an eye disease.
- There is increased risk of side effects, such as gastrointestinal upset and allergy.

Initially azithromycin was only given to patients with clinically obvious active disease. However, it was realised that this would miss patients with asymptomatic infection, leaving a large reservoir of infection. A huge donation of azithromycin (Zithromax) by the drug's manufacturer (Pfizer Inc.) has allowed mass treatment of whole endemic communities. For example, in Ethiopia, many millions of doses of azithromycin are given out each year with the intention of giving treatment to every single member of the community irrespective of clinical signs. There is no doubt that this allowed huge progress in combating trachoma. However, we do not yet know how frequently and for how long treatment needs to be given in different communities with different prevalences of trachoma. Mathematical models and clinical programmes suggest that high prevalence areas require treatment twice yearly and those with moderate prevalence, once yearly. Fortunately, although millions of azithromycin tablets are taken each year, there is no evidence of the development of resistant strains of *C. trachomatis*.

Trachoma frequently co-exists with other diseases. For example, vernal conjunctivitis is also common in trachoma endemic communities. These patients may require antibiotic and a topical steroid. The effects of steroid on trachoma are unclear. There are theories both in favour and against using them; trachoma is a grossly inflammatory disease and much of the damage may result from the inflammation rather than the actual infection, in which case steroids may dampen this down. However, *C. trachomatis* may survive and replicate more easily in an immune-suppressed environment. Therefore steroids should be used with caution and only under the direct supervision of a specialist and at present should not be used for trachoma alone.

Vaccination has been tried in the past, but without success probably because much of the damage is done by the inflammation rather than the organism. In fact the trial vaccinations appeared to provoke increased inflammation and scarring.

Surgery

Trichiasis and entropion are by far the most common and important complications of trachoma. When these occur the patient has already suffered from quite severe scarring trachoma and it is too late for public health measures or antibiotics to make much difference. However, surgery must be carried out as soon as possible. Otherwise, the inturning eyelashes will continue to damage the cornea, causing keratitis, corneal ulcers, progressive corneal scarring and visual loss. Corneal scarring is basically irreversible, although after successful eyelid surgery the cornea can become a little clearer. This is probably because active keratitis can get better and also because corneal scars fade slightly over time. In some high prevalence areas it is estimated that as many as 5% of the population have trachomatous trichiasis. For example, in Ethiopia, there are thought to be 1.2 million people requiring lid surgery.

Over the last century many different procedures have been described for the treatment of TT. Trachoma control programmes in endemic countries currently routinely use some of these. Others are only used by specialists in oculoplastic surgery and others have been superseded or shown not to work well and should not be used. The variety of options suggests that on the one hand, the 'perfect' surgical procedure does not exist and that the treatment should ideally be tailored to the individual clinical problem. However, on the other hand, the huge prevalence of TT and limited surgical services in most trachoma endemic countries demands a simple, quick procedure that can be taught to and carried out by non-ophthalmologists with the most basic equipment in the most basic locations. Treatment options broadly divide into those that only treat the lashes and those that also correct the underlying anatomical eyelid abnormality.

Eyelash removal

1. *Epilation.* The eyelashes can be pulled out with tweezers (**Figure 8.19**). In some places the majority of patients self-epilate. The eyelashes will of course grow again, but many patients, particularly those with milder disease prefer this regular but simple treatment to eyelid surgery. It is

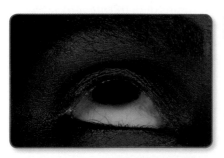

Figure 8.19 All of the upper lid eyelashes have been epilated.

important that the lashes are removed completely from their follicle and not broken or cut, so as not to leave short, sharp lashes. This just makes the situation worse. It is helpful to teach a relative or friend of the patient how to perform careful epilation (**Figure 8.20**). There is now randomised controlled trial evidence that epilation is an effective alternative treatment to surgery for milder disease (less than five trichiatic lashes). It is particularly useful in patients with metaplastic lashes and no/minimal entropion.

2. *Eyelash destructive procedures*. Electrolysis and cryotherapy have been used to try to destroy the root of one or more trichiatic lashes in order to prevent the lash regrowing. Although these procedures are widely used in rich countries there are problems with using them in poor countries where trachoma is prevalent.
   - The equipment required is expensive, requires maintenance and is dangerous if misused.
   - Considerable experience is required to conduct these procedures
   - There is the possibility that although the treatments may destroy offending lashes, they stir-up inflammation, which worsens conjunctival scarring.

3. *Excision*. If only a small area of eyelashes is misplaced, it is possible to excise individual eyelashes together with their roots. This can be a time consuming surgical procedure and requires an operating microscope and considerable surgical experience.

Surgical procedures to correct entropion

Multiple different operations have been used for trachomatous trichiasis. In most of these the principle is to mobilise the entropic component of the eyelid and reposition and suture this in the correct orientation, i.e. to rotate the lower end of the upper lid outwards to prevent eyelashes scratching the cornea. The two most widely used procedures are:

1. *Bilamellar tarsal rotation* (**Figure 8.21**): a full thickness cut is made through the upper lid before placing everting sutures to roll out the portion of the eyelid with the eyelashes.

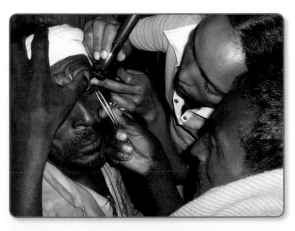

Figure 8.20 A patient's relative is taught to epilate by a health worker.

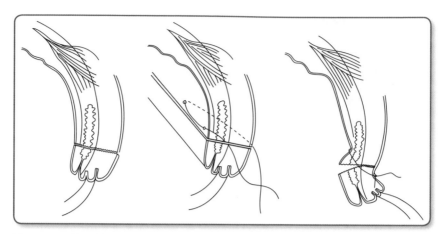

Figure 8.21 Bilamellar tarsal rotation surgery.

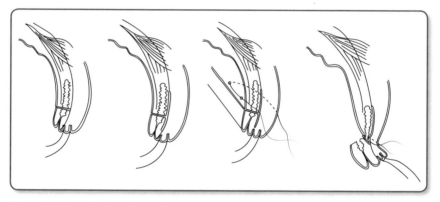

Figure 8.22 Posterior lamellar tarsal rotation surgery.

2. *Posterior lamellar tarsal rotation* (also known as the Trabut procedure)
    (**Figure 8.22**): the posterior lamella is incised and dissected away from
    the anterior lamellar and everting sutures are inserted to hold it.

These procedures can be very challenging because in more severe cases of
trachoma, the eyelid is often very scarred and deformed and without the
usual tissue planes within it. In general the aim of surgery is to overcorrect
the entropion (making the lid turn outwards more than normal), as it is likely
to turn back inwards over time (**Figure 8.23**).

The vast majority of patients with trachomatous scarring live in remote
locations where there are few ophthalmologists and therefore the operation
is done by ophthalmic assistants and nurses. However with appropriate
training very high quality and high volume surgery can be achieved in even
the most remote locations (**Figure 8.24**).

For any reader who plans to do trachoma surgery, detailed descriptions of
techniques are available. These references are in the reading list at the front of
the book.

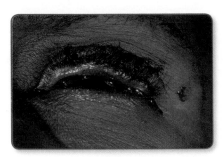

Figure 8.23 The appearance of the eyelid after trachomatous trichiasis surgery. The eyelid looks 'over-corrected'.

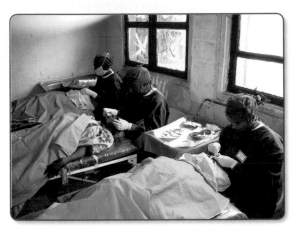

Figure 8.24 Nurses conducting trachomatous trichiasis surgery in rural Ethiopia.

The prevalence of active trachoma has reduced markedly in recent years, probably because of changes in society and the implementation of the A, F and E components of the SAFE strategy. However, the estimated number of people requiring lid surgery worldwide has actually increased from 7.2 million to 8.2 million between 2003 and 2009. Although in part this may reflect more accurate prevalence surveys, it is probably more an indication of the enormous problems with providing trachomatous trichiasis surgery. These include:

1. *Surgical provision.* Patients with trachoma often live in poor and remote places. These places are much less likely to have practising surgeons. Even when surgeons that can perform trachoma surgery are placed in remote clinics they frequently move on to other jobs or locations or have other obstacles, such as lack of surgical equipment and not enough time, to provide surgery.
2. *Surgical recurrence.* Patients have very damaged and scarred eyelids, the procedure is challenging and the surgeons can be of very variable ability. Sometimes over half of the patients undergoing surgery subsequently have recurrence of their trichiasis.
3. *Patient barriers to receiving surgery.* Even when free surgery is provided in rural locations, patients often do not attend. Many reasons have been found for this including, indirect costs (the costs of lost employment, travel, additional childcare, accommodation), concerns about the quality of surgery and preference for epilation.

Corneal scarring and corneal blindness

Corneal scarring is the most significant complication of trachoma, and is the reason that people go blind. Corneal transplant is the only remaining option for visual rehabilitation, but this is not widely used or recommended for the following reasons.

- This operation requires resources, expertise and intensive follow-up that are rarely available in areas with trachoma.
- Trachomatous corneas are usually vascularised, which puts the patient at high risk of transplant rejection.
- The scarred conjunctiva and tear film apparatus puts the graft at high risk of failure.
- If corneal transplant is going to be undertaken it is essential that entropion and trichiasis are fully corrected beforehand.

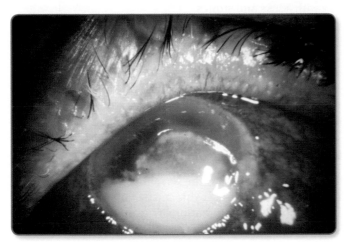

Corneal ulcers are very common. Prompt, correct and intensive treatment can often save sight, but wrong treatment or no treatment at all often leads to blindness.

The cornea is the most important of the anterior structures in the eye. The only purpose of the eyelids, conjunctiva and lacrimal apparatus is to protect the cornea and keep it healthy and transparent. If they are diseased or damaged, inflammation or scarring in the cornea often follows. The cornea has an especially close relationship with the conjunctiva, and sometimes suffers from the same disorders. This is because the epithelium of the cornea is directly continuous with the epithelium of the conjunctiva.

The cornea is a fascinating and atypical organ because it has no blood supply. It obtains its metabolic needs from the blood vessels of the limbus and from the aqueous fluid in the anterior chamber. When the eyelids are open, oxygen from the atmosphere diffuses through the tear film into the cornea. When the eyelids are closed, the conjunctival blood vessels also nourish the cornea. The cornea has a very good nerve supply, which makes it extremely sensitive to both touch and pain. A tiny foreign body in the cornea will cause a lot of pain, but would not be felt anywhere else. The structure of the cornea is described in Chapter 2 in **Figures. 2.1** and **2.2** and the technique of examining the cornea has been described in Chapter 3.

Patterns of corneal disease

The cornea is a very sensitive and specialised organ, which must retain its clarity despite being exposed to the atmosphere. It is at significant risk of suffering injury, inflammation or infection. Major risks to the cornea in tropical and poor countries include:

- Hot, dry air, dust or sand particles in the atmosphere, and smoke all irritate the corneal and conjunctival epithelium. This may increase the risk of corneal trauma and infection.

- Poor hygiene promotes the spread of ocular infections.
- Vitamin A deficiency specifically targets the cornea (see Chapter 10)
- Eye trauma is more common in agricultural workers and where children play more freely with sticks and stones.
- Ultraviolet light exposure may harm the cornea and conjunctiva.

Therefore almost all corneal diseases are particularly common in the tropics and poor countries. Indeed, the prevalence of corneal scars and corneal blindness in any community is a good indication of the general health, hygiene and nutrition of that community. For example, vitamin A deficiency and trachoma are major causes of preventable corneal blindness that are both entirely associated with poverty.

Terminology

It is helpful to run through and define the terminology that is frequently used when describing corneal disease, as this can be quite confusing.

- *Keratitis:* any type of corneal inflammation. If the inflammation is in the epithelium and Bowman's membrane, it is called 'superficial keratitis'. If the inflammation is superficial, but only occurs in certain, small discrete spots on the cornea, it is called 'superficial punctate keratitis' (SPK). If the inflammation is in the stroma, it is called 'deep', 'stromal' or 'interstitial' keratitis. If it occurs in both the conjunctiva and the cornea, it is called keratoconjunctivitis.
- *Corneal ulcer:* disruption of the corneal epithelium with involvement of the underlying stroma. There are many possible causes but ulcers are often either infective or inflammatory.
- *Corneal scar:* white or hazy corneal stromal opacity that results from any significant stromal inflammation, trauma or infection. Scars are usually permanent although they may they fade with time. Because the cornea is such a specialised structure, any inflammation or injury that is deeper than just the epithelium, is likely to cause some permanent damage or scar. The pattern of scarring will vary according to the nature of the original inflammation.

The principles of diagnosis of corneal ulcers

Corneal ulcers are usually easily identified with fluorescein and a blue light (**Figure 9.2**). Corneal ulcers are a very common cause of visual impairment and blindness. Prompt treatment is essential. However, in order to give the correct treatment, the cause of the ulcer must also be identified. Even if the exact cause of the ulcer is unknown, it is essential to try to answer three questions:

1. *Is the ulcer infective or non-infective?* Infective ulcers require urgent treatment that will kill the infection, while non-infective ulcers require assessment and then treatment of the cause, and may need steroid treatment.
2. *If the ulcer is infective, is this bacterial, fungal, viral or protozoal (particularly acanthamoeba)?* Bacterial and fungal ulcers need urgent

and intensive treatment to prevent blindness. Other ulcers may become secondarily infected with bacteria. It is therefore wise to give prophylactic topical antibiotics for most corneal ulcers. The likelihood of different types of infection is very different in different locations. For example, fungal infection is more common in poor and tropical countries than rich countries or in cooler climates.

3. *Is it safe to use steroids?* Herpetic ulcers need antiviral treatment and get much worse if steroids are used. Steroids should not be used in the early stages of treating bacterial or fungal ulcers.

A summary of the common causes of corneal ulcers and their treatment is given in **Table 9.1**. Each type is then discussed in more detail in this chapter.

Table 9.1 Common causes and main features of corneal ulcers			
Cause of ulcer	**Predisposing factors**	**Clinical appearance**	**Treatment**
Herpes simplex (**Figures 9.2** and **9.3**)	Can occur in anyone Recurrences are common	Irregular edge, superficial, 'dendritic' (branching)	Antiviral agents Debridement *Not* steroids
Bacterial infection (**Figure 9.6**: suppurative corneal ulcer)	Injury, poor corneal health, contact lenses	Round, central cornea, slough and infiltrate around ulcer, hypopyon	Intensive topical antibiotic drops. *Not* steroids until clearly improving
Fungal infection (**Figure 9.9**)	Injury with vegetable matter, poor corneal health, agricultural work, tropical climates	Similar to bacterial infection, but more chronic course	Intensive antifungal agents. *Not* steroids until clearly improving
Nutritional ulcers (xerophthalmia) (**Figures 10.11** and **10.12**)	Malnourished children, particularly in areas with vitamin A deficiency, measles	Xerosis (dryness) of conjunctiva and cornea, usually central and lower half of cornea, often bilateral	Vitamin A supplementation. Topical lubrication and antibiotics *Not* steroids
Inflammatory marginal ulcers (marginal keratitis, peripheral ulcerative keratitis, Mooren ulcers, phlyctenular keratitis) (**Figures 9.12–9.16**)	Can occur in anyone, but different inflammatory ulcers associated with different conditions such as blepharitis and autoimmune disease	At or near limbus, often long and thin following limbal curve	Topical steroids and/or systemic immunosuppression depending on cause and severity
Vernal ulcers (Figure 7.18)	Children and adolescents, particularly if history of atopy/allergy	Central oval-shaped ulcer, conjunctival inflammatory changes, itching	Topical antihistamines and/or topical steroids Debridement (removal of slough often helps)
Exposure ulcers (**Figure 9.17**)	Facial nerve palsies/poor lid closure (including leprosy), proptosis, unconsciousness	Lower half of cornea, just below lowest point of upper lid	Closure of eyelids, lubricants
Neuropathic ulcers	Herpetic corneal infections, diabetes, chronic corneal damage	Very variable	Topical antibiotics, lubricants, lid closure

Corneal infections

Many types of micro-organisms can invade the cornea including viruses, bacteria, fungi and parasites. Most of these organisms come from outside, through the epithelium and into the cornea. However, a few may already be in the body, and migrate through the limbus.

- Viruses can invade a healthy cornea through the epithelium. They often also infect the conjunctival epithelium, and so viral infection often presents as superficial punctate keratoconjunctivitis and/or corneal ulcers.
- Bacteria and fungi cannot normally penetrate a healthy cornea. Therefore, they can only enter if the defences are disturbed, or if there is a break in the epithelium. The bacteria and fungi often produce toxins, which cause tissue death (called necrosis) and pus formation in the corneal tissue (suppurative keratitis).
- Leprosy, syphilis and onchocerciasis all enter the cornea from infection elsewhere in the body via the limbus. Therefore, they are mainly found in the stroma, and cause stromal keratitis.
- *Acanthamoeba* is a protozoal parasite which is typically associated with contact lens wear and appears to need a break in the epithelial surface after which it can cause a slow growing, severe stromal ulcer.

Symptoms of corneal ulcers

There are many different types of corneal ulcer, but the extreme sensitivity of the corneal epithelium causes a fairly uniform set of symptoms: pain, blurred vision, photophobia and watering. The important exception to this is people who have lost their corneal sensation ('anaesthetic cornea' or 'neuropathic cornea'). This often occurs following herpes simplex or herpes zoster infections and masks the usual symptoms.

Pain

Corneal pain is sharp and severe, because of the very good sensory nerve supply to the cornea.

Blurred vision

Corneal ulcers both obstruct the usually clear cornea and make the surface irregular, thereby interfering with the usual optics of the cornea. The degree of visual impairment depends upon the size, density and position of the ulcer. Obviously, a central ulcer will affect the vision more than a peripheral ulcer. Also a large deep ulcer with inflammation in the surrounding cornea affects the vision more than a superficial ulcer.

Photophobia

Patients with corneal disease and corneal pain almost invariably have light sensitivity and increased pain with light. It is not precisely clear why this occurs, as there is no proof that corneal nerve fibres are also light sensitive. However, light sensitivity decreases with topical anaesthetic, suggesting they are at least in part responsible for this.

Watering
Increased tear production is a reflex response to the corneal damage.

Signs of a corneal ulcer

Examination of an eye with a corneal ulcer shows the following features:

Conjunctival and ciliary vessel dilatation – a 'red' eye
Although the whole eye can become red, the most intense inflammation is usually of the ciliary vessels, i.e. near the limbus and the intensity decreases towards the fornices (**Figure 9.1**).

Opacity
Larger ulcers may be visible to the naked eye, but smaller less deep and dense ulcers usually require magnification and ideally a slit lamp. The lesion is seen much more clearly with fluorescein and blue light (**Figure 9.2**). There may also be inflammation or infiltrate in the corneal stroma around the ulcer.

Anterior chamber inflammation and/or hypopyon (Figure 9.5)
Larger more inflamed ulcers can cause anterior uveitis. Severe ulcers may cause pus to accumulate in the anterior chamber: hypopyon. Pus is composed of white cells mixed with fibrin, dying cells and tissue debris. Often this pus will settle with gravity to the bottom of the anterior chamber.

Pupillary constriction
The pupil is often slightly constricted, perhaps because of the increased light sensitivity

Viral Infections

Herpes simplex corneal disease

Herpes simplex virus (HSV) is a double-stranded DNA virus, which can cause pathology in most of the ocular and periocular tissues. Almost the

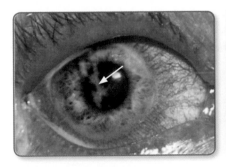

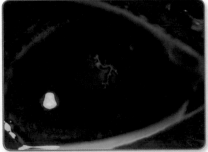

Figure 9.1 Ciliary dilatation in a patient with a herpetic corneal ulcer (arrow). The 'white' of the eye is inflamed and red, but this is most intense near the limbus, where the ciliary vessels are very dilated.

Figure 9.2 A dendritic herpes simplex corneal ulcer with fluorescein stain. The cornea looks normal to the naked eye before adding fluorescein which shows up the branching pattern of the ulcer.

entire adult population carries HSV, although the vast majority are asymptomatic. There are two main subtypes of HSV (HSV 1 and 2). HSV 1 mainly causes ocular, oral and facial disease and HSV 2, mainly causes genital disease, although there is some overlap. The initial infection (primary infection) comes from contact with an infected person. The majority of primary infections take place during infancy and adolescence, but infection can happen at any time including in-utero and during delivery. Primary infection is usually either asymptomatic or mild with acute follicular conjunctivitis, a few vesicles on the lids and regional lymphadenopathy. Occasionally it is quite severe with multiple large vesicles on the face, mouth or eyelids, and also some general malaise. The symptoms then resolve completely. However, the virus is not eliminated and instead remains dormant in the body and can then reactivate to cause recurrent episodes of ocular disease. Immunecompromised individuals are at particular risk of recurrent episodes. HSV infection can cause pathology in the lids (HSV blepharitis, Chapter 7), the conjunctiva (HSV conjunctivitis, Chapter 7), the cornea (HSV ulcers and disciform keratitis), the anterior chamber (anterior uveitis, Chapter 11), and the retina (HSV retinitis, Chapter 20). We will consider HSV corneal disease in this chapter.

HSV corneal infections occur more frequently in men, seem to reactivate in periods of stress, or during other illnesses, and are more common in autumn and winter. However, they can occur at any time, especially if steroids are being used as these reduce the cell-mediated immunity which is suppressing the virus. Patients who have ocular HSV often report also having cold sores, which are peri-ocular herpetic vesicles.

HSV epithelial keratitis

Epithelial disease is the most common manifestation of HSV. Although the ulcers are very characteristic in shape (dendritic, meaning 'tree-like' - see Figure 9.2), they can be confused with healing corneal abrasions that have 'tongues' of epithelium extending into the defect making the remaining area look dendritic ('pseudodendritic'). Occasionally, in immune-compromised individuals, the ulcer is larger and deeper. This is referred to as an 'amoeboid' ulcer (**Figure 9.3**). Herpetic corneal ulcers are usually only found in the epithelium and superficial layers of the stroma. This is why they are only visible with fluorescein dye. Herpetic corneal ulcers can usually be diagnosed by their typical appearance. The virus can be identified in a virology

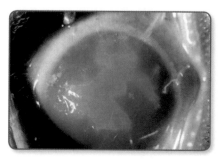

Figure 9.3 A severe 'amoeboid' herpes simplex ulcer. The ulcer is visible even without fluorescein. The patient was a young child recovering from measles.

laboratory quite easily by modern techniques such as immunofluorescence, but this is rarely necessary.

HSV ulcers must not be treated with mixtures of topical antibiotics and steroids (it is unfortunately a very common practice to treat red painful eyes with these combination drops). The antibiotics will not stop the virus, and the steroids will only depress the immune defences of the body, allowing the virus to proliferate rapidly, causing a much more serious infection. Therefore, the cornea must always be examined very carefully with fluorescein dye before using steroid drops.

Stromal inflammation and disciform keratitis

HSV epithelial keratitis can cause stromal inflammation, which is seen as opacity or cloudiness in the stromal layers (**Figure 9.4** and **Figure 9.14**). This is caused by the body's immune reaction to the viral infection. The cornea swells with inflammatory fluid, so it appears hazy. There may be both stromal keratitis and ulceration of the corneal surface. However, sometimes the inflammation occurs without epithelial disease, which is called disciform keratitis, because there is a central 'disc-shaped' area of inflammatory oedema. After the initial inflammation has settled, stromal keratitis often leaves a vascularised stromal scar.

Although stromal inflammation is commonly caused by herpetic infections, it can occur in other infective conditions and inflammatory diseases. The specific cause should be identified and treated.

Anterior uveitis and secondary glaucoma

Anterior uveitis is very common when stromal inflammation is present. It is clear that steroid treatment is required, but there can be a difficult balance between avoiding steroids during the infective stage and using them in the inflammatory stages of the disease.

Perforation

This does not occur with the natural history of the disease, but is occasionally seen if topical steroids are inappropriately used and continued without checking the cornea, or in immunosuppressed patients.

Longer term - sequelae

Corneal anaesthesia

Herpes virus causes reduced corneal sensation. This may continue for months or even years and can result in other infections or injuries presenting

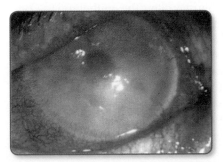

Figure 9.4 Stromal keratitis. The cornea appears hazy, which is due to corneal oedema. Note the dilatation of the ciliary blood vessels.

late as they are not felt by the patient. Also, the lack of sensation impairs the normal healing of corneal lesions.

Recurrent and chronic ulceration

Recurrences of HSV keratitis are common. They occur at very irregular intervals, usually in the same eye as the first ulcer. After several attacks of herpes simplex, the corneal stroma may become quite scarred and Bowman's membrane destroyed. At this stage there is no active virus present but the epithelial cells cannot grow over the irregular ulcer bed, and the ulcer will not heal, especially if the cornea is anaesthetic. A tarsorrhaphy or conjunctival flap procedure (see page 195) may help to heal these chronic ulcers.

The treatment of herpetic corneal ulcers

Antiviral drugs are the most effective method of treating herpetic ulcers. They inhibit the metabolism of viruses. However, viruses spend nearly all of their life cycle inside the host cells where they are relatively resistant to any chemotherapy. When the virus is dormant, oral antivirals reduce the frequency of infective episodes but do not eliminate the virus.

Acyclovir (Zovirax) is the most affordable and effective topical antiviral agent and is prescribed as an ointment to be used five times per day for 10 days. Oral acyclovir can be also be used to treat infective episodes (400 mg, five times per day for 10 days) or long-term at a lower dose to reduce the frequency of relapses (approximately 400 mg, twice a day for 6–12 months). Idoxuridine is another topical antiviral agent, which is available both as drops and ointment. It can be toxic to the corneal epithelium. There are also other topical antiviral agents available, but these are not widely used. Cycloplegic drops should also be given while the eye is painful. An ulcer that has also affected the stroma will leave a scar, but the epithelium itself regenerates without scarring.

Before the development of antiviral treatments, the main treatment was to remove diseased epithelium. This can still be done where antiviral drugs are not available. Two methods are used:

1. **Debridement**

   Debridement is a simple technique. The cornea is anaesthetised with local anaesthetic drops and the epithelium gently wiped off the area over and around the ulcer with a sterile cotton wool bud. After debridement, antibiotic and mydriatic drops or ointment (e.g. chloramphenicol and atropine) should be applied every day until the ulcer has healed. Some people recommend keeping the eye padded with the eye shut underneath after debridement, as this may allow the epithelium to regenerate more quickly.

2. **Chemical cauterisation**

   Chemical cauterisation is another traditional technique. Phenol is probably the best agent, but alcohol and iodine can also be used. First anaesthetise and dry the cornea. Then moisten a wooden stick in 10% phenol and touch the edges of the ulcer with this stick. Phenol makes the epithelium turn white. This must be done with great care, as these chemicals are very toxic.

The treatment of stromal keratitis

Herpes stromal keratitis is often difficult to treat. Topical steroids will suppress the inflammation very quickly and effectively, and also prevent corneal scarring. As long as the corneal epithelium is intact and there is no fluorescein staining ulcer, it is safe to give topical steroids in moderate doses (one drop 3 times daily). If the cornea is ulcerated as well, then antiviral treatment should be given and topical steroids started at a very low dose (e.g. one drop once daily). These patients must be observed carefully in case the ulcer enlarges whilst taking topical steroid drops.

Treatment of chronic infections

Occasionally, particularly in immunocompromised individuals, the disease does not respond to conventional treatment or resolve on its own. In these situations, consider the possibility of another cause, such as low grade fungal infection or acanthamoeba (see page 209). Then the following treatments may be considered:

- *Tarsorrhaphy* (suturing some or all of the upper and lower eyelid together to partially or totally close the eyelids temporarily): this prevents exposure, allows the tear film to coat the ulcer at all times, and reduces lid movement over the ulcer, all of which may encourage the epithelium to heal.
- *Conjunctival flap* (**Figure 9.5**): a flap of conjunctiva is mobilised to cover the defect. This often resolves the condition, but will definitely leave a scar.

Treatment of inactive scars

Corneal grafting can be used for a dense residual corneal scar, or to replace chronically diseased corneal tissue with healthy cornea. These grafts often have relatively low success rates, because of the risk of recurrent HSV infection and because the cornea is often already vascularised.

Suppurative keratitis: bacterial and fungal infections

The healthy cornea can resist invasion by pathogenic micro-organisms. If the natural corneal defences are weakened by disease or injury, bacteria or fungi can penetrate from outside and cause an acute, infective corneal ulcer (see **Figures 9.6 and 9.7a–c**). These acute and severe infections are called

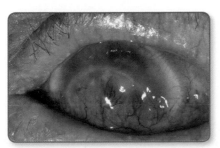

Figure 9.5 A conjunctival flap used to cover a corneal ulcer that would have penetrated. This has saved the eye and a little bit of vision.

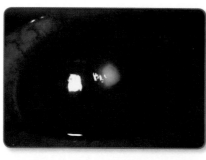

Figure 9.6 Bacterial corneal ulcer (suppurative keratitis). White-yellow pus in the ulcer bed and inflammation in the cornea around the ulcer, is just visible as a faint haze.

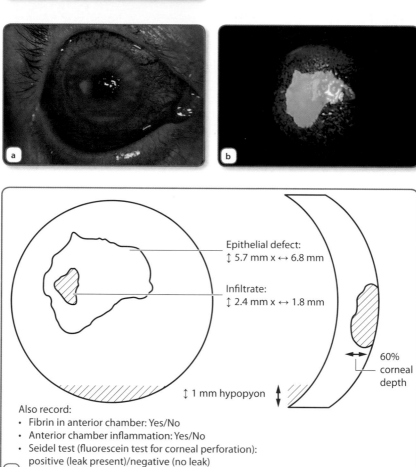

Epithelial defect:
$\updownarrow$ 5.7 mm x $\leftrightarrow$ 6.8 mm

Infiltrate:
$\updownarrow$ 2.4 mm x $\leftrightarrow$ 1.8 mm

60% corneal depth

$\updownarrow$ 1 mm hypopyon

Also record:
- Fibrin in anterior chamber: Yes/No
- Anterior chamber inflammation: Yes/No
- Seidel test (fluorescein test for corneal perforation): positive (leak present)/negative (no leak)

Figure 9.7 Suppurative keratitis from bacterial infection. (a) The corneal ulcer and hypopyon. The white area of infiltrate has a ragged edge. (b) The same corneal ulcer as in (a) stained with fluorescein. The area of epithelial defect is much larger than the area where there is pus in the cornea. (c) How the appearance of this ulcer would be recorded, to assess its progress. If possible a record of this sort should be made every day.

'suppurative ('pus forming') keratitis' because there is pus formation in the surrounding tissue. Suppurative keratitis is common in tropical climates and frequently leads to blindness. It requires very urgent treatment. In rich countries and colder climates, nearly all cases of suppurative keratitis are caused by bacteria and around 1% or less are caused by fungi. However, the situation is very different in the tropics and poor countries, where fungal infections may be responsible for up to 50% of cases. The key points on suppurative keratitis are summarised in **Box 9.1**.

Risk factors for suppurative keratitis

Our eyes are all exposed to potentially pathogenic bacteria all the time. However, we rarely get corneal infections, because of the unbroken, well-protected ocular surface. Certain factors increase the risk of micro-organism entering the cornea, or decrease the host's defence systems:

- *Trauma*, e.g. foreign body, abrasion, inturning eyelashes (e.g. in trachoma) or other injury. This causes breaks in the corneal epithelium, allowing micro-organisms to enter, settle and grow in the cornea. Ocular trauma is particularly common in poor countries and with agricultural work. Trauma is associated with up to 90% of cases of fungal keratitis, with 60% of these being vegetative matter trauma.
- *Defective eyelid closure or proptosis*, which causes corneal exposure (see **Figure 19.16** and **Figure 19.17**).
- *Dry eye or tear film abnormalities*: this reduces the natural defences of the eye.
- *Reduced corneal sensation*: this reduces the protective response to damage to the cornea.
- *Vitamin A deficiency*: this causes both dry eye and probably reduces ocular immune protection.
- *Contact lenses*: these are a particular risk if they are poorly cleaned, poor fitting or washed in water rather than sterile solutions. They are associated with bacterial, fungal and acanthamoeba keratitis.
- *The prolonged use of topical steroid drops*, as this suppresses the immune system.
- *Immune compromise*: patients taking immune suppressing drugs or with immune compromising disease, as well as newborn infants who

---

Box 9.1 The key points on suppurative keratitis
- Suppurative keratitis is a common problem especially in tropical climates and frequently leads to blindness.
- A Gram stain is a great help in identifying the cause so that the right treatment can be given.
- Urgent and intensive treatment with topical antibiotics or antifungals may save the eye.
- The treatment has two distinct aims: (1) to sterilise the tissues by killing the organisms and (2) afterwards to promote healing.
- Fungi, which are a common cause in the tropics, are particularly hard to treat.

have less developed immune systems are more susceptible to corneal infection than healthy adults.

Bacterial or fungal corneal ulcers produce the same general symptoms as any corneal ulcer. The two ways of recognising suppurative keratitis are by its position and its appearance.

Position

Suppurative keratitis is nearly always at the centre of the cornea or just below the centre, because this is the most exposed part. It is also farthest from the blood supply and the immune defences of the body.

Appearance

The appearance of the ulcer reflects the acute inflammatory reaction to the bacterial or fungal toxins in the surrounding tissues. All the constituents of pus are present (protein exudate, large number of neutrophils, dying cells and tissue debris), and the ciliary blood vessels are dilated. The ulcer has a yellow, rough appearance from the pus and tissue debris (**Figure 9.6**) and in advanced or severe cases there will be inflammation and pus in the surrounding cornea. In these severe cases there will also be inflammatory cells in the anterior chamber, which sink to the bottom to form a hypopyon (**Figure 9.7**).

Because the cornea has no blood supply, it is difficult for the body to mobilise its immune defences against the invading micro-organisms. If suppurative keratitis is not treated, it often progresses rapidly with serious complications, and frequently blindness (some of these are shown in the diagrams and pictures of **Figure 9.8**).

Other clinical consequences of suppurative keratitis

Iritis and secondary glaucoma

Some degree of iritis is always present. If this iritis is severe it may obstruct the flow of aqueous fluid, causing raised intraocular pressure.

Perforation and endophthalmitis

Untreated ulcers may perforate right through the cornea into the anterior chamber. Aqueous leaks out of the eye. If the perforation is only small it may help the infection to heal. This is because antibodies and cells from the vascular iris will come into contact with the infected cornea. In this case, the iris will stick to the back of the cornea, to form an *anterior synechia*. However, sometimes infection spreads inside the eye (endophthalmitis), which is a very serious complication. This nearly always results in blindness, and possibly loss of the globe. If the eyeball does survive, it often becomes shrunken and atrophic and with low pressure (phthisis bulbi).

Long-term sequelae of suppurative keratitis

Corneal scars

After resolution of the infection, a scar almost inevitably remains in the area where the bacterial ulcer has destroyed the corneal stroma. Even if the infection resolves in the early stages, either spontaneously or with treatment, some degree of corneal scarring is likely. The scar is often dense and causes profound and permanent visual impairment. They can fade slightly with time.

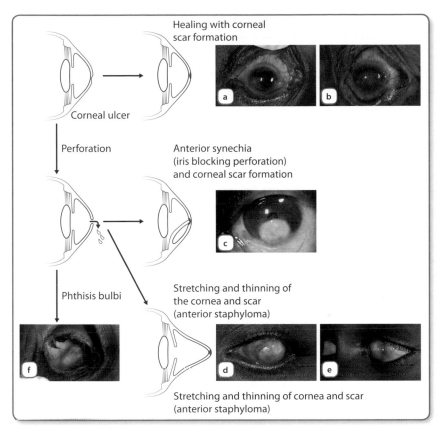

Figure 9.8 The complications of corneal ulcers. (a) Faint non-central corneal scar. (b) Severe vascularised corneal scar. (c) Corneal scar and anterior synechiae. (d) Corneal staphyloma front. (e) Corneal staphyloma from the side. (f) Phthisis bulbi.

Staphyloma

A corneal staphyloma (Greek: grape) is a bulging out of the cornea in an area of severely thinned cornea, or an area that perforated, but formed a thin fibrous scar across the defect. The scar then bulges as the pressure in the eye rises.

Distinguishing bacterial and fungal keratitis

Bacterial keratitis

Bacterial keratitis usually progresses very rapidly with a clinical course of only a few days. Almost any pathogenic bacteria can cause corneal ulcers, but the most common are *Pseudomonas*, *Staphylococcus*, *Streptococcus*, *Pneumococcus*, *Meningococcus*, *Gonococcus* and *E. coli*. It is not possible to tell from the appearance of the ulcer which bacteria are the cause, but there may be some pointers. For example, *Pseudomonas* is particularly common in contact lens wearers and can enlarge and destroy the cornea quickly, while gonococcus predominantly occurs in neonates, within the first days of life. Furthermore, different bacteria are more likely in different locations, e.g. *Streptococci* are the most common cause of suppurative keratitis in South India, but *Pseudomonas* is a far more common cause in Ghana.

Fungal keratitis

The known risk factors for fungal keratitis are:

- Hot climates
- Humid climates
- Injury with vegetable matter

In tropical climates, studies have found 50% of ulcers to be fungal. However this is likely to be even higher in rural areas.

There are a great variety of fungi found in nature and they vary greatly in their virulence. Most fungi are not pathogenic at all, and some are only very weakly pathogenic. The infections that these cause are therefore mild, and may recover spontaneously. Most of the pathogenic fungi, which do infect the eye, have a chronic and slowly progressive course with ulcers developing over a few weeks. However there are a few fungi, which can produce an acute ulcer, which looks like a bacterial infection. Fungi cannot penetrate a healthy, uninjured cornea.

The most common pathogenic fungi in the cornea are *Fusarium, Aspergillus* and *Candida*. Fusarium is found especially in moist climates and is more invasive. *Aspergillus* is more common in drier climates, and *Candida* often occurs in immunesuppressed patients and in patients with corneal graft.

Sometimes fungal corneal ulcers have the same clinical appearance as bacterial ulcers. However, the following are clinical features that make an ulcer more likely to be fungal (**Figure 9.9**).

- A rough raised 'shaggy' or 'sloughy' surface, and an irregular or serrated edge. Fungal ulcers can also have localised extensions into the surrounding corneal stroma ('satellite' lesions). However, these can occur in ulcers caused by other infections as well.
- Both fungal and bacterial suppurative ulcers are usually a yellow-white colour. If the colour is anything other than yellow, then a fungal infection is much more likely.
- Hypopyon and anterior chamber fibrinous exudates occur in both fungal and bacterial corneal ulcers, but they have been shown to occur significantly more frequently in bacterial suppurative keratitis.

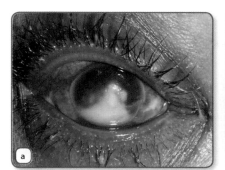 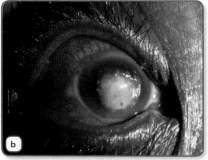

Figure 9.9 Two cases of severe fungal keratitis. Although these two ulcers look different they both have 'feathery edges' and are raised a little above the surface of the cornea. These features are strongly suggestive of fungal ulcers. The satellite lesions (areas of infiltrate separate from the main ulcer) can occur in non-fungal corneal ulcers.

- Fungal ulcers usually progress more slowly and there may also be a history of the symptoms improving for a time and then becoming worse again. Therefore, the longer the ulcer has been present, the more likely it is to be fungal. Some fungal corneal ulcers have had weeks of intensive treatment for bacterial ulcers, without showing any clinical improvement.

Diagnosis and identification of the organism

It is usually fairly easy to make a diagnosis of suppurative keratitis from the symptoms and clinical appearance of the ulcer. However, suppurative keratitis is one of the few eye diseases where laboratory tests are very helpful and can make a big difference. If the organism can be identified, there is a much better chance that the correct treatment will be given. There are two ways of identifying the organism, direct examination with a microscope and culture.

Direct examination with the microscope

This has several advantages:
- The only equipment needed is a microscope, some slides and bottles of tissue stain.
- It is quick to do and gives an almost immediate result.
- External laboratory expertise is not required. Anyone can learn how to prepare microscope slides and how to look at them.

The technique for microscopy and a stain is as follows, and the whole process takes about 5 minutes.

1. Apply local anaesthetic drops to the eye.
2. Scrape the edge of the ulcer quite firmly with the edge of a hypodermic needle or the side of a scalpel blade. Most of the bacteria are found at the edge of the ulcer, not the centre. If it has almost perforated this must be done with great care. If culture facilities are available, then half the specimen is used for microscope examination and the other half is put straight on to culture plates for incubation.
3. Spread out on a glass slide as thinly as possible or cigarette lighter, and allow to air dry.
4. Fix by gently warming with a spirit lamp or cigarette lighter, allow to cool and stain with Gram stain (crystal violet) for 1 minute. Rinse the slide in running water and then stain for another 1 minute in Gram's iodine. Then rinse the slide again in running water.
5. Pour acetone over the slide and rinse in running water immediately so that the time in contact with acetone is less than 2 seconds. Counterstain with carbol fuchsin for 30 seconds. Rinse again in water, and dry in the air or with blotting paper.
6. Examine the slide under the low power of a laboratory microscope. When everything is focused and centred, then change to the oil immersion lens (see **Figure 9.10**).

Stains for fungi

The exact choice of stain for specific fungi is beyond the scope of this book, but most fungi will stain with a Gram stain, although they will show up particularly well with lactophenol cotton blue.

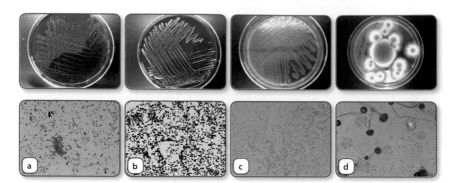

Figure 9.10 The microscopic identification of organisms causing suppurative keratitis. Culture (top row) and microscopy (bottom row). (a)*Streptococcus pneumoniae* ('pneumococcus'): alpha-haemolytic colonies on blood agar showing characteristic 'draughtsman' morphology, staining as Gram positive diplococci. (b) *Staphylococcus epidermidis* (a typical coagulase-negative staphylococcus): characteristic white colonies on blood agar, staining as Gram positive cocci in grape-like clusters. (c) *Pseudomonas aeruginosa:* mucoid colonies on MacConkey agar, staining as Gram negative bacilli. (d) *Aspergillus fumigatus:* downy colonies on Sabouraud agar, staining with Lactophenol cotton blue stain to show characteristic morphology.

Culture

A culture of bacteria or fungi will give a more specific diagnosis and will allow the organism(s) to be fully identified. It can also be used to determine the antibiotics to which the bacteria are sensitive to. There are, however, certain practical problems, which limit its usefulness as a test:

- It requires a moderately well-equipped laboratory and staff trained in using the equipment.
- Bacteria take time to grow in culture. Results may not be available for two or more days.
- The ulcer sample needs to get to the laboratory. Ideally, the material should be put directly onto culture slides and transferred to the laboratory. Alternatively it can first be put in special transport media before being plated out in the laboratory. If culture is planned it is best not to put fluorescein drops or preserved anaesthetic in the eye until the corneal scrape has been taken as they may inhibit the growth of the organism. However, non-preserved anaesthetic can be difficult to obtain in many areas.
- Fungi are extremely difficult to grow. Most of them need to be incubated at room temperature as well as 37°C. They may require a special growth medium. They will take much longer to culture, often several weeks, and may be hard to identify. Fortunately most fungi can be detected with a careful microscopy of corneal scrapings.

Treatment of suppurative keratitis

Treatment has two aims:

1. Sterilisation: killing the organisms responsible for the ulcer.
2. Healing: the cornea must recover, with epithelium regrowing and scarring ideally minimised in order to get the best possible visual outcome.

Treatment of bacterial ulcers

Bacteria are sterilised or killed with antibiotics. Antibiotics may be given topically as drops or ointment, by subconjunctival injection and occasionally intravitreally and systematically if endophthalmitis is occurring. However, drops are the most effective and therefore most widely used route. These are initially given very intensively in order to kill the bacteria and then the frequency tapered as some antibiotics are quite toxic to the corneal epithelium and so while they are effective at sterilising the ulcer, they can slow down the healing.

Antibacterial treatment is obviously needed if the Gram stain shows bacteria. If microscopy is not available, or if the result will be delayed or is inconclusive, antibacterial treatment should still be started immediately because bacterial corneal ulcers are extremely destructive and may progress rapidly with a great risk of blindness.

1. **Drops**

   Drops are the best treatment for bacterial ulcers that are confined to the cornea, as the normal cornea has no blood vessels, so penetration from the circulation is usually poor and slow. The drops should be given hourly throughout the day and night (or at least two hourly at night) for the first two days if possible. They can then be reduced to two to four hourly (day-time only) as this allows the cornea to recover from the potentially toxic drops and the patient to get a good night's rest.

   The choice of antibiotic drop depends on what if any bacteria are identified and on the availability and local bacterial sensitivities and resistance and therefore it is not appropriate to be prescriptive in this book. However, at present the fluoroquinolones (e.g. levofloxacin, ofloxacin, and moxifloacin) are widely used and effective for a wide range of bacteria and in particular the pseudomonal infections that commonly occur in contact lens wearers. They are also a good choice of antibiotic when treatment is being given 'blind' (without microbiological results) as they are well tolerated, have good corneal penetration and are broad spectrum. In many situations there are high levels of resistance to chloramphenicol drops and this is very unlikely to be the first line of treatment.

   In some cases it may be appropriate to give two antibiotic drops, e.g. if an ulcer appears to be only partially responding to the first drop, or if two different bacteria are identified. If two antibiotics are being given hourly a few minutes or more gap should be left between them.

   Stronger (fortified) drops are also available, typically gentamycin and cefuroxime. These are often very effective at killing bacteria and are often used together as gentamycin is particularly effective for gram-negative organisms like *Pseudomonas* and cefuroxime for gram positive ones like Meningococcus and Gonococcus. They must be used with caution as they are toxic to the corneal epithelium. Gentamycin is particularly toxic. If the epithelium has not healed over after 3 or 4 days treatment, then they should be given less frequently or standard strength topical antibiotics given instead. If concentrated drops are not commercially available, they can be prepared fairly easily in a number of ways so as to make a solution that will be stable for about 4 days. This is long enough to provide treatment.

There are three methods of making strong antibiotic solutions:

- Antibiotic powder can be added to a bottle of artificial tear-drops containing hypromellose. The hypromellose produces a viscous solution, which allows the antibiotic to be in contact with the ulcer for a little longer.
- A bottle of ordinary strength antibiotic can be fortified with more antibiotics. The best example of this is gentamicin. The commercially available gentamicin contains 3 mg/mL in a 5 mL bottle. If an ampoule of gentamicin for injection (containing 80 mg in 2 mL) is added to this, the result is 95 mg of gentamicin in 7 mL of fluid (approximately 14 mg/mL gentamycin)
- If neither of the above are possible, the antibiotic powder can just be added to 5 mL of water or saline for injection.

The recommended strengths of these concentrated antibiotics solutions and their antibacterial activity are shown in **Table 9.2**.

Remember that very high local antibiotic doses are achieved with drops and, therefore, the laboratory sensitivities are not always borne out clinically. For example, the laboratory may find an organism to be resistant to a particular antibiotic, but when this is given hourly, it is still an effective treatment.

The patient must be monitored frequently. If there is worsening or no improvement after about 3 days the organism is probably not sensitive to the treatment. Further samples should be taken if possible, the treatment should be changed, and reconsider whether this could be a fungal infection.

If after a period of treatment, the infection looks to be resolving, e.g. the stromal infiltrate and hypopyon has reduced, but the epithelial defect remains, it is likely that drug toxicity is becoming a problem and the frequency of instillation should be reduced.

2. **Ointments**

Ointments are useful at night, but they are not as effective as drops for intensive use. This is because it is uncertain how well the active

Table 9.2 Concentrated antibiotic drops for suppurative keratitis			
Antibiotic	**Strength**	**Dilution**	**Bacterial activity**
Aminoglycosides Gentamicin Amikacin	14 mg/mL 50 mg/ mL	95 mg in 7 mL 250 mg in 5 mL bottle	Gram-negative organisms especially *Pseudomonas* and *E. coli*
Cephalosporins Cefuroxime Ceftazidime Cephazolin, etc.	50 mg/mL	250 mg in 5 mL bottle	Gram-positive organisms + Gram-negative cocci meningococcus gonococcus
Penicillins Penicillin Ticarcillin	10 mg/mL	50 mg in 5 mL bottle	Streptococcus especially Pseudomonas especially

ingredient comes out of the ointment base, and dissolves into the tears. Concentrated ointments are not available. They should only be used by day if drops are not available.

3. **Subconjunctival injections**

   These provide reasonable drug levels in the cornea (see page 84 and Table 4.1 for technique and antibiotic dosages). However, the length of action is variable and they can be painful even with topical anaesthetics in an inflamed eye. They are useful when the patient cannot be observed on a daily basis.

4. **Systemic antibiotics**

   The indications for systemic antibiotics are:
   - Perforated ulcers
   - Associated infection in peri-ocular tissues
   - Ulcers that are close to the limbus

Additional treatment

Dilating drops

Mydriatics, such as cyclopentolate 1% three times/day or atropine 1% once/day should also be given to reduce the pain a little and prevent iris posterior synechiae forming if there is significant anterior chamber inflammation.

Steroids

It is unclear if steroids are beneficial for treating bacterial keratitis. It is possible that the long-term visual outcome for some ulcers caused by some bacteria is slightly better if steroids have been used, although it is not known when the best time to introduce them is. The potential advantages are that they reduce inflammation and resultant scarring. However, they inhibit the host's immune system which may reduce their ability to clear the infection and they can increase stromal thinning, which may increase the risk of perforation.

If they are going to be used, one must be certain that the keratitis is not caused by fungal, viral or acanthamoeba infection. They should probably only be used after several days of intensive antibiotic treatment, when it is clear that the infection is not getting worse, they should be used cautiously (perhaps three times per day) and the patient must be monitored regularly.

The treatment of fungal ulcers

The correct treatment can stop a fungal infection before it totally destroys the cornea and some fungal infections may even heal slowly without treatment. However, fungal ulcers are very difficult to treat and the results of treatment are often disappointing for a number of reasons:

- The diagnosis is frequently delayed as patients often live in remote, rural communities with very poor access to specialist healthcare.
- Fungi respond much more slowly to treatment than bacteria.
- Drug availability: although several fungicidal drugs are available, many pharmacies and shops do not stock them, and they may be very expensive and not prepared in an ocular form.
- Fungi sensitivities: it can be difficult to determine which anti-fungal to use, particularly if the causative organism has not been identified.

- Prolonged treatment is required: this requires excellent patient compliance, consistent supplies of antifungal drops and regular review by an eyecare worker.

The situations in which fungal treatment is likely to be appropriate are:

- Fungal hyphae or spores seen on microscopy or culture.
- Clinical appearance and history are suggestive of fungal infection.
- Full course of antibacterial treatment without improvement. Although this could represent resistant bacteria, it is crucial to consider fungal infections at this stage.

Topical treatment (Table 9.3): Topical antifungal drugs should be applied frequently, ideally initially hourly and then every 2 hours, until there is no clinical evidence of infection. Prolonged treatment, for a month or more may be required. There has not been nearly enough research into fungal keratitis to give definitive treatment guidelines and therefore several different drops are widely used with different success rates in different situations and for different fungal species. However it is thought that the drugs in **Table 9.3** are effective in approximate order of preference.

Antifungal eye drops are not available in many places. However, antifungal skin and vaginal preparations are often widely available. If nothing else is available it is possible to use these in the eye, although it is obviously not ideal and they may be painful to instil and toxic to the epithelium. Sometimes antifungals are available in tablet form, or as powder in an ampoule for systemic use, and will need to be dissolved (although many fungicidal drugs are not soluble in water). Again this is far from the ideal way of giving topical eye medication, but may be the only option for a potentially blinding infection.

Another treatment for fungal ulcers that is currently being investigated is corneal crosslinking. With this treatment, the cornea is infused with a drug called riboflavin and is then crosslinked under an ultraviolet light. It causes the cornea to become stiffer and is therefore being increasingly used for keratoconus (see below), but may also help treat fungal infections. The efficacy and safety are currently unknown.

Systemic treatment: This is only indicated in desperate cases with huge or penetrating ulcers, or if topical treatment is not available. The drugs of choice are ketoconazole or itraconazole because they both have a broad spectrum of activity and are well absorbed by mouth. If these are not available, other azole drugs can be tried. All these drugs have a slight risk of liver toxicity, and can be expensive. Other systemic drugs with antifungal activity, which have been tried, are thiabendazole (25 mg/kg/day orally or prepared as a 4% suspension topically), which is primarily an anthelminthic drug, but has antifungal properties and flucytosine (200 mg/kg/day), which is relatively non-toxic and is especially effective against *Candida*.

Suppurative keratitis and HIV infection

There is no definite evidence yet that suppurative keratitis is linked with HIV infection. However, HIV positive patients have depression of their cellular immunity, which is particularly involved in overcoming fungal

Table 9.3 Topical antifungal drugs		
Drug (class)	Dose and formulation	Uses, advantages and disadvantages
Natamycin (Polyene)	5–10% suspension, or ointment	Wide range of antifungal activity. It is the treatment of choice for filamentous fungi. It may not penetrate to the stroma as well as econazole or the other azole drugs and therefore periodic epithelial debridement can be considered to improve penetration. Natamycin is a useful prophylactic treatment for corneal abrasions with vegetable matter in hot humid climates, which helps to prevent fungal keratitis developing. It is probably not as effective as econazole in treating established fungal infections. Randomised controlled trials have shown no difference in outcomes between natamycin 5% and econazole 2% and natamycin to be more effective than itraconazole for fusarium keratitis.
Amphotericin B (Polyene)	0.15%	Water soluble and can be prepared from powder for intravenous injection. It is particularly effective for *Candida* and *Aspergillus*, but like natamycin, corneal penetration is poor through an intact epithelium. In severe cases, amphotericin can also be given subconjunctivally, intracamerally, intravitreally or intravenously.
Econazole (or cloterimazole/ miconazole/ (Imidazole)	1%	Good spectrum of activity and reasonable penetration but possibly less effective than the polyenes and therefore often used in combination. They can only be dissolved in oily solutions and not aqueous ones, which limits their effectiveness. A 1% solution in arachis oil (peanut oil) can be made up by grinding and dissolving a tablet and given as hourly drops. They are much more commonly found as skin or vaginal creams (see below).
Fluconazole, itraconazole (Triazole)	1%	Very effective against *Candida* but less effective against *Aspergillus* and *Fusarium*. Although this is commercially available as 0.3% strength, some people recommend it being fortified to 1.0%.
Voriconazole (Triazole)	1%	Better broad-spectrum activity than the other triazoles, and therefore effective against filamentous fungi and yeast, including *Fusarium*, *Aspergillus* and *Candida*. Good stromal penetration.
Nystatin		This is usually quite ineffective and has poor penetration compared to the other antifungals. It does not dissolve very well but can be made up in a suspension of 100,000 units per mL.
Chlorhexidene 02% Povidone iodine (antiseptic)		Very effective in the laboratory but possibly less effective in patients. They are painful to instil and quite toxic to the epithelium. It is very useful if no other antifungals are available. It is recommended as 0.2% chlorhexidene gluconate drops and is useful for acanthamoeba infections at the weaker strength of 0.02% (see below).

infections. If a patient appears to have an unusual ulcer, either in appearance, response to treatment or the causative organism, the possibility that the patient has immune-compromising disease, such as HIV, must be considered.

Surgical treatment for suppurative keratitis

Sometimes, in spite of the best of efforts, suppurative keratitis fails to respond to medical treatment and there are some situations in which the following surgical options need to be considered. The surgical techniques for these procedures are described in *Eye Surgery in Hot Climates, 4th edition*. London: JP Medical, 2014.

Evisceration

If the infection has spread into the eye causing endophthalmitis, and this cannot be controlled with systemic antibiotics, and there is no perception of light in the eye, the eye should be eviscerated to prevent long and unsuccessful treatment and possible further complications. Untreated, uncontrolled endophthalmitis can lead to infection in the cavernous sinus and very occasionally is fatal.

Conjunctival flap

This procedure is beneficial for non-healing ulcers that are confined to the cornea. The conjunctival flap covers the ulcer with an epithelial surface and brings blood vessels to the site, to allow the patient's immune system to kill the bacteria or fungi and heal the defect. A successful conjunctival flap operation requires extensive mobilisation of the conjunctiva, which is then sutured securely to cover the ulcer. This procedure can be used as a last ditch emergency attempt to save an eye and is surprisingly effective at treating a persistent or nearly perforating ulcer, but will leave a vascularised scar.

Tarsorrhaphy

This is joining the upper to the lower eyelid. The whole of both lids can be joined – complete tarsorrhaphy. However, it is more common just to join the outer part of the upper and lower lids, which may be enough to help the ulcer heal. A conjunctival flap is probably a more effective procedure for grossly infected eyes that are near to perforating.

Charting the progress of an ulcer

Suppurative keratitis is always very difficult to treat. The appearance of the eye and its treatment needs to be reviewed, every day if possible. The best way to assess progress is to photograph the ulcer. However, this is not possible in most places and therefore thorough clinical documentation is essential. This should include sketches and recording of the depth of the ulcer, the amount of epithelial loss, the state of the surrounding cornea and the size of any hypopyon (See **Figure 9.7c**).

Acanthamoeba

Acanthamoeba is a widespread protozoan organism found in most tap water. Very occasionally it can invade the cornea to produce severe corneal ulcers that are very difficult to treat. The diagnosis of acanthamoeba keratitis (AK) is frequently missed and mistreated as fungal or bacterial ulcers or as herpes simplex keratitis.

Diagnosis

Clinical history

Acanthamoeba infection must be considered in the differential diagnosis in any patient with any of the following:
- Contact lens wearers who have poor lens hygiene, particularly if their lenses are exposed to water.
- Corneal trauma, which may have been contaminated with soil or water.

- Ulcers that are failing to respond to conventional treatment.
- Ulcers with atypical features.

Clinical appearance (Figure 9.11)

AK can present with a very varied clinical appearance. This is one of the reasons it is so difficult to diagnose. Apart from the typical history, the following features should make you suspicious:
- Limbitis: inflammation at the corneal limbus
- Perienural infiltrate: the corneal nerves become inflamed and larger, and easier to see than normal
- Punctate keratitis and corneal epithelial loss

In more advanced cases you may also see (**Figure 9.11b**):
- A large chronic central corneal ulcer
- A ring of inflammatory infiltrate around this ulcer
- Uveitis

Microbiological

In most places laboratory resources and expertise are inadequate to make a formal diagnosis of AK. However, if a suitably equipped laboratory is available the following methods can be used:
- Corneal scrape onto an *E. coli* inoculate agar plate.
- Histological examination of corneal specimen to look for organisms and cysts.
- Staining with specific stains such as Calcofluor white.

Treatment

Early diagnosis is the key to successful treatment as the outcomes worsen the longer the infection is not treated. The primary treatment is hourly polyhexamethylene biguanide (PHMB) 0.02% for 48 hours and then gradually reduced over the next few weeks. This can be replaced with chlorhexidene drops if PHMB is not available. Treatment is often supplemented with Brolene, which is another antiseptic. Once the infection is under control, topical steroids may be very gradually introduced to try to minimise scarring.

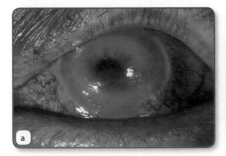
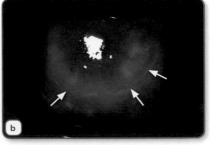

Figure 9.11 (a) Acanthamoeba. The large corneal ulcer causes extensive haziness of the cornea and the vigorous anterior uveitis causes endothelial inflammatory precipitates. (b) Acanthamoeba ring infiltrate (arrows).

Inflammatory corneal disease

Sometimes the cornea is the site for non-infective inflammation. It can be difficult to distinguish inflammatory corneal conditions from infective ones. Moreover, there can be considerable overlap between the two, with infections provoking an inflammatory keratitis. In general, inflammatory conditions, tend to occur near the corneal margin, close to the limbal blood vessels, while infective conditions are often more central, further away the immune defence at the limbus.

Peripheral corneal inflammatory ulcers

An individual's immune system is able to create large and painful peripheral ulcers. Unlike primary infective ulcers, these are not usually circular, but instead are curved, following the curve of the peripheral cornea.

When a peripheral ulcer is seen, the first question that must be asked is: what has provoked it? Although sometimes there is no clear provoking disease or condition, there often is and these may require treatment, either to reduce the risk of the inflammatory ulcers continuing to occur, or because there is a significant systemic disease that can be damaging elsewhere in the body. Some of the predisposing systemic diseases are complex or rare autoimmune diseases (diseases in which the body's own immune system 'attacks' its own tissues) that may be difficult or impossible to treat in poor countries, but it is still prudent to try and make the diagnosis.

The following conditions frequently predispose to inflammatory ulcers.

Blepharitis

Blepharitis is inflammation of the eyelids (**Figures 6.4** and **6.5**). This is discussed in more detail in Chapter 6. Patients with blepharitis are at much greater risk of developing peripheral inflammatory corneal ulcers. These ulcers are often called *marginal keratitis* (**Figure 9.12a** and **b**). There are sometimes multiple ulcers in the peripheral cornea. It is unclear if the agent that provokes the immune response is the abnormal debris, the secretions, or bacteria (and the toxins they produce) that accumulate in the secretions, or

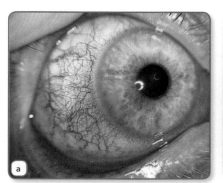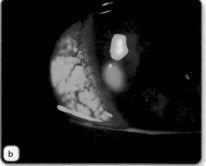

Figure 9.12 Marginal corneal infiltration or marginal keratitis. (a) There is a peripheral, white infiltration just inside the limbus with dilatation of the limbal blood vessels mainly in the area next to the opacity. (b) Fluorescein has been instilled which stains the ulcer.

perhaps most likely, all of these factors. Marginal inflammatory ulcers generally heal without intervention, although leave a white marginal stromal opacity. However, they do respond very quickly to steroids or steroid/antibiotic drops (approximately four times/day and then reducing over 1-4 weeks depending on severity), which can be very useful as they can be painful.

Phlyctens

Phlyctenular keratoconjunctivitis usually starts as an inflamed nodule in the conjunctiva and is described in Chapter 7. They may also cause inflammation in the peripheral cornea causing a localised ulcer with surrounding intense inflammation. Phlyctenular corneal ulcers are raised and have a fan of blood vessels entering them from the conjunctival side (**Figure 9.13**). Phlyctens respond well to topical steroids.

Stromal keratitis

Stromal keratitis causes area(s) of haziness in the corneal stroma (**Figure 9.14**). The haziness is caused by inflammation and infiltration of the cornea by immune cells. The immune response is most commonly provoked by herpes viruses, but can also be caused by other infections such as syphilis, mumps, measles, Lyme disease and *Acanthamoeba*. Stromal keratitis usually responds well and quickly to topical steroids. However, try and identify and treat the cause if you can. Also, remember that steroids will suppress the patient's immune system and carry the risk of making an infection worse.

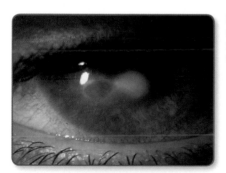

Figure 9.13 Phlyctenular corneal ulcer. This ulcer is gradually advancing from the limbus towards the centre of the cornea and leaving a vascularised scarred area behind it.

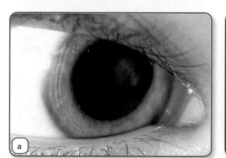
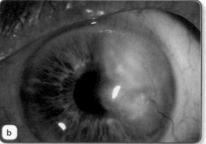

Figure 9.14 Stromal keratitis. (a) Early stromal keratitis. A circle or 'disc' shaped patch of stromal inflammation can be seen. This patient had chicken pox. (b) Recurrent severe stromal keratitis. This patient had herpes simplex keratitis. As well as the active stromal keratitis, there is also corneal vascularisation and scarring from previous episodes. Courtesy of Dr N Rogers.

Peripheral ulcerative keratitis (PUK) (Figure 9.15)

PUK is deep ulceration in the peripheral cornea that usually occurs in association with a systemic autoimmune disease. The most commonly associated diseases are collagen vascular diseases like rheumatoid arthritis, polyarteritis nodosa, polyangiitis with granulomatosis (previously known as Wegener granulomatosis) and systemic lupus erythematosus. The ulcers may be deep and may even perforate. They are often very painful. In cases of PUK, the clinician should, not only focus on the eye but also consider the possible systemic disease. PUK is also treated with steroids, but much more intensive and prolonged treatment is required, as well as treating any associated systemic disease.

For systemic immunosuppression the first line of treatment is systemic steroids. This is the only immune-suppressing agent that is available in most parts of the world. A fairly high dose (e.g. 60 mg of prednisolone daily) can safely be given for a week or even two weeks, but then the dose must be reduced as there are many dangers of long term systemic steroids (see page 91).

Other immunosuppressive drugs are the cytotoxic drugs such as azathioprine, cyclophosphamide and cyclosporin. These are all powerful and toxic drugs and they must be given under supervision, preferably by someone who is familiar both with their use and complications such as bone marrow and kidney depression. However, these ulcers may be severe and blinding and may need treatment with these drugs.

Mooren ulcer or ring ulcer

This is a severe and persistent type of peripheral ulcerative keratitis, which can cover a large part of the corneal margin, and sometimes the whole limbus (**Figure 9.16**). Hence they are sometimes called ring ulcers. Unlike peripheral ulcerative keratitis, Mooren ulcer is not associated with any systemic diseases. In addition to spreading around the cornea, these ulcers may spread slowly towards the centre of the cornea. They cause necrosis and loss of the superficial layers of the cornea, and leave a vascularised and opaque scar when they heal. They are usually unilateral but occasionally

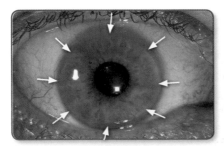

Figure 9.15 Peripheral ulcerative keratitis, showing a peripheral ring of thinned cornea. The arrows show the thinned area.

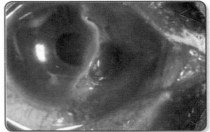

Figure 9.16 A severe Mooren's ulcer. The ulcer has eroded half the circumference of the cornea and has an overhanging edge. This particular ulcer has perforated and the iris prolapsed through the hole. Perforation is not common with Mooren's ulcers.

occur in both eyes. They can be very deep, although it is unusual for them to perforate. Mooren ulcers cause severe pain and photophobia. The cause is unknown, but is probably some kind of abnormal autoimmune reaction in which the body destroys its own corneal collagen tissue. There may be a local 'trigger' such as an infection or trauma, which starts the process. Mooren ulcers are fairly uncommon, but they are much more frequent in the tropics, and are particularly common and severe in young males from Africa and the Indian subcontinent. They are often very difficult to treat and can progress to destroy the entire cornea. Topical steroids are the first line of treatment, but the response can be very poor and slow. Therefore accurate and frequent assessment and drawing of the ulcer is important (Figure 9.7). Systemic immunosuppression is required in severe cases.

Surgical treatment of peripheral inflammatory ulcers

Wide excision: Several reports have suggested that excision of the conjunctiva around the ulcer is beneficial. The technique is to excise about 5 mm of conjunctiva and Tenon layer around the ulcer to leave bare sclera. The theory behind this is that the antibodies provoking the inflammatory response are brought to the cornea by the limbal conjunctival vessels. This may be a helpful technique if powerful immunosuppressive drugs are unavailable or causing side effects, or not working.

Treatment of perforation: If an ulcer perforates, and there is an aqueous leak, the eye is at great risk of destruction as although the ulcer was initially inflammatory, bacteria can enter the eye and cause endophthalmitis. Every possible attempt must be made to urgently seal the opening. Some possible techniques are:

- A conjunctival flap can be used to cover the hole (see above).
- Cyanoacrylate glue will stick to tissues and cover a small hole until the tissues heal. The glue must be applied to a dry surface, and works better if a soft contact lens is then placed over the cornea.
- Amniotic membrane if available is very effective at sealing these holes and restoring the surface epithelium of the cornea.
- Corneal grafting if available.

At the same time medical treatment should be continued.

Other causes of corneal ulcers

Exposure corneal ulcers

The health of the cornea depends on having normal eyelid closure and a healthy tear film. If tears and frequent blinking do not adequately cover the cornea, corneal ulcers develop from the exposure and drying. Conditions that should be considered in cases of exposure ulcer include:

- Facial palsies and other causes of lagophthalmos.
- Proptosis, e.g. from thyroid eye disease and orbital masses.
- Severe dry eye, e.g. Sjögren syndrome and thyroid eye disease.
- Prolonged unconsciousness, e.g. in intensive care.

Exposure corneal ulcers are often located centrally in the lower third of the cornea as this is the most exposed part of the cornea (**Figure 9.17a–c**). These

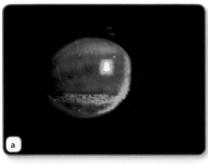
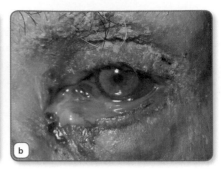
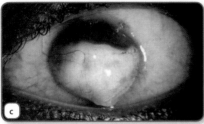

Figure 9.17 Corneal exposure. These pictures show a sequence of events but are from different patients. (a) Corneal exposure causing superficial punctate keratopathy in the exposed inferior cornea. (b) The prolonged exposure allows the cornea to become infected and an ulcer to form. There is extensive purulent discharge which is stained with fluorescein dye. (c) The infection clears but the exposure and infection cause a dense corneal scar to form. Note the fatty deposits in the cornea and the flat top to the scar from the line of the upper eyelid. The upper part of the cornea protected by the eyelid has remained clear.

ulcers often become complicated by secondary bacterial infection. It is very important to try to restore adequate eyelid cover for the cornea, and to keep the cornea well lubricated with tear substitutes. This is particularly important in unconscious patients, when it is essential to check that the eyelids are shut, and to use a viscous lubricant gel.

Neuroparalytic keratitis

Neuroparalytic keratitis is similar to exposure corneal ulceration, and it occurs when the cornea loses its sensation and therefore its protective reflexes. Neuroparalytic keratitis is common in leprosy and herpetic keratitis, which disable the corneal sensory nerves.

Vitamin A deficiency and measles

Vitamin A deficiency and measles are very important causes of severe corneal ulceration in young children (see Chapter 10).

Vernal eye disease

Vernal eye disease may cause corneal ulceration in children and adolescents (see page 152 and **Figure 7.15–7.18**).

Superficial punctate keratitis

Superficial punctate keratitis (SPK) is the general name for localised punctate lesions (small spots) on the epithelial surface of the cornea. These can be caused by many different ocular conditions. The eyes feel gritty, uncomfortable and light sensitive, and there may be a reflex increase in tear production. There is usually some slight blurring of the vision. The individual lesions are not usually visible to the naked eye. However, with fluorescein

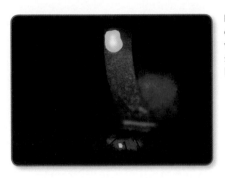

Figure 9.18 Superficial punctate keratitis. The cornea looked normal until fluorescein drops were instilled. With blue light, the fluorescein stain is obvious and the punctate pattern can be seen.

stain, a faint green haze appears on the surface of the cornea (**Figure 9.18**) and if a slit lamp is used, the multiple individual epithelial lesions can be seen. The distribution and character of the lesions should be noted and also the conjunctiva carefully examined. This often helps to determine the specific cause. There are many different causes of superficial punctate keratitis, but the following is a list of the more common causes:

- *Dry eye* (keratoconjunctivitis sicca) is caused by diminished tear production and is quite common in old people. It is described in more detail in Chapter 7.
- *Exposure.* If for any reason such as proptosis or a facial palsy the cornea becomes exposed, then punctate keratitis will often develop (see above).
- *Adenovirus infection* (epidemic keratoconjunctivitis, see Chapter 7 Figure 7.12). Adenovirus is extremely common. It usually clears quickly. However, in some patients (or perhaps with some strains of adenovirus) it causes SPK. The lesions are in the epithelial and subepithelial layers, and are usually all over the cornea. Characteristic changes also occur in the conjunctiva. They can persist for weeks or months after the initial infection, but resolve quickly with a weak topical steroid such as fluorometholone.
- *Trachoma* (see Chapter 8). The lesions are mainly in the subepithelial layers and are near the upper limbus. There are also characteristic conjunctival changes.
- *Vernal conjunctivitis* (see Chapter 7). The lesions are superficial and are especially noticeable near the limbus. Again, there are characteristic conjunctival changes.
- *Onchocerciasis* (see Chapter 16). The lesions are mainly beneath the epithelium, and all over the cornea.
- Leprosy (see Chapter 17). Punctate keratitis may rarely occur in lepromatous leprosy. There will usually be other signs of leprosy in the skin.

Degenerative corneal disease

Ageing and sunlight associated corneal degeneration

Degenerative changes are also quite common. Some of these are ageing changes like *arcus senilis* (**Figure 19.19**) while others are caused by excess exposure to sunlight like *pterygium* and *solar keratopathy* (**Figure 9.20**).

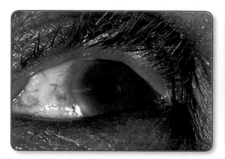 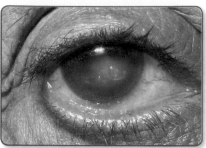

Figure 9.19 Arcus senilis. A white ring is present in the peripheral cornea.

Figure 9.20 Solar keratopathy. The yellow vesicles are localised to the exposed part of the cornea.

Arcus senilis appears as a white ring just inside the limbus. It is very common in old people but does not affect the vision.

Solar keratopathy

Excessive exposure to ultra-violet sunlight sometimes causes changes in the cornea called 'solar keratopathy' or 'climatic droplet keratopathy' (**Figure 9.20**). This condition occurs as a horizontal band in the most exposed part of the cornea just below the centre. In the early stages, there are fine subepithelial droplets and a fine 'frosting' at the level of Bowman membrane, but there is no significant visual loss. In the advanced stages, however, yellow nodules and cysts are visible to the naked eye, and the vision may deteriorate. Solar keratopathy is especially common in people who live by the sea in desert climates, probably because of UV light reflecting off the water. In severe cases the superficial layers of the cornea affected by solar keratopathy can be removed by excising the superficial part of the cornea. This is not always easy and the patient may not end up with a completely smooth clear corneal surface, but in bad cases it should produce a significant improvement in the vision. In very well resourced eye clinics this excision can be performed with a laser.

Corneal dystrophies

Corneal dystrophies are degenerative diseases of the cornea, and are nearly always bilateral. Some of these dystrophies are essentially premature ageing changes and others hereditary, and therefore can start affecting the vision in a young person. Fortunately, the corneal dystrophies that seriously affect the vision are not common. We will discuss the two most common: keratoconus and Fuchs endothelial dystrophy.

Keratoconus

Keratoconus is the most common corneal dystrophy and is a condition in which the cornea gradually becomes more cone-shaped and thin at the centre (**Figure 9.21**). It is usually bilateral (although often asymmetrical) and typically first starts causing symptoms between 15–25 years of age. Initially the patient may develop myopia and astigmatism, which may be corrected with glasses but as the disease progresses glasses are not effective at correcting the vision.

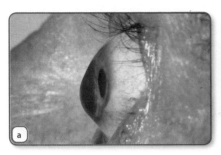 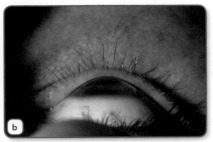

Figure 9.21 Keratoconus. (a) The cornea has deformed and become more 'pointed' or 'cone-shaped'. (b) This can be seen very clearly when the patient looks down and the conical shape of the cornea distorts lower eyelid.

Keratoconus frequently occurs in otherwise entirely healthy individuals, but is more common in association with atopic diseases like asthma and eczema, and especially in patients with vernal conjunctivitis and in patients with Down's syndrome. It is possible that eye rubbing contributes to the disease progression. There is also a racial predisposition, with keratoconus being more common in people from the Middle East and the Indian subcontinent. In the early stages, keratoconus is easy to diagnose with a slit lamp or a retinoscope ('scissors' reflex), or distortion of the red reflex with a direct ophthalmoscope, but without these tools, it is often missed. As the disease progresses, the cone becomes more obvious and when the patient looks down, the cone of the cornea can be seen distorting the lower eyelid (Munson sign, Figure 9.21b). Sometimes there is a sudden split in the corneal endothelium and Descemet's membrane so that the aqueous fluid rapidly enters the corneal stroma. The cornea will then become oedematous and opaque with sudden further deterioration of vision. This is called 'hydrops' (**Figure 9.22**). In a few weeks the hydrops usually resolves as the endothelium heals again and the corneal oedema disappears. Some people treat acute hydrops with injections of sterile air in the anterior chamber; this speeds up the recovery, but carries a small risk of introducing infection into the eye and it is not clear that the long term outcomes are significantly different to conservative management.

Many cases of keratoconus can be treated with hard contact lenses but these require expertise in fitting and can be difficult for the patient to manage. Advanced cases of keratoconus are treated with a corneal graft. In recent years there have been promising results with a treatment called crosslinking, in which the cornea is infused with a light sensitive dye (riboflavin) and an ultraviolet light directed over the cornea. This is thought to stiffen, or age the fibres in the cornea, which appears to slow down or even stop the progression of the disease. However, this treatment requires expensive equipment and training.

Fuchs endothelial dystrophy (Figure 9.23)
Fuchs endothelial dystrophy is the premature degeneration of the corneal endothelial cells. They become less able to maintain the correct corneal hydration and the cornea becomes oedematous, causing significant loss of vision (see below).

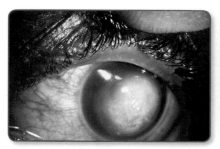

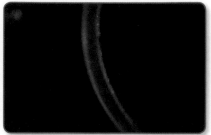

Figure 9.22 Acute hydrops in keratoconus. There is a sudden loss of vision as the cornea suddenly swells and becomes opaque.

Figure 9.23 Fuchs endothelial dystrophy. The endothelial layer of the cornea (the right side of the cornea as you look at) is irregular and has some pigmentation in it.

Corneal oedema

In a normal cornea, the endothelial cells transfer fluid out of the stroma into the anterior chamber, and so keep the cornea dehydrated. If the endothelial cells cannot function properly for any reason, the cornea thickens and becomes oedematous. Special instruments are necessary to detect this increased thickness, but the oedema gives the cornea a hazy appearance, which is visible to the naked eye. The earliest symptoms of corneal oedema are blurred vision, and seeing coloured rings (or haloes) around white lights. Small drops of fluid in the oedematous cornea split white light into the colours of the spectrum, and so a rainbow halo is seen. If the corneal epithelium is also oedematous, superficial blisters will develop in the epithelium. These blisters are usually very painful.

The three major causes of corneal oedema are:
- *Stromal keratitis*. The inflammation of the cornea also causes corneal oedema (Figure 9.3).
- *Corneal endothelial cell damage*. This is usually secondary to either a disease process (e.g. Fuchs endothelial dystrophy, see above) or from cataract surgery (see Figure 12.26) damaging the endothelial cells
- *Very raised intraocular pressure*. The high pressure prevents the corneal endothelial cells from transferring fluid from the cornea into the anterior chamber (see Figure 15.19). Corneal oedema is only a symptom and can occur in many diseases. Treatment will depend on the diagnosis you make. It can be a sign of angle closure glaucoma. It is therefore very important to check the intraocular pressure of any patient with corneal oedema.

Pterygium

A pterygium (from the Greek for 'wing') consists of hypertrophic conjunctival epithelium (**Figures. 9.24** and **9.25**). It grows from the limbus towards the centre of the cornea in the shape of a wedge. A pterygium only occurs in the exposed part of the cornea between the eyelids. It usually develops on the nasal side at the 3 o'clock position but occasionally temporally at the 9

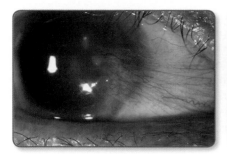

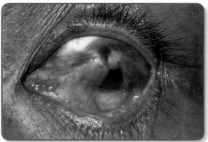

Figure 9.24 This pterygium has just started to grow onto the cornea. It may not advance any further or it may take many years before it affects the vision. This pterygium is inflamed. This can occur occasionally causing some discomfort and can be treated with mild steroid drops or will settle without intervention in time.

Figure 9.25 Blinding pterygium. There is medial and lateral pterygium that has grown right across the pupil and has blinded the patient.

o'clock position. The main part of the pterygium (nearer the limbus) is more vascular than the surrounding conjunctiva, and has blood vessels, which run radially towards the tip of the pterygium. At the tip of the pterygium there is degeneration and opacification of the superficial cornea. The whole of the pterygium is raised above the corneal surface.

Excessive exposure to ultraviolet sunlight is the main stimulus for the growth of a pterygium. Other, but probably less important factors include dry, hot and dusty conditions. Therefore, pterygia are particularly common in people who live in sunny areas and spend a lot of their time outdoors. Pterygia usually grow slowly and steadily over many years. However, they are normally more active, vascular and fleshy in young people, and become thin and atrophic in old people.

Symptoms of a pterygium

Patients present with several different symptoms:
1. *Cosmetic.* Many patients complain of the change in appearance of their eye.
2. *Inflammation.* Pterygia are prone to recurrent episodes of mild inflammation, possibly because they are vascular and raised above the corneal surface. The patient may complain of irritation to the eye, and dilated blood vessels may be visible on the pterygium. Attacks of intermittent inflammation may be treated with short courses of topical steroids.
3. *Loss of vision.* A large pterygium may reach the pupil, and partially blur or obstruct the vision, and a very large pterygium may completely cover the pupil (**Figure 9.25**). In these cases surgery is the only treatment.

Treatment of pterygium

The only accepted successful treatment for pterygia is surgical excision. However, unless the pterygium is in danger of obscuring the vision, conservative management (no treatment, just observe) is a better choice, as there is a high risk of recurrence particularly in younger patients living in hot climates who have 'active' fleshy pterygia. The principle of surgery is to excise the conjunctival portion of the pterygium and to gently try to 'peel away' the corneal portion, doing as little damage as possible to the underlying cornea. The risk of recurrence is much lower if an autograft of healthy conjunctiva is taken from elsewhere on the patient's eye, usually the superior bulbar conjunctiva. Post operatively frequent topical steroids should be used in order to suppress inflammation. Topical cytotoxic drugs (e.g. mitomycin) have been tried as a way of reducing the recurrence, but the results have been mixed, and they are not generally used except for challenging recurrences.

It is possible that sunglasses may give the cornea some protection against ultraviolet light, and so reduce the incidence of pterygium.

Band keratopathy

Band keratopathy (or band corneal degeneration) is a fine layer of calcium salts, which are laid down at the level of Bowman membrane in the exposed part of the cornea (**Figure 9.26**). It sometimes occurs after chronic uveitis, or several surgical procedures in an eye, but may develop for no obvious cause. Band keratopathy can be treated fairly easily. First the corneal epithelium should be removed under local anaesthetic drops. The calcific deposit can then be removed by gently scraping the corneal surface whilst applying drops of a chelating agent such as sodium versenate, which dissolves calcium.

Corneal scars

The epithelium is the only part of the cornea, which can regenerate easily. Therefore, damage to just the epithelium will heal without scarring. Any deeper damage or inflammation of the corneal stroma is likely to leave a scar (**Figure. 9.8**). In areas where there is a high incidence of corneal diseases, such scars are very common. A corneal scar has two basic clinical features: vascularisation and opacification. Corneal scars are caused by all the conditions discussed above which affect the deeper layers of the cornea but three of the major tropical eye disease – trachoma, xerophthalmia and

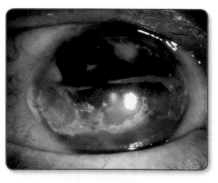

Figure 9.26 Band keratopathy.

onchocerciasis – must be considered when one sees corneal scarring. The pattern of corneal scars varies with each of these diseases and is discussed more in the relevant chapters.

Vascularisation

Vascularisation is the growth of blood vessels into the cornea, as a response to inflammation (**Figure 9.27**). When the inflammation subsides, the vessels slowly regress and eventually empty altogether. It is sometimes still possible to see these 'ghost vessels' with a slit lamp. However, obvious vascularisation of the cornea may indicate that the original inflammatory process is still active.

Opacification

Opacification occurs because the collagen fibres are arranged irregularly in the scar, and are therefore opaque. In the normal healthy cornea the collagen fibres are all arranged in a regular pattern, which makes them transparent. Scars may very gradually fade slightly over many years, but they generally leave some degree of permanent opacity. Lipid, calcium or amyloid deposits may occasionally develop in some scars. A nebula (which means cloud) is a name for a faint, corneal scar and a leucoma (which means white spot) is a name for a denser, localised scar.

The treatment of corneal scars

The aim of treatment is firstly to improve the vision and secondly to improve the cosmetic appearance of the patient. However, it is important to assess several factors before deciding what treatment, if any, to give.

- Is the original disease active? For example, if trachoma is still causing tarsal conjunctival inflammation, or if there is irritation to the cornea from trichiasis, these conditions must be treated first. When the inflammation and vascularisation in the cornea subside, the opacity may gradually become less dense.
- Where is the scar and how large, dense and vascular is it? The scar may cover the pupil totally, partly or not at all. The iris may adhere to the back of the cornea, and so distort the pupil.
- At what age did the scarring occur? Corneal scarring occurring before the age of about five is likely to make the eye amblyopic (see page 438)

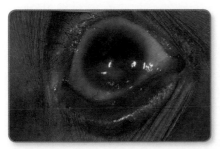

Figure 9.27 Corneal vascularisation. This patient has a corneal ulcer that is becoming scarred. Superficial vessels are growing into the ulcerated, scarred area of the cornea. This ulcer looks actively inflamed, as the eye is red and the opacity has a hazy, poorly defined margin.

and the visual potential much poorer. The earlier the scarring occurred, the denser the amblyopia will be. If the damaged eye also has a squint or there is nystagmus, and if the other eye has normal vision it is even more likely that the damaged eye will be amblyopic.

- How healthy is the rest of the eye? If there has been significant pathology inside the eye, such as intraocular infection, the visual potential is likely to be very poor.

There are several possible ways to improve the vision of patients with corneal scars:

1. Spectacles

If the scar does not totally cover the pupil, spectacles may help. The scar may distort the cornea to produce a high degree of astigmatism and this astigmatism can sometimes be corrected with spectacles.

2. Mydriatic drops

These may improve the vision by dilating the pupil and allowing the patient to see round the corneal scar.

3. Optical iridectomy

This can be a very effective and permanent method of enabling the patient to see round the corneal scar (**Figure 9.28**). The iridectomy alters the position of the pupil aperture so that it is in line with the clear cornea. In an abnormal eye, an iridectomy is usually a fairly straightforward operation, as the iris easily prolapses through a limbal incision. However, the iris of a diseased eye may stick both to the lens and to the back of the cornea, making the operation much more challenging and with greater potential to cause further intraocular damage. After a successful optical iridectomy, patients usually have considerable astigmatism because they are not looking through the centre of the cornea.

4. Corneal grafting

Corneal grafting (keratoplasty) is the removal of the central part of the cornea (usually about 7 mm in diameter) and replacing this with a donor cornea, which normally comes from someone who has recently died (**Figures 9.29** and **9.30**). Grafting can markedly improve vision, but also has a significant risk of complications. The major complications are infection, rejection and recurrence of the original disease process, all of which may significantly

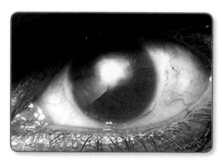

Figure 9.28 Optical iridectomy. This patient has a central corneal scar, but the surgical iridectomy has created a new 'pupil' that he can see through to a certain extent.

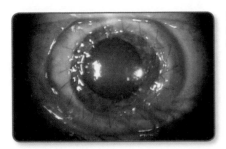

Figure 9.29 A corneal transplant. The sutures are only removed at least a year after the surgery.

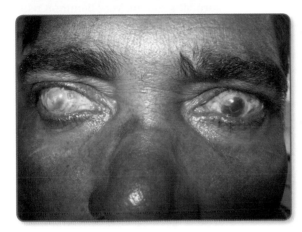

Figure 9.30 A successful corneal graft. This patient was blind with right optic atrophy and left bullous keratopathy. A corneal transplant was performed by taking the healthy right corneal and transplanting it in the left eye. The unhealthy left cornea was replaced in the right eye.

worsen the visual outcome. It is a major surgical procedure and requires corneal banking (storage) facilities, great surgical expertise, and long-term post-operative topical treatment and follow-up.

Nowadays corneas can be stored for up to a month in tissue culture medium. However, this requires a well-run, well-equipped 'cornea bank' with experts managing it. This is not available in most areas of poor countries. Where corneal graft material is very hard to obtain, it may be possible to rotate some healthy clear cornea into the pupillary area to improve the vision of a patient with a large corneal scar. This is called a rotation autograft. However, it is much easier and almost equally effective to do an optical iridectomy. Rarely, a patient may be blind in the other eye but still have a healthy cornea. It is possible to graft corneal tissue from one eye to the other, but this of course creates significant risk to the healthy eye (**Figure 9.30**).

Corneal grafting can be the whole thickness of the cornea (penetrating keratoplasty) or partial thickness. Dense deep scars would require the whole thickness to be transplanted. However, for more anterior scars a partial thickness graft has significant benefits. In this type of graft, which is called deep lamellar keratoplasty, the anterior layers are removed and replaced, and the deeper layers (Descemet's membrane and endothelium) remain. This reduces the risk of intraocular infection and rejection. If the primary problem is of the endothelium, e.g. Fuchs endothelial dystrophy (see above), it is now possible to do an endothelial cell layer graft (endothelial keratoplasty).

Many people who are blind from corneal disease could see again if they received a corneal graft. Unfortunately, the medical services in most poor countries are not sophisticated enough to give these people the treatment they need. In these places only about 1% of patients who might benefit from a corneal graft ever receive one, and many are not successful. However, most of this corneal blindness is preventable before the stage of ever needing a graft. Efforts to prevent corneal scarring in the whole community are much more cost effective and worthwhile than the very expensive treatment of a few individuals.

Unfortunately, those places where corneal scars are very common usually have very little specialist eye care. These are also often the areas where people are usually least willing to donate eyes for grafting after death. Furthermore, the patients who most need corneal grafts because they have very dense corneal scars are the ones most likely to develop graft rejection or graft failure. Severely scarred corneas usually also have extensive vascularisation. Blood vessels from the patient's cornea will therefore invade the graft, and allow an immune response to be mounted. Other patients who would not benefit from a corneal graft are those with extensive conjunctival disease or a significant eyelid abnormality because normal healthy eyelids, conjunctiva and tear film are essential for a corneal graft to stay clear. The only option for these patients is a keratoprosthesis (see below) or limbal transplants, which are both highly specialised procedures that are only available in a few places in the world.

5. Keratoprosthesis (Figure 9.31)

Keratoprosthesis is the placement of a small, clear plastic disc or cylinder into the centre of the patient's scarred natural cornea. It can restore sight, but also carries high risks of serious complications and requires intensive and expert follow-up. This advanced, high technology surgery shows what modern science is able to do, but is very rarely carried out.

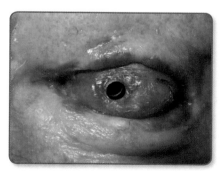

Figure 9.31 A successful keratoprosthesis. This totally blind patient from advanced corneal disease was able to see extremely well for 10 years with this prosthesis inserted in the left eye.

Cosmetic treatment of corneal scars

The cosmetic appearance of an eye with a corneal scar may be improved by tattooing the cornea (**Figure 9.32**). The method is to shave off the superficial cornea and then scratch pigment into the corneal stroma. The pigment should be of the same colour as the iris or pupil. Tattooing the cornea is only recommended when the vision is very poor in the damaged eye, and the other eye is normal. Corneal grafting will also improve the cosmetic appearance of the eye. However, in most poor countries, corneal graft material is much too precious to be used for cosmetic reasons alone. If a corneal scar is so large that the eye has no vision, and if it is ugly or painful, then it is better to eviscerate (remove) the eye and replace it with an artificial eye (**Figure 9.33**).

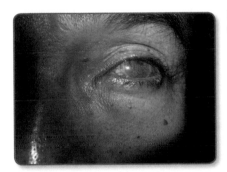

Figure 9.32 Corneal tattooing to hide a corneal scar.

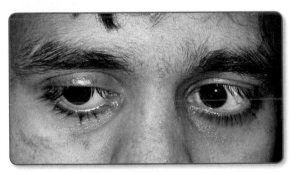

Figure 9.33 A prosthetic right eye. This was a cheap prosthesis that is available and affordable in poor countries. It was not custom-made to match the other eye, but still looks very good. As the patient looks to the right, the prosthetic eye moves in this direction.

10 Xerophthalmia and nutritional corneal ulceration

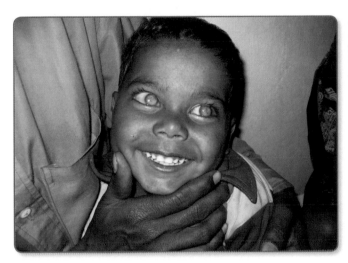

A young child who has recovered from xerophthalmia. But what sort of a future does he have?

Visual loss from vitamin A deficiency affects young children only. It is completely preventable. Every child with xerophthalmia and nutritional corneal ulceration therefore means that the parents have been unable to feed their child properly. The local community has failed to help one of its poorest and weakest members. Doctors and politicians have failed to give basic health care where the need is greatest.

Even in areas of known poverty and malnutrition, it is common for senior doctors and specialists to never see children with xerophthalmia and sometimes not even be aware that there is a problem, although the disease may be quite common. The families of these children are certainly too poor to go to private clinics and often too poor or live too far even to go to public hospitals. These families are mostly found in isolated rural villages or inner city slums.

For more than 50 years we have known basically why malnourished children go blind from vitamin A deficiency associated corneal ulcers. Every year new research brings more knowledge on subjects such as the prevalence of vitamin A deficiency, and the best ways of preventing and treating it. Furthermore, we know that both prevention and treatment is cheap and very effective and even reduces childhood death rates. However, vitamin A deficiency and its devastating complications are still very common.

The WHO estimates that approximately 190 million preschool age children and 19 million pregnant women have low vitamin A levels. Of these, over 5 million preschool children and nearly 10 million pregnant women have vitamin A deficiency night blindness. Most of these people are in Africa (**Figure 10.1**). Every year between a quarter and half a million children are blinded by xerophthalmia. The majority of these children die before long, although some do survive to make xerophthalmia by far the commonest cause of childhood blindness in the world. Only about a quarter of these children recover with reasonable eyesight.

However, this is a disease of poor people in which great progress has been made. It has become a much higher priority disease in the WHO and in health programmes. Vitamin A supplements, food fortification and education are occurring much more widely. In spite of this many countries still have huge numbers of vitamin A deficient children, and it remains a major cause of visual loss and death.

Terminology

The medical words used to describe vitamin A deficiency associated eye disease are confusing. The eye disease is often called *xerophthalmia*. This simply means 'dry eyes' in Greek. However, xerophthalmia has now come to mean eye disease from vitamin A deficiency. Dry eyes, is in fact just one small part of this blinding disease. There are also changes in the cornea and conjunctiva that cause them to resist wetting and then corneal ulcers start to develop, which ultimately can be blinding. These children live in poverty, and there are several other factors that contribute to the risk of

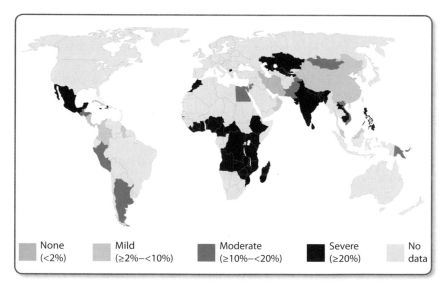

| None (<2%) | Mild (≥2%–<10%) | Moderate (≥10%–<20%) | Severe (≥20%) | No data |

Figure 10.1 Vitamin A deficiency around the world. There are countries, such as Somalia and Indonesia, that have many children with vitamin A deficiency, but as there is no data for these countries they are not marked on this map.

corneal ulceration (**Figure 10.2**). But, remember that there are numerous other causes of corneal ulcers (see Chapter 9) in young children, which are not related to malnutrition and require completely different treatment. However vitamin A deficiency is the most important cause and must not be missed.

In xerophthalmia, perhaps more than any other eye disease, one must take a step back and look at the health of the whole patient, and of the whole community. Vitamin A deficiency is a severe systemic disease that causes ill health and even death. It causes:

- Poor physical and mental growth and development.
- Multiple systemic problems including of the eyes, skin, nails and bones.
- Increased risk of contracting other diseases or allowing other diseases to have much more severe consequences.

Vitamin A deficiency is also an indicator that these patients are likely to have other significant health problems associated with severe poverty:

- Generalised malnutrition. These children are very likely to have very poor diets and in particular they may also have protein energy malnutrition (PEM).
- Poor sanitation and hygiene, and vitamin A deficiency are both independent causes of gastrointestinal disease.
- Missing vaccinations. These children are unlikely to have received a measles vaccination. Children with vitamin A deficiency are much more at risk of the severe blinding complications of measles.
- Poor education. Parents of these children are less likely to recognise the signs of vitamin A deficiency and will be less able to seek help. The disease is therefore often seen much too late by health professionals. For example, they might not be able to get antibiotics for the corneal ulcers.

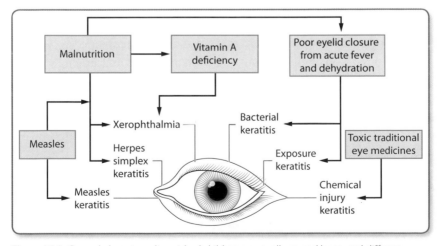

Figure 10.2 Corneal ulcers in malnourished children are usually caused by several different factors working together to damage the cornea. This diagram highlights some of the more important causes and how they combine together to damage the cornea.

- Traditional eye medications (see page 244). The lack of access to government clinics (or the poor quality of government clinics) means these patients are much more likely to use traditional eye medications. Some of these medications are very toxic, particularly in vitamin A deficient patients, who have much weaker defences.

The interactions of factors associated with poverty that cause xerophthalmia are very complex, but the remedy is simple. A proper diet of cheap, nutritional foods, which even the poorest families could buy, would greatly reduce the incidence. Failing this, supplementation with vitamin A is effective. A basic child welfare scheme with immunisation against measles would probably eradicate childhood corneal blindness. Programmes to eradicate vitamin A deficiency have a very high priority in WHO and in the 'VISION 2020 The Right to Sight' programme, for two good reasons:

1. Vitamin A deficiency causes extreme personal suffering and economic loss all over the world.
2. Vitamin A deficiency is completely preventable.

The epidemiology of xerophthalmia

Xerophthalmia is very closely associated with poverty. The reasons for this are:
- Poor people generally eat vegetable foods because they are cheap. However, the best sources of dietary vitamin A (e.g. liver, butter, cheese, kidney, eggs and milk) are all expensive animal foods.
- Vitamin A compounds are fat soluble, but poor people usually eat very little fat therefore the small amount of vitamin A they do eat, is absorbed less well.
- Some vegetable foods are excellent sources of vitamin A in the form of carotene (**Figure 10.3**). However, most starchy white foods, which are the staple diet of many poor communities, contain very little vitamin A (**Figure 10.4**). For example, there is a high incidence of xerophthalmia in areas of South India, Bangladesh and Indonesia, where rice is the staple food. Conversely in some poor areas the staple food is rich in vitamin A, e.g.red palm oil on the West African coast and cow's milk among some nomadic tribes. In these areas, vitamin A deficiency is very uncommon.

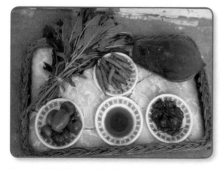

Figure 10.3 Vegetable foods rich in vitamin A include red palm oil, carrots, spinach, papayas and tomatoes.

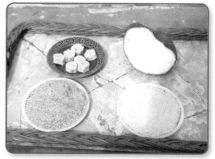

Figure 10.4 Rice and other (pale coloured) vegetable foods like plantain, cassava and yam are the staple diet in many communities; they are very low in vitamin A.

One useful guide to finding out if vitamin A deficiency is a problem in any particular community is to ask if the local language has special words for night blindness or for a Bitot spot. The existence of these words indicates that the community is traditionally prone to vitamin A deficiency.

Vitamin A deficiency sometimes occurs even when foods rich in vitamin A are cheap and easily available. There may be taboos, religious customs or cultural reasons why children do not eat these foods, or the child may simply not like the taste of them. In some communities, it is customary to wean small children with starchy cereals and root crops. In some cultures the father is given the best food or eats first before the children. This is particularly ironic and sad because the father does not need the vitamin A but the child does.

In some areas, xerophthalmia is especially common at certain times of the year. These are the times when fruits and green vegetables rich in vitamin A are not available, or when there are seasonal epidemics of acute infection.

Young children between 6 months and 3 years are the ones most at risk from acute xerophthalmia in its blinding and life-threatening forms. Young children often have evidence of protein malnutrition and they are particularly susceptible to acute illnesses, especially measles, which exacerbate the disease. They are much more likely to develop severe corneal ulcers. From the age of about four, children may have mild conjunctival changes and night blindness, but are less likely to develop ulcers or life-threatening illnesses.

Breast-feeding generally protects against xerophthalmia as breast milk should contain maternal vitamin A. However, in communities where xerophthalmia is common, the mother's diet may be so poor in vitamin A, that her milk is deficient in it. Therefore, the weaning child cannot build up adequate stores of vitamin A in the liver. Mothers should be encouraged to continue breast-feeding for longer in poor communities in order to continue giving the child vitamin A (and for the many other health benefits to the child of breast milk). Although most countries now insist that formula milk contains vitamin A, these 'milks' are expensive. Poor families may replace the breast milk with simple dried skimmed milk or sweetened condensed milk (which might contain little or no vitamin A), or even just water.

Poor people who live in city slums are sometimes at even more risk than people living in villages. They are less likely to eat fresh vegetables and milk products, and more likely to wean their children earlier. In theory they should be more accessible to government health programmes, although such programmes are often very unsuccessful in slums.

Vitamin A deficiency has sometimes been described as being like an iceberg (see **Figure 10.5**). The corneal ulcers and scarring is the tip of the iceberg which is easy to see. The burden of malnutrition and deprivation is much less obvious just like most of an iceberg which is invisible under this sea.

The biochemistry and physiology of vitamin A

Vitamin A is what is called an 'essential micronutrient'. This means it cannot be made by our bodies and must come from our diet. **Figure 10.6** shows the metabolism of vitamin A and how it passes from food to the

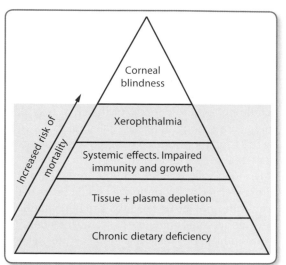

Figure 10.5 The iceberg of vitamin A deficiency. The corneal ulcers are the visible tip of the iceberg, but the malnutrition and its severe damaging effects are hidden beneath.

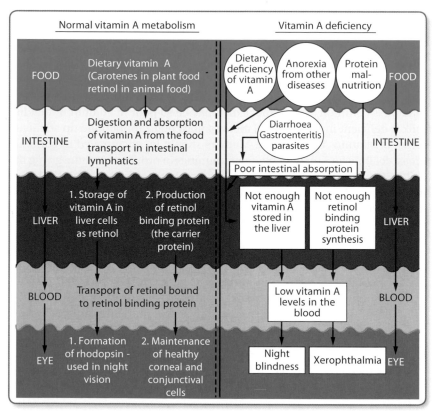

Figure 10.6 An outline of vitamin A metabolism and vitamin A deficiency. The left side of the diagram shows normal vitamin A metabolism in a healthy person and how it passes from food (green) to the intestine (yellow), the liver (brown), the blood (pink) and finally, to the eye (blue). The right side of the diagram shows the main causes of vitamin A deficiency (circles) and their effects (rectangles).

eye, and the factors that cause vitamin A deficiency. This is a rather complicated diagram, but the basic principle of how we get vitamin A is that we eat foods with vitamin A in them and it goes from our intestine to our liver where it is stored. It then leaves the liver, bound to a protein, and goes to the bodily tissues that require it. Almost all tissues require vitamin A for normal functioning.

The earliest records of the clinical appearance of xerophthalmia and resulting corneal ulceration are in ancient Egyptian and Chinese texts. However, the cause of the disease remained unclear until relatively recently. An experiment 100 years ago showed that animals develop a condition similar to xerophthalmia if they are fed a diet deficient in fat. Then, in 1921, xerophthalmia was diagnosed in children in an orphanage in Denmark whose diets were deficient in milk. During the last 50 years, our knowledge of the biochemistry and physiology of vitamin A has greatly increased. The chemical name for vitamin A is retinol. It is a fat-soluble unsaturated alcohol and is an essential vitamin for most animals.

Dictary sources of retinol

Dietary retinol comes from two groups of foods: plant foods and animal foods. Plant foods are particularly important because they are the staple diet for poor people; most poor people rarely eat meat. **Table 10.1** lists the concentration of vitamin A in some of these foods.

Animal foods contain the active vitamin retinol, but some foods are much richer in retinol than others. The liver (including fish liver), which stores retinol, is the best source. Milk products are also very rich in retinol. Meat (animal muscle) is a less good source of retinol.

Table 10.1 The concentration of vitamin A in different foods

Animal Foods	Retinol (IU per 100 g or 100 mL)	Plant foods	Carotene (IU per 100 g or 100 mL)
Fish liver oil	100, 000	Red palm oil	50,000–100,000
Animal liver	10,000	Carrots	10,000
Butter	3000	Spinach	10,000
Cheese	1500	Sweet potatoes	5000
Kidney	1000	Apricots, mangoes	2000
Eggs	1000	Tomatoes	1000
Fish	200	Green beans	1000
Fresh milk	150	Yellow maize	350
Meat (mutton, beef, etc.)	20	Wheat	Slight
Lard	Negligible	Rice Potatoes White maize Cassava	Negligible

Adapted from Moore, T. Vitamin A. Elsevier; Amsterdam, 1957.

Plant foods contain carotene pigment, which is chemically related to retinol. There are many different carotene pigments. They are converted into retinol in the wall of the intestine, but some are converted more effectively than others. Carotene is the pigment that gives the highest yield of retinol. Although beta-carotene by weight is half as active as retinol, it is in fact only one sixth as active because it is not so well absorbed and not all of it is converted into retinol.

On a walk round a village market in the tropics one will find vegetable foods that are both rich and poor in vitamin A. The best source of vitamin A is red palm oil. Green leafy vegetables (e.g. spinach) and orange coloured fruit and vegetables (e.g. carrots, mangoes, papayas) are also very good sources, although spinach is harder to digest and therefore less vitamin A may be extracted. The vitamin A rich foods are either pigmented or are eaten as leaves (**Figure 10.3**). Many cereals and root crops (e.g. rice, cassava, yams and white maize), which are often the staple diet of poor people, contain little or no vitamin A. Foods with little vitamin A are usually white and starchy (**Figure 10.4**).

The quantity of vitamin A (as retinol or carotene) in foods is still widely measured with the international unit (IU) despite this scale being discouraged.

International units

1 IU is equivalent to 0.3 µg of retinol or 0.6 µg of beta-carotene or 1.2 µg of other carotenes

1 µg (microgram) = 1/1000 000 of a gram

Absorption and storage

Retinol and the carotenes are fat-soluble. During digestion in the intestine, they are broken down (emulsified) and absorbed. Retinol is more effectively emulsified and absorbed than the carotenes. In ideal conditions, about 90% of ingested retinol, and about 70% of ingested carotene is absorbed. However, if the intestine is diseased or has a heavy load of parasites, absorption may be much less (see **Figure 10.6**). Cooking improves the absorption of carotenes, although food must not be overcooked, as this reduces the vitamin A levels. The best way to prepare vegetables to get the maximum absorption of carotenes is to fry them. Frying both breaks up the cells and provides fat in which the carotene dissolves. If plants are eaten raw, or not ground up enough, or not cooked enough, the carotene pigments may not be released from the plant cells. These carotenes may then pass undigested through the alimentary tract. Dietary fat is essential for the absorption of carotenes. However, foods containing fat are often more expensive, which further disadvantages poor families. It is also important that food is stored in the dark as ultraviolet light reduces the vitamin A content. This is further disadvantage to poor families who may not have good food storage facilities.

Carotenes are slowly converted to retinol in the wall of the intestine. All the absorbed retinol is then transported in the intestinal lymphatics to the bloodstream. Most of this retinol is taken up and stored in the liver. The rest of the retinol is either conjugated with glucuronic acid and excreted in the bile, or metabolised and excreted as degradation products in the urine. The liver stores retinol very effectively, and it can maintain adequate serum levels for up to 6 months. This is why vitamin A deficiency can be prevented with only infrequent doses of retinol. **Box 10.1** shows what happens to a single dose of vitamin A.

Transport from the liver to the tissues

For retinol to go from the liver to the tissues where it is used, the following must be present:

1. There must be some retinol stored in the liver.
2. The carrier protein, retinol binding protein (RBP) must be synthesized in the liver, because retinol must be bound to RBP before it can be released into the plasma.

In a healthy individual, retinol and RBP are both present in the liver. However, in vitamin A deficiency, there is not enough retinol stored in the liver and the RBP therefore remains in the liver, and does not enter the circulation. In protein deficiency malnutrition, the opposite is true. There is not enough RBP synthesised in the liver. The retinol therefore remains stored, and does not enter the circulation.

Functions of vitamin A

Vitamin A has several different biochemical functions in the body.

The maintenance of healthy epithelial tissues

This is the most important function of vitamin A, but the biochemical mechanism of this is not clearly understood. Vitamin A deficiency is important for all the epithelial surfaces in the body; the conjunctiva/cornea is of course one of the most important of these surfaces, but these lining tissues are also essential for the function of the intestine, lungs and urinary tract. There are two specific changes noted in epithelial tissues in vitamin A deficiency:

Keratinisation of the epithelium

Keratin is a hard protein present in the skin. In xerophthalmia it develops on the surface of the mucous membranes as well. These then become harder and resist wetting. A skin condition called 'perifollicular hyperkeratosis' is the result of vitamin A deficiency. In this condition, keratin tissue builds up around the hair follicles.

Loss of goblet cells

The goblet cells secrete mucus, which helps to maintain the moistness and health of mucous membranes. This is reduced in xerophthalmia. These changes occur in mucous membranes all over the body and not just the eye, but they are most obvious in the conjunctiva and the cornea.

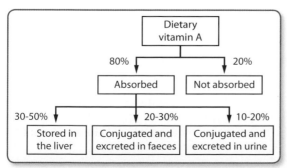

Box 10.1 The fate of a single dose of vitamin A.

Formation of rhodopsin (visual purple)

Vitamin A is needed for the formation of rhodopsin. This pigment is found in the photoreceptor rods in the retina, which are essential for vision in poor light conditions. This is the only function of vitamin A for which the precise biochemistry has been worked out. The aldehyde form of vitamin A is called 'retinal'. Retinal combines with opsin (a protein found in the photosensitive part of the rods) to form rhodopsin. When the retinal molecule is exposed to light, it changes from one chemical form (isomer) to another. Further chemical changes then produce the electrical impulse, which the brain eventually interprets as light. Vitamin A deficiency produces a condition called 'night blindness'. In night blindness, dark adaptation and the ability to see in poor light conditions (evening, early morning and night) are specifically impaired.

Measuring vitamin A levels

There are many ways to measure vitamin A levels and the best method varies depending on the available facilities and on whether one is trying to assess levels in a community or in a specific individual:

1. Dietary analysis: this is an important way to study the community, but it is not a useful way to study an individual patient.
2. Biochemical tests: these give a good indication of vitamin A levels. Spectrophotometry or fluorometry is used to assay vitamin A or retinol, and immunodiffusion is used to assay the serum retinol binding protein (RBP). RBP is easier to measure but retinol levels give a more accurate assessment of vitamin A deficiency. However, both these methods are much too complex for ordinary use and are only used in research.
3. Clinical assessment of the eye: this is the best and easiest way to diagnose vitamin A deficiency in an individual. It is also very valuable in community surveys. However relying on clinical examination alone may occasionally be misleading. For example:
    –   Conjunctival xerosis and Bitot's spot (see below) are relatively common signs, but they do not always progress to blindness and may indicate previous rather than current vitamin A deficiency. On the other hand, active corneal signs are much less frequent, and therefore harder to assess in a survey. However, they are much more likely to indicate a severe risk of blindness.
    –   Xerophthalmia corneal scars give a good indication of the incidence of blindness in a community. However, there may be many different reasons for a corneal scar.

Vitamin A deficiency in young children

Young growing children are at much greater risk of vitamin A deficiency than adults (**Table 10.2**). There are two reasons for this:

1. The vitamin A requirement per unit of body weight is much greater for a child than an adult. The recommended daily intake of vitamin A per kg

Table 10.2 Examples of vitamin A sources and the suggested quantity of each food to reach adequate daily vitamin A

| Age group | Suggested quantity of food-types, one of which to be consumed each day | | | |
	Carrots	Sweet potatoes	Dark green leafy vegetables	Mango
Children:				
6–11 months	1.5 tablespoon	1 tablespoon	1/3 cup	1/2 medium sized
1–2 years	1.5 tablespoon	1 tablespoon	1/2 cup	1/2 medium sized
2–6 years	2 tablespoon	1.5 tablespoon	1/2 cup	2/3 medium sized
Females:				
Non-pregnant	¼ cup	2.5 tablespoon	1 cup	1 medium sized
Pregnant	¼ cup	2.5 tablespoon	1 cup	1 medium sized
Lactating	¼ cup	1/4 cup	1.5 cup	2/3 medium sized

Adapted from Sommer A. Vitamin A deficiency and its consequences, 3rd edition. World Health Organization; Geneva, 1995.

body weight is 65 μg (125 IU) for an infant, but only 12 μg (36 IU) for an adult, i.e. the total requirements for infants is about half that of an adult, despite them being much less than half the weight, and eating much less than half the volume of food.

2. A child cannot store vitamin A in the liver as well as an adult. Clinical complications of vitamin A deficiency are common in children with inadequate vitamin A in their diets, but extremely rare in adults. Even if adults are deprived of vitamin A in experimental conditions, it is many months before any signs of vitamin A deficiency appear.

As well as visual impairment, vitamin A deficiency is also thought to cause 1 million child deaths each year, because of its debilitating effects on young children who become generally weak and unable to resist infection.

The signs and symptoms of vitamin A deficiency in the eye

Classification

Table 10.3 shows the WHO classification system of the signs of vitamin A deficiency in the eye. Everyone who is concerned either with child welfare or eye disease in areas where malnutrition is common should be familiar with these basic signs of xerophthalmia.

Table 10.3 The WHO classification systems of xerophthalmia

Signs of chronic vitamin A deficiency	Signs of acute vitamin A deficiency
Conjunctival xerosis (X1A)	Corneal xerosis (X2)
Bitot's spot (X1B)	Corneal ulceration with less than 1/3rd of cornea affected (X3A)
Night blindness (XN)	
Xerophthalmic scars (XS)	Keratomalacia, i.e. corneal ulcers with more than 1/3rd of cornea affected (X3B)
Xerophthalmia fundus (XF)	

There are two very important points to remember:
1. The signs are not a sequence in which problems develop and may occur at different stages of the disease or after the acute disease has resolved.
2. Many vitamin A deficient children will not have any of the eye signs, but still urgently require vitamin A treatment.

Conjunctival xerosis – XIA

Changes occur on the bulbar conjunctiva, especially the exposed parts. Look for the following features, which may be widespread, or localised to small patches of the conjunctiva (**Figures 10.6–10.8**):

Dryness

This causes the conjunctiva to lose its normal, shiny lustre and instead, look like wax or paint. When the eye moves, it is sometimes possible to see wrinkles and folds in the thickened conjunctiva (**Figure 10.7**). It also becomes 'unwettable', so that the tear film breaks up and leaves dry patches. As the conjunctiva thickens and loses its transparency, the underlying blood vessels are more difficult to see.

Increased pigmentation

This gives the conjunctiva a fine, diffuse, smoky grey-brown appearance, especially near the limbus in the interpalpebral fissure. This pigmentation is common in xerophthalmia, but it is also a feature of vernal conjunctivitis.

Creamy, white debris

This is sometimes found, especially where the upper and lower eyelids meet, the lower fornix, or the lid margins around the openings of the meibomian glands. This debris is a feature of advanced conjunctival xerosis.

All these changes can be difficult to detect in the early stages. For this reason, it is not easy to diagnose vitamin A deficiency on the basis of conjunctival

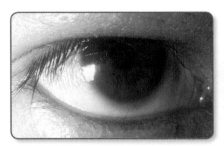

Figure 10.7 Conjunctival xerosis. There is waxiness, wrinkling and dryness of the conjunctiva, but these early changes can be very difficult to detect.

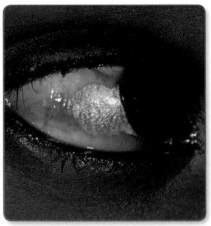

Figure 10.8 Conjunctival xerosis and a Bitot spot. The area around the Bitot spot is pigmented and there is a creamy, foamy deposit on its surface.

xerosis alone. Conjunctival xerosis is fully reversible with vitamin A treatment, which must be given urgently.

Bitot spot – XlB

A Bitot spot is a small, oval or triangular (pointing away from the cornea) plaque of material on the surface of the bulbar conjunctiva. It is nearly always located in the interpalpebral fissure (**Figure 10.8**), usually on the temporal side but occasionally nasal. The material is usually foamy, but may look waxy or greasy, and may contain pigment from eye make-up. If the material is wiped away, it leaves a dry conjunctival bed with a rough surface. There is often increased pigmentation of the conjunctiva around the Bitot spot.

A Bitot spot probably forms because the eyelids do not wipe the abnormal bulbar conjunctiva properly. The conjunctival cells start to become more like skin than mucous membrane (squamous metaplasia). Sometimes a structural defect (e.g. a squint or an eyelid abnormality) causes a different part of the conjunctiva to be more exposed than normal. A Bitot spot is likely to form on this exposed area.

A Bitot spot is a very obvious clinical sign. If it is seen with other conjunctival signs, vitamin A deficiency is very likely. However, Bitot spots do not always indicate vitamin A deficiency and are sometimes seen in older children and adults who appear to be well-nourished. In these cases it is quite likely that the child was vitamin A deficient when younger.

Night blindness – XN

Vitamin A is necessary for the light sensitive rods in the retina to function properly. Vitamin A deficiency therefore causes poor dark adaptation and poor night vision. This is called *nyctalopia*. Night blindness is the most sensitive sign of vitamin A deficiency, and usually appears before any conjunctival or corneal changes. It is possible to detect night blindness either by electroretinography or dark adaptation tests. However, both these methods require sophisticated equipment and a co-operative patient and are therefore not widely available. In practice, it is usually best to question the parents carefully about the child's behaviour in the evening and early morning and to explain to them what night blindness is (**Figure 10.9**). Parents will often tell you that their child can see in the daytime, but seems to be blind when the sun goes down. The child may become much less sociable in the evening and prefer to stay inside or near the fire as this provides some light. In areas where xerophthalmia is common, pregnant women and nursing mothers will sometimes complain of night blindness. A study from Indonesia showed that children with night blindness were three times more likely to die than those without, while children with night blindness and Bitot spots were nine times more likely to die.

There are other diseases that affect the retinal rods, such as retinitis pigmentosa (see page 341). These can also cause night blindness. Therefore, if possible the retina of these children should be examined, particularly if there are no conjunctival signs of vitamin A deficiency and the child appears well nourished.

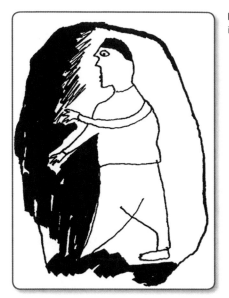

Figure 10.9 This child's drawing shows what it is like to have night blindness.

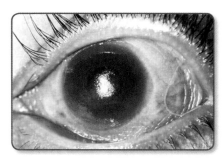

Figure 10.10 Corneal and conjunctival xerosis. The light reflection from the cornea is altered because it is dry. The conjunctiva is also dry, thickened and slightly pigmented. Some frothy tears and a thick string of mucus can also be seen.

Corneal xerosis – X2

Corneal xerosis is an extension of the conjunctival signs onto the cornea (**Figure 10.10**). It is much less common than conjunctival xerosis, but it is a highly specific sign for acute vitamin A deficiency. The surface of the cornea looks rough, dull and irregular. The break up time of the pre-corneal tear film shortens to less than 10 seconds. To measure the break up time:

1. Instil a fluorescein drop into the eye.
2. Wait until the patient blinks.
3. Measure for how many seconds the fine tear film remains intact on the surface of the cornea before it breaks up (measuring the break up time of the tear film is in fact much easier said than done!).

Eyes with corneal xerosis are at great risk of developing serious corneal damage and visual loss from non-infective and infective corneal ulceration. However, one of the remarkable features of xerophthalmia is that the changes up to this stage are rapidly and completely reversible if vitamin A treatment is given without delay. After only 3 or 4 days the conjunctival and corneal xerosis and night blindness can be completely cured. Many Bitot spots will also disappear, although less quickly.

Corneal ulceration – X3A

There are many causes of corneal ulceration (see Chapter 9), but **Table 10.4** identifies features that make xerophthalmia more likely to be the cause (see **Figures. 10.11** and **10.12**):

Corneal ulceration is not fully reversible. It will always leave some corneal scarring which is likely to impair the vision and severe cases will be destructive to the eye (see below). However, surprisingly, there can be a great reduction in corneal destruction and corneal scars can be minimised with vigorous and urgent treatment.

Keratomalacia – X3B

Keratomalacia is the most severe consequence of xerophthalmia. Part (>1/3rd), or all of the cornea quickly degenerates and melts away (**Figure 10.13**) because the cornea becomes necrotic. A mass of white or yellow gelatinous, necrotic matter replaces the normal cornea. Keratomalacia has two striking features:

1. The onset is very rapid. The cornea can be destroyed in a few days.

Table 10.4 Features that suggest vitamin A deficiency is more likely than other causes of corneal ulceration	
From the history	**From examination**
• History of recent illness such as measles, diarrhoea or other illness associated with fever • No medication of any kind has been put in the eye(s) • No history of eye injury • Surprisingly little pain, tissue reaction and inflammation (unless also infected) • Child not adequately breast fed • The mother is poor and malnourished.	• Conjunctival and corneal xerosis present • Bilateral disease • The ulcer has a punched out appearance, or may even be full thickness with protrusion of the iris • Ulcers typically central and inferior

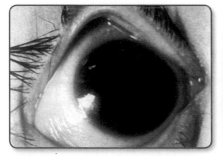

Figure 10.11 Corneal xerosis with ulceration. The eye is not inflamed, as the conjunctiva is white. The dry, wrinkled conjunctival changes confirm the ulcer is caused by vitamin A deficiency; it's position on the upper half of the cornea is unusual.

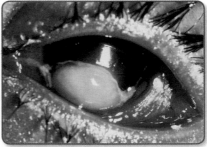

Figure 10.12 This eye has corneal xerosis with a severely infected corneal ulcer.

2. There is surprisingly little tissue reaction or inflammation.

Very often the intraocular contents extrude through the corneal defect. In many cases, the end result is either a shrunken blind eye (phthisis bulbi), or to staphyloma formation (see page 199). The exact mechanism of the sudden corneal 'melt' is not really understood although it is thought that collagenase enzymes are formed that dissolves and destroy the cornea. Secondary infection of the ulcer does not seem to be necessary to start the ulceration, although this is very likely to occur and cause more complications. A study from Bangladesh found that two thirds of children with keratomalacia had died within a few months.

Xerophthalmic corneal scars – XS

There are many causes of corneal scarring. Therefore, it is impossible to be sure if a corneal scar is from a previous episode of xerophthalmia. Xerophthalmic scars vary from a very faint scar to total destruction of the eye. Corneal scars from xerophthalmia are usually in the central or lower part of the cornea, and they are usually bilateral (**Figure 10.14**). One eye may, however, be much more scarred than the other. Corneal scarring in a malnourished child with no history of trauma or other eye infections strongly suggests xerophthalmia.

Xerophthalmia fundus – XF

Vitamin A deficiency can produce a characteristic change in the retina. Pale yellow spots appear, especially near the retinal vessels, and also in the retinal periphery (**Figure 10.15**). This is a rare finding and is not blinding.

Geographic patterns in xerophthalmia

The clinical pattern of xerophthalmia is very variable. In Africa, the early signs of xerophthalmia are uncommon, but the late and devastating signs are seen frequently, probably because of the high prevalence of measles. In India and Indonesia, conjunctival and corneal xerosis is much more common, but measles is a less important factor.

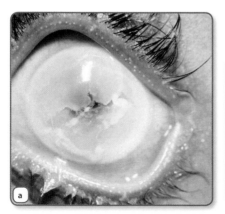
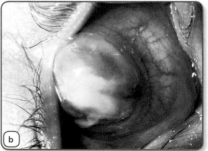

Figure 10.13 Keratomalacia. (a) The cornea has completely dissolved away and a thin sheet of fibrin covers the eye. (b) The intra-ocular contents are beginning to protrude and become covered with pus.

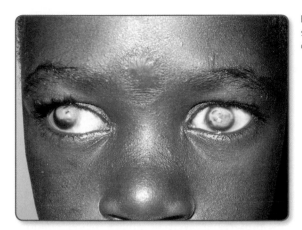

Figure 10.14 Bilateral corneal scarring from vitamin A deficiency.

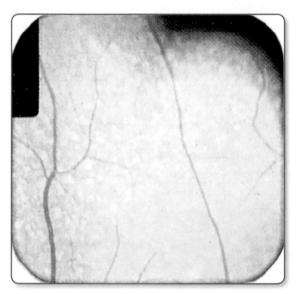

Figure 10.15 Xerophthalmia fundus.

Other causes of corneal ulcers in xerophthalmia

Exposure ulcers

Acutely ill, malnourished children often lie exhausted and dehydrated with their eyelids not properly closed. The blink reflex, which helps to protect the cornea and wet it with tears, is often reduced. Therefore, the exposed part of the cornea becomes dry and ulcerated. It is one reason why xerophthalmia ulcers are found particularly in the lower part of the cornea. **Figure 9.17c** shows a very severe example of this: the patient was unconscious for a long time, and the cornea ulcerated and became very scarred. Only the top part under the eyelid was preserved intact.).

Herpes simplex virus (HSV)

Secondary HSV infections of the cornea are common after measles. HSV lies dormant in the nerve endings. Malnutrition and measles together depress cellular immunity, so that HSV can becomes active and cause a severe infection. In a healthy person, HSV causes a localised superficial ulcer in the cornea, or a 'cold sore' on the lip. However, after measles in malnourished children, severe ulcers may develop especially in the eye and in the mouth (see Figure 9.3 and **Figure 10.16**). These are often much larger and deeper than the usual herpetic ulcers. Also, they may be bilateral and the mouth and eyelids may also be ulcerated.

'Treatment' by traditional healers

In many parts of the world, sick children are taken to traditional healers and often have various traditional medicines applied to their eyes. All sorts of substances may be used, such as mixtures of herbs, urine, kerosene and euphorbia sap. Many of these are toxic and dangerous to an already unhealthy cornea and conjunctiva. However other traditional healers are able to diagnose vitamin A deficiency and give appropriate advice. Other children may be treated with 'conventional' but completely inappropriate medicines, such as steroids, that have been bought from a market stall or pharmacist, without any medical advice.

Other systemic factors in patients with vitamin A deficiency

Protein energy malnutrition

Protein energy malnutrition (PEM) causes widespread and complex changes in the body. In general, PEM retards growth and development, and weakens a child's resistance to infection. More specifically, it upsets the metabolism

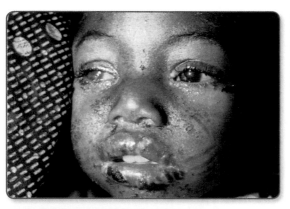

Figure 10.16 A perforating ulcer in the right eye and severe ulceration around the mouth. The child had measles and the measles rash can be seen on the face.

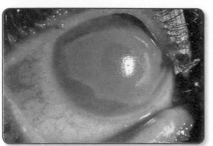

Figure 10.17 A measles ulcer. A large, superficial ulcer stained with fluorescein. The child had measles and the conjunctiva is inflamed probably from measles keratoconjunctivitis.

of vitamin A. In protein deficiency, there is not enough RBP synthesized in the liver (**Figure 10.6**). Less retinol can enter the bloodstream, and so the body tissues are deprived of vitamin A. This is why children with both vitamin A deficiency and PEM have more severe eye lesions than children with vitamin A deficiency alone.

There are many ways to assess PEM in young children. It is usual to measure either the arm circumference or the child's weight for age, and to look for any signs of oedema.

A child who receives treatment for PEM often has a sudden 'growth spurt'. This sudden growth increases the utilization of any vitamin A stores. Appropriate action will then be necessary to replace these stores, so that there is no danger of vitamin A deficiency.

Infection

Vitamin A helps prevent infection, by maintaining intact surfaces, membranes and protective mucus on top of them, and possibly also by having a fundamental role in the immune system itself. Therefore children who are vitamin A deficient are more likely to get infection. These infections can precipitate corneal ulcers and the other acute complications of vitamin A deficiency because:

1. A child's vitamin A requirements increase when they have an infection.
2. A child's food intake usually decreases when they are ill.
3. Gastrointestinal infections are likely to reduce the absorption of vitamin A.
4. Ill children may be lying in bed, sick, exhausted and with their eyes open (see above).

Measles

Measles hugely increases the body's need for vitamin A to repair damaged cells in tissues throughout the body. It rapidly depletes the stores of vitamin A in the liver, which may already be low. It is therefore one of the most important, avoidable and devastating causes of corneal ulceration in children. It is a common causes of death and children that survive are at risk of many other health problems but in particular visual loss and hearing loss. Indeed, in many parts of Africa, more than half of all cases of child blindness are from corneal ulceration following measles.

Measles is more damaging to the eye than other childhood infections, because the measles virus actually invades the conjunctival and corneal epithelium. During an attack of measles, even healthy and well-nourished children develop superficial keratoconjunctivitis. Normally, this resolves completely, but in malnourished children it may progress to severe corneal ulceration (**Figure 10.16**).

Intestinal parasites

Intestinal parasites may lower the absorption of carotenes and retinol from the intestine.

The treatment of xerophthalmia

The treatment of vitamin A deficiency requires:

- Treatment of the eye and systemic illness
- Correction of the vitamin A deficiency and other nutritional deficiencies
- Treatment of the community that the patient lives in.

In other words, it is not enough just to dispense injections, tablets and eye ointment. The social, economic and family problems that have caused the disease must also be recognised. One expert in xerophthalmia said: 'first the eye, second the child and third the kitchen.' There is a fourth aspect – the community.

Nutritional and general treatment

Children with vitamin A deficiency need multiple large doses of vitamin A. Children (aged 6 months to 5 years) who receive vitamin A supplements have a 24% lower mortality risk than those who do not receive supplements. Vitamin A supplements are estimated to have now prevented 1.25 million deaths since the WHO and its partners started distributing them in 1998. Furthermore these children also have a reduced risk of diarrhoea, measles and of course xerophthalmia. Supplementation should be considered for the following groups:

- All children with active corneal ulceration that is suspicious for vitamin A deficiency. It can be difficult or impossible to determine the precise cause of a corneal ulcer, but if there is even the slightest suspicion of vitamin A deficiency, treatment should be given (**Table 10.5**).
- All children with measles in areas of likely vitamin A deficiency.
- All children with any of the signs of xerophthalmia.
- All severely ill or malnourished children from areas where xerophthalmia occurs, even if there is no clinical evidence of xerophthalmia.

It is very important to explain to the mother that three doses are required in children with ophthalmic signs. Therefore one must watch the first dose being taken and give the mother the other two doses with clear instructions that these should be taken on day 2 and day 14.

Table 10.5 shows the doses of vitamin A that the WHO recommends. Most preparations of vitamin A also contain small doses of vitamin E (tocopherol). Vitamin E seems to improve the absorption and utilisation of vitamin A. Treatment for pregnant woman is only recommended in areas of severe vitamin A deficiency (night blindness levels greater than 5% in children aged 6 months to 5 years). The doses should be much smaller, but given more frequently, as it is possible that high doses of vitamin A can harm a developing fetus. Babies that are younger than 6 months and immediately postpartum mothers should not be given vitamin A supplements, as it is possible high doses of vitamin A are harmful to the baby (occasionally vitamin A supplementation can cause bulging of the fontanel). However, is very important that the mothers are encouraged to eat a healthy diet.

If vitamin A capsules are not available, the child must eat foods that are rich in vitamin A. If the child is unable or too sick to swallow, intramuscular preparations are available. It is also important to correct any PEM. Many malnourished children also need treatment for dehydration, pyrexia, bronchopneumonia, gastroenteritis, measles or intestinal parasites.

Table 10.5 Treatment of children with any ophthalmic signs of vitamin A deficiency			
Age of child	**Oral dose**		**Dosing schedule**
	mg	**IU**	
<6 months	27.5	50,000	
6–12 months	55	100,000	Day 1, day 2 and day 14
>12 months	110	200,000	
Preventive treatment in the community			
Patient group			
Neonates	Supplementation not recommended: encourage exclusive breast-feeding		
Children aged 6–11 months	55	100,000	One dose, oral liquid
Children aged 12–59 months	110	200,000	Repeat every 4–6 months
Pregnant mothers (only in areas where vitamin A deficiency is a severe public health problem (prevalence of night blindness in children age 6–59 months >5%)	Either 5.5 Or 13.75	10,000 25,000	Daily for 12 weeks until delivery Weekly for 12 weeks delivery
Post-partum mothers	Supplementation not recommended		
IU, international units of retinal palmitate.			

Topical treatment to the eye

All eyes with evidence of corneal ulceration need topical treatment. Even eyes without ulcers may need treatment to prevent ulcers forming. Eyes with advanced ulceration must be handled very gently, so that the ulcer does not perforate. It is advisable to try to cover the eye with a plastic shield at all times because of the risk of them rubbing the eye and causing or worsening a perforation and it may even be necessary to restrain their hands to protect the eyes.

Antibiotics

Bacterial infection is probably not a primary cause of these corneal ulcers. However, bacteria are certainly very common secondary invaders. If there is a hypopyon or pus in the cornea around the ulcer, this is evidence of secondary bacterial infection. These patients will need intensive topical antibiotic drops (see page 203). Subconjunctival and systemic antibiotics may also be helpful in severe cases. Antibiotic ointment 3 or 4 times a day can also help to prevent corneal infection in more mild cases.

Antiviral agents

Herpes simplex infection may cause many of these ulcers, especially after measles. The treatment for herpes simplex is topical and systemic antiviral agents every 2 hours (see page 194).

Closing the eyes

Any severely ill, young child who has poor eyelid closure is at risk of developing corneal ulceration. It is very important and very easy to prevent this. It is so simple just to teach the parents to keep the eyelids closed while the child is sick, and yet many children go blind from exposure ulceration. It is also helpful to apply plenty of antibiotic ointment, which will lubricate and protect the cornea.

Padding an eye

Padding, if done properly, may help because it prevents dehydration and exposure of the cornea. It also helps the epithelium to heal, and reduces pain and photophobia. However, the eye must be closed under the pad. If it is not, padding can be harmful as it will rub against the cornea or prevent the lids closing and cause further damage. Padding may also allow bacteria to breed in the warmer, contained area. Therefore, padding is only recommended where there is excellent nursing and the pad can be changed regularly.

Mydriatics

These are advisable for all cases of active corneal ulceration. The most common treatments are atropine 1% drops once a day or cyclopentolate 1% two or three times a day.

Steroids

Normally steroid drops or ointment should never be applied to these ulcers. It is especially dangerous for the many eyes that may have herpes simplex infection. The one circumstance in which they may be useful is when children have burns to the eyes from toxic traditional eye medicines. However, one must be sure of the history, and steroids should be used with very great care and frequent observation.

Surgery

In the acute active stage of the disease when the cornea is ulcerated, surgery has no part to play. These children are very sick and would not tolerate the anaesthetic. When the child has recovered, the eye is not inflamed and the ulcer has become a corneal scar, it is possible that optical iridectomy surgery or even a corneal graft will improve the vision. The treatment of corneal scars is discussed on page 221.

Community treatment: the prevention of blindness from xerophthalmia

'Prevention is better than cure.' This old saying is truer of xerophthalmia than any other eye disease. Prompt, effective treatment may save either the sight or the life of some children. Sadly, however, there are many more who are permanently blind when they first seek medical treatment, and even more who never receive any treatment at all. The WHO has established certain criteria, which indicate whether xerophthalmia is a serious problem in the community (**Table 10.6**).

Any prevention programme must have two essential features:
1. It must be based in the community, rather than the hospital or clinic.
2. It must have the cooperation of and coordination between different groups of people who are all critical for educating and treating individuals and communities. This includes public health doctors,

ophthalmologists and eye care practitioners, local government, people in charge of agricultural policy and nutrition and school teachers. Xerophthalmia is a complex problem, and there is no simple remedy. Measures for prevention are possible at different levels in the community. The government may intervene to improve the health of the nation as a whole. Or else individual mothers may receive nutritional advice and support. A preventive measure that is appropriate in one community may not be appropriate in another. The following list describes some of the measures that different communities have taken.

1. **Distribution of massive dose capsules**

    Vitamin A capsules containing 55 mg (100 000 IU) are easy to obtain and very cheap. In fact, the biggest expense in these programmes is the distribution, and not the cost of the capsules themselves. A single dose of 55 mg for children under 1-year-old, and 110 mg for children over one, can protect against vitamin A deficiency for up to 6 months. It is important not to give more than one dose of vitamin A/month. Children who have had more than one dose a month sometimes show signs of vitamin A toxicity: headaches, vomiting and nausea.

    Pregnant women and lactating mothers also need vitamin A. However, it is advisable to give small doses more frequently. If the woman is pregnant, there is in theory a very small risk that a single massive dose might damage the fetus.

    Children at risk need vitamin A capsules for the first 5 years of life. The community must therefore be well-organised to make capsule distribution effective. The most common reason for capsule distribution programmes failing is that they do not reach the very children who are most in need of protection.

2. **Fortification of foods**

    Some foods can be fortified with vitamin A, without changing their taste or appearance. However, for this to be successful, one must identify foods that all the children in the community eat, and which are processed at one or two central factories where vitamin A could be added. This method has been successful in countries in Central America where, in the 1970s they started to fortify sugar with vitamin A. This led to a marked decrease in xerophthalmia. In Guatemala and

Table 10.6 The diagnosis of xerophthalmia in the community	
Criterion	Minimum % of the population at risk
Clinical	
XN: Night blindness	1.0
X1B: Bitot's spot	0.5
X2 + X3: Corneal xerosis	0.01
XS: Xerophthalmic scars	0.05
Biochemical	
Serum retinol (vitamin A) less than 10 µg/100 mL (0.35 µmol/L)	5.0

Nicaragua they also introduced vitamin A supplementation to children aged 6 months to 5 years and xerophthalmia has virtually disappeared in Guatemala, and low serum retinol levels (<0.7 µmol/L) are found in less than 2% of Nicaraguan school children. Other countries such as South Africa and Zambia have had less success with programmes of food fortification and vitamin A supplementation, but this has been because of much lower coverage than was achieved in the Central American countries.

3. **Horticulture and agriculture**

   It is often difficult to persuade members of a community to change their diet and agricultural methods. However, in order to treat vitamin A deficiency at source, it is necessary to encourage people to grow and eat the right sorts of food. Green leafy vegetables (e.g. spinach) and orange coloured fruit and vegetables (e.g. carrots, mangoes, papayas) are very rich in carotene. They are also cheap and easy to grow, particularly in the hot climates where vitamin A deficiency is most common and severe. Even seemingly small changes can make a big difference, such as changing from growing regular sweet potatoes to the orange-fleshed sweet potato, which has a higher vitamin A content. A more complicated but potentially very effective way of increasing vitamin A intake is to genetically modify seeds, in order to increase the vitamin A content of the fruit and vegetables that will grow. Finally, improved methods of food preservation could make vitamin A rich foods available throughout the year.

4. **Nutrition and health education**

   Nutrition and health education is possible in many ways and at many levels, e.g. radio, television, schools, adult education classes, hospital out-patient waiting areas and community outreach programmes. It is only young children who are at risk from xerophthalmia, and they are totally dependant on their mothers and/or carers. For this reason, the aim of any programme must be to educate the mothers and future mothers of young children. These mothers will need advice about:

- Breast-feeding and weaning and which weaning foods to choose and how to prepare them.
- Selecting cheap but nutritional foods. The parents must learn that it is the children who need the few bits of milk, meat, fish or eggs that the family can afford, and not the father who will be fine with mainly starchy foods.

   It is preferable if nutritional advice about how to wean a child off breast milk is part of a comprehensive programme of child-care. Some hospitals have special nutritional rehabilitation centres for malnourished children and their mothers. The children receive treatment, and the mothers receive advice and guidance. The treatment of a malnourished child should always include some sort of nutritional advice and counselling of the mother.

   Some communities rely on or use traditional healers. These healers are often much more accessible to patients in remote areas, and therefore co-operation between traditional healers and 'conventional' health practitioners is essential. Wherever possible, local health workers should try to maintain good relations with local healers, as they are often very receptive to health education. Some suggestions about cooperation are made in Chapter 1.

5. **Immunisation**

Immunisation programmes can prevent many serious childhood illnesses, especially measles. The measles vaccine is a living, but attenuated virus, and it needs very careful cold storage. Unfortunately, many vaccine schemes for measles have failed because the vaccine has died, due to the cold chain not being effective. A heat stable effective measles vaccine has not yet been produced, although there are hopes for the future. The eradication of measles would, of course, be a huge achievement in itself, but it would also be a major advance in the prevention of nutritional corneal blindness in children.

Xerophthalmia in children is a very complex disease. There remain numerous unanswered questions about many parts of the disease and the interaction between malnutrition, vitamin A deficiency and measles. However, it is a tragic disease that really should not be allowed to continue causing devastating consequences. Effective action could prevent this disease. Surely this is not too much to hope?

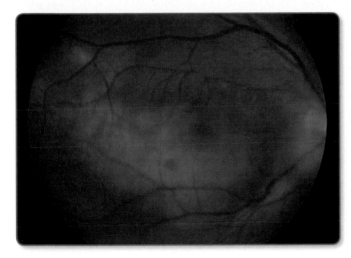

Uveal diseases are not very common. However, they may be the clue to important systemic diseases; this patient with choroiditis has tuberculosis.

The uvea is the middle layer of the eye and consists of the choroid, the ciliary body and the iris. These are very different tissues; the choroid is a vascular layer that supplies nutrition to the outer retina; the ciliary body produces aqueous and controls accommodation, and the iris is a pigmented tissue that controls light entry. Therefore, they are affected by varying diseases. However, there are also similar conditions that affect the uveal layer and in particular inflammatory and some infective conditions. We have therefore included tuberculosis and syphilis in this chapter, although both of these infections can affect any bit of the eye and periocular tissues.

Uveitis

Inflammation is by far the most common disease of the uvea, and this is called 'uveitis'. Uveitis is divided into different types depending on which part of the uvea is involved.
*   Anterior uveitis (or iritis/iridocyclitis): inflammation of the iris and ciliary body (i.e. anterior uvea). Clinically, it is seen as inflammation in the anterior chamber.
*   Posterior uveitis (choroiditis): inflammation confined to the choroid. Clinically, it is seen as inflammation in the choroid and usually the retina as well. There may be some extension of the inflammation in to the posterior vitreous.
*   Intermediate uveitis: inflammation in the peripheral choroid and the ciliary body. Clinically it is seen as inflammation in the vitreous gel.
*   Panuveitis: inflammation of the whole uveal layer.
Anterior uveitis is the commonest type of uveitis. Intermediate and posterior uveitis are less common.

Acute anterior uveitis (AAU)

Symptoms and signs

AAU is one of the commonest causes of a painful, red eye. It typically presents with pain, photophobia, blurred vision and a red eye. The severity of each of these signs is quite variable. An acute attack occurs much more commonly in one eye but can occasionally occur in both simultaneously. The patient may report having had similar episodes previously.

The signs of AAU are very distinctive (**Table 11.1**). They are best seen with a slit lamp, but some signs can be seen with an ordinary magnifying lens, or even the naked eye. The signs are:

- *Ciliary vessel dilatation*: these radial vessels around the cornea are usually more dilated than the rest of the anterior surface vessels. (**Figure 11.1**).
- *Anterior chamber cells* (**Figure 11.2**): during the acute attack, the anterior chamber contains white blood cells and inflammatory protein exudate, which come from the iris and ciliary body. It takes practice to see these signs with the light from the slit lamp. A bright, focussed,

Table 11.1 Signs of acute anterior uveitis	
Location	**Sign**
Limbus	Ciliary vessel dilatation
Cornea	Keratitic precipitates
Anterior chamber	Cells Flare Hypopyon
Iris and pupil	Constricted with poor dilatation Irregular shape Posterior synechiae

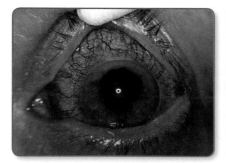

Figure 11.1 Ciliary vessel dilatation and posterior synechiae from acute anterior uveitis. The episcleral and scleral vessels are generally inflamed and dilated, but this is particularly prominent near the limbus. The posterior synechiae have prevented the pupil dilating and have made it irregular in shape. They are more obvious on attempting to dilate the pupil.

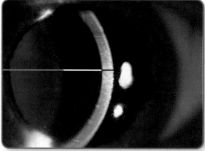

Figure 11.2 Anterior chamber (white line); cornea (red line); lens (blue line). The tiny bright dots in the anterior chamber are the inflammatory cells.

small beam of light from the slit lamp is required to hit the anterior chamber at an angle. The white blood cells will appear like particles of dust in a beam of sunlight, or like stars twinkling in the night sky. The protein exudate appears as a smoky appearance, which is sometimes described as 'flare' (**Figure 11.3**). In severe inflammation, white cells and fibrin exudate may collect at the bottom of the anterior chamber to form an inflammatory hypopyon (**Figure 11.18**).

- *Keratic precipitates:* these are clumps of white blood cells from the anterior chamber that have stuck to the posterior surface of the cornea (the endothelium) (**Figures 11.4** and **11.5**).
- *Small pupil and posterior synechiae:* The iris constricts and adheres to the anterior capsule of the lens (posterior synechiae) (**Figure 11.1**). The pupil therefore appears small and irregular, even to the naked eye. If the pupil is dilated with mydriatic drops, these adhesions between the iris and the lens may become more noticeable. Dilatation sometimes breaks these adhesions, but deposits of iris pigment remain stuck to the lens surface. Even when the inflammation subsides, these adhesions between the iris and the lens persist. There may be evidence of adhesions from previous episodes of anterior uveitis (**Figure 11.6**).

If a slit lamp is not available, AAU can usually be detected with an ophthalmoscope alone. A strongly positive lens should be used in the ophthalmoscope

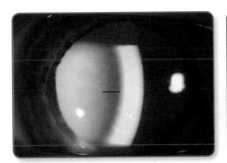

Figure 11.3 Acute iridocyclitis to show the aqueous flare. Note the reflection of the beam of light from a slit lamp as it passes through the anterior chamber (red line). The flare in this case is particularly obvious.

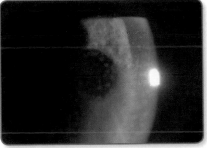

Figure 11.4 Chronic iridocyclitis causing large 'mutton fat' keratic precipitates.

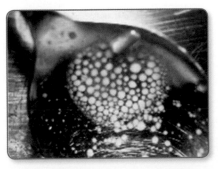

Figure 11.5 Actual mutton (sheep fat). This spoon of mutton fat shows how similar the keratic precipitates can be. Uveitis is often described as granulomatous when there is an inflammatory reaction producing isolated nodules of inflammation like this; or non-granulomatous when white cells and/or protein are found in the anterior chamber or vitreous and there are no large inflammatory nodules.

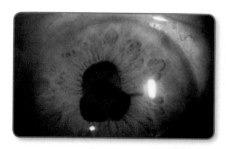

Figure 11.6 Old, inactive anterior uveitis. The posterior synechiae have left deposits of the iris on the lens surface and the pupil is irregularly shaped because the iris is stuck to the lens.

(between +10 and +20), which must be held close to the patient's eye. The following signs may then be visible:

- The shadows of the keratic precipitates against the red reflex (**Figure 11.7**).
- The irregular pupil and pigment deposits from the iris on the lens surface.

The course of the disease

After the inflammation subsides, the ciliary vasodilatation and the anterior chamber inflammatory exudate both disappear. The keratic precipitates shrink and become pigmented, and eventually they too usually disappear. These improvements can happen quite quickly with steroid treatment (see below). Sometimes, without treatment the disease slowly resolves but sometimes, serious ocular complications can occur (see below). Any adhesions between the pupil margin and the lens or any deposits of iris pigment on the lens surface are both permanent. Recurrences in the same eye or the other eye are common.

Chronic anterior uveitis (CAU)

In chronic CAU, the onset of the disease is usually much more gradual. There is often a specific cause, such as herpes zoster virus inflammation, sarcoid or juvenile idiopathic arthritis, which is known to cause more chronic disease. There is usually little or no pain, and often the only significant symptom is blurred vision. There are often more prominent keratic precipitates, which are sometimes large and pale, when they are called ('mutton fat' precipitates (**Figure 11.4** and **Figure 11.5**). Occasionally one can also see inflammatory granulomatous nodules on, or beneath the surface of the iris.

Complications of anterior uveitis

Complications are frequent, especially if no treatment is given, and may cause permanent blindness.

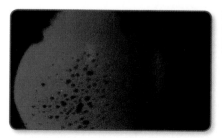

Figure 11.7 Anterior uveitis seen with an ophthalmoscope. The shadows of the keratic precipitates can be seen against the red reflex. The pupil is also irregular.

Secondary glaucoma

This is the most common cause of permanent visual loss and blindness in patients with anterior uveitis. Therefore, the intraocular pressure of any patient with anterior uveitis must be checked, both at presentation and during treatment. There are three possible mechanisms of glaucoma in patients with anterior uveitis:

1. Obstruction of aqueous drainage at the trabecular meshwork by the inflammatory exudate and cells in the anterior chamber. The pressure can rise very high, but as the inflammation subsides, it usually returns to normal. However, any damage to the optic nerve and loss of vision is permanent.

2. Pupil block glaucoma (**Figure 11.8a–c**). If the entire pupil margin of the iris has adhered to the lens, the passage of aqueous between the posterior and anterior chamber is completely obstructed. Pressure then builds up behind the iris causing it to bow forwards into the anterior chamber (this is sometimes called 'iris bombé'). The pressure rises very high. Fortunately this is rare.

3. Steroid treatment (see below). The intraocular pressure of some patients rises in response to steroid treatment. Therefore, the intraocular pressure

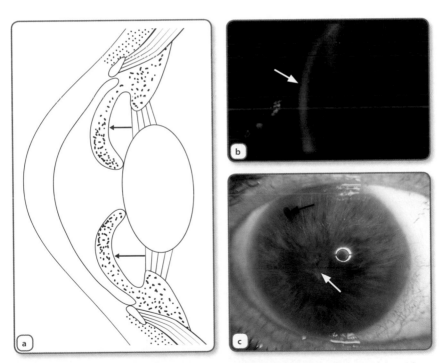

Figure 11.8 (a) A diagram of pupil block glaucoma. The iris is completely adherent to the surface of the lens right round the pupil margin. The arrows show how the pressure of the aqueous pushes the iris forwards. This is called iris bombé. (b) Iris bombe. The iris can be seen bowing forward (red arrows) towards the cornea (white arrow). (c) An eye that has had pupil block glaucoma. The entire pupil margin of the iris is adherent to the lens. The peripheral iridotomy (red arrow) has been made superiorly to allow aqueous to move from the posterior chamber to the anterior chamber. A fibrinous membrane also covers over the pupil (white arrow). This has been caused by old episodes of inflammation.

must always be measured during any follow-ups. The pressure usually returns to normal after stopping treatment, although very occasionally does not, and glaucoma treatment is required (see Chapter 15).

Reduced intraocular pressure

A small reduction in the intraocular pressure during an episode of anterior uveitis is also common. This is probably caused by the inflammation affecting the ciliary body's ability to produce aqueous. Occasionally, severe and persistent inflammation can cause permanent damage to the ciliary body and its processes. The intraocular pressure will then be very low, called hypotony and in bad cases the eyeball may shrink with the low pressure. This is called 'phthisis bulbi'.

Cataract

Cataracts are common in patients with recurrent or persistent anterior uveitis (**Figure 11.9**). The actual mechanism is unclear; the intraocular inflammation probably upsets the metabolism of the lens and the steroids used in treatment may cause cataract. When the inflammation has subsided, cataract surgery can be done to restore the sight. However, extra treatment with steroids at the time of surgery should be considered to prevent the uveitis recurring.

Iris atrophy

Iris atrophy may follow inflammation. The iris becomes thin and depigmented (**Figure 11.10**). Examination of the red reflex with an ophthalmoscope is a very good way of detecting iris atrophy. The glow of the red reflex will be seen through the atrophic iris.

Band degeneration (Figure 9.26)

This is the development of a band of opaque calcific deposit under the corneal epithelium. It sometimes occurs in chronic anterior uveitis and often in patients with phthisis.

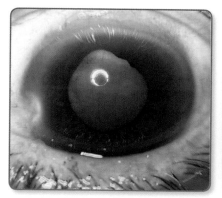

Figure 11.9 Dense cataract after anterior uveitis. The irregular pupil margin shows that this patient has had anterior uveitis in the past.

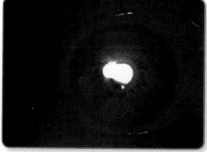

Figure 11.10 Iris atrophy from previous inflammation. This picture is taken with a slit lamp. The narrow beam of light enters through the pupil and the reflected light is seen coming through the thin iris.

Posterior uveitis (choroiditis)

In posterior uveitis, the choroid is the main focus of the inflammation. However, the retina is frequently affected as well (chorioretinitis or retino-choroiditis) and often there is some inflammation in the vitreous or even anteriorly in the eye. It can be very helpful for making a differential diagnosis to try and determine if the primary inflammation is choroidal, which might make one consider conditions such as toxoplasmosis, or retinal when viral retinitis should be considered.

Symptoms and signs

The main symptoms of posterior uveitis are floaters and visual loss. Posterior uveitis is not usually very painful, but a severe attack often causes some discomfort or ache behind the eye. The pattern of visual loss depends on which part of the choroid is affected, but the following features are typically seen:

- In almost all cases of posterior uveitis, inflammatory cells and debris are released into the vitreous. These will cause some blurring of vision or produce moving shadows in the vision called 'floaters' (**Figure 11.11**).
- Posterior uveitis located at or near the macula will cause loss of visual acuity by affecting the function of the macula. Sometimes the macula may be damaged by inflammation in other parts of the choroid or retina, because choroidal and retinal inflammation can cause retinal oedema to develop in the macula. This affects the function of the tightly packed cone cells.
- Posterior uveitis near the optic disc will usually damage the optic nerve fibres, and cause a corresponding visual field defect.
- Posterior uveitis in the periphery of the choroid may cause very little visual loss in itself, although large areas of choroidal inflammation will impair the peripheral visual field, and lots of small spots of choroidal inflammation may be seen as dark areas in the vision.

On fundus examination, inflammation of the choroid appears as greyish-yellow or greyish white opacities. When the inflammation is active, these areas are often oedematous, making them a little raised and giving them a soft fluffy edge (**Figure 11.12**), unlike the clearly demarcated flat and pigmented scarred

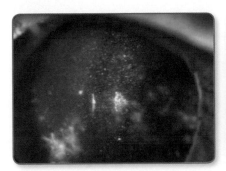

Figure 11.11 Vitreous cells. The many collections of inflammatory cells that can be seen are in the vitreous behind the lens.

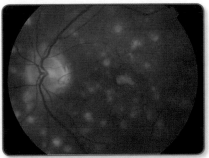

Figure 11.12 Multifocal choroiditis. There are many fluffy white areas of active choroidal inflammation.

areas that remain after the acute episode has resolved (**Figure 11.13**). The retinal blood vessels can be clearly seen overlying the opacities, although the view of the fundus itself may be hazy because of vitreous inflammation, which can make fundus examination difficult. There may be one area of inflammation, large or small, or several small areas, which is sometimes called multifocal choroiditis. The appearance is sometimes described as looking like 'car headlights in fog'. Sometimes there may be generalised inflammation spread over the entire choroid. Occasionally, an inflammatory exudate may develop between the choroid and the retina. This is called an exudative retinal detachment. This type of detachment is usually found at the periphery of the retina.

Old, inactive choroiditis

After the inflammation has subsided, a characteristic localised scar remains. There is usually a mixture of dark and pale areas of atrophy and hypertrophy of the retinal and choroidal pigment (**Figures 11.13**). The scars may be large or small, single or multiple.

Course of the disease

As the disease resolves, the vision usually improves. However, there will always be a permanent defect in the vision corresponding to the area of the choroidal scar. There is often permanent damage to the macula. In severe cases the scar tissue may spread into the vitreous, and later on cause a traction retinal detachment.

Intermediate uveitis (pars planitis)

In intermediate uveitis the inflammation comes from the pars plana of the ciliary body. It is more common in children and young adults and is bilateral in 80% of cases. Patients usually describe 'floaters' and some blurring of vision from inflammatory cells in the vitreous. Sometimes the vitreous inflammatory cells clump together to form white balls, which are referred to as 'snowballs' or collections of white exudate over the inferior pars plana, which is referred to as 'snow banking' (**Figure 11.14**). Cystoid macular oedema and lens opacities are common complications. These both cause loss

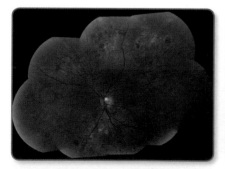

Figure 11.13 Inactive choroiditis. Areas of inflammation have become pigmented scars.

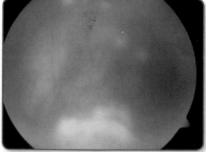

Figure 11.14 Severe vitreous inflammation. White balls of inflammatory cells ('snowballs') and a collection of vitreous inflammation inferiorly ('snow banking') are visible. There is a very hazy view of the retina because of all the inflammatory cells.

of visual acuity which may be how the intermediate uveitis is first diagnosed. On examination of the eye some inflammatory changes and white exudates may be seen in the peripheral retina.

Causes of uveitis (Table 11.2)

There are many possible causes of uveitis. The cause will not be found in most patients, particularly those with anterior uveitis. However, it is important to consider infections, inflammatory disease, autoimmune disease, trauma and cancer. A careful history must be taken and a thorough examination performed (think about diseases like tuberculosis, syphilis and leprosy) in all cases of uveitis as the cause is frequently missed. Health practitioners are often too quick to label it 'idiopathic' (i.e. no clear cause). Routine investigations such as urine testing (for associated kidney disease), a chest X-ray (e.g. for pulmonary tuberculosis) and blood test (e.g. for syphilis) may help to diagnose these diseases.

Some systemic and ocular conditions are more typically associated with anterior inflammation and others with intermediate and posterior inflammation. **Table 11.2** classifies the different groups of diseases that cause or are associated with uveitis and identifies the typical location in the eye of the inflammation. However, there is great variation in the inflammatory presentation of many diseases, and particularly for systemic diseases such as tuberculosis and sarcoid. We will discuss some of these conditions in more detail in this and other chapters.

Infective causes of uveitis

The eye has a very active and responsive immune system. It is therefore not surprising that many ocular and systemic conditions can provoke a vigorous immune response. These include: worms, protozoan parasites, fungi, bacteria and viruses. The incidence of these infective causes varies greatly from country to country and even village to village. Some of these systemic infections are severe, chronic and even fatal.

The relationship between infection and uveitis has changed dramatically in recent years because of the HIV/AIDS epidemic. In those areas where HIV/AIDS is prevalent, several well-known infectious causes of uveitis have become both much more common and much more severe, e.g. toxoplasmosis, tuberculosis, candidiasis, cytomegalovirus and the herpes infections. The most significant infective causes of uveitis in poor and tropical countries are described below.

Leprosy

Leprosy is an important cause of both acute and chronic anterior uveitis but does not invade the choroid. The effects on the eye are described in Chapter 17.

Tuberculosis

Tuberculosis is not a common cause of uveitis. It is discussed in detail at the end of this chapter.

Syphilis and other spirochaete infections

Syphilis can cause almost any ocular inflammatory and infective signs. It is discussed in detail at the end of this chapter.

Table 11.2 Ocular and systemic diseases associated with or causing uveitis

Associated/causative disease	Typical location of uveitis
Ocular disease	
Infection	
Viruses, e.g. HSV, HZV, CMV	Anterior or posterior
Protozoa, e.g. toxoplasmosis	Posterior
Fungi, e.g. *Candida*, histoplasmosis	Posterior
Parasites, e.g. onchocerciasis, toxocara, cysticercosis, myiasis	Mainly posterior
Post-surgical/penetrating injury infection	Pan uveitis
Inflammatory disease	
HLA-B27 related uveitis	Anterior
Sympathetic ophthalmitis	Pan uveitis
Birdshot chorioretinopathy and other white dot syndromes	Posterior
Fuchs heterochromic iridocyclitis	Anterior
Post-surgical non-infective	Anterior
Glaucomacyclitic crisis (Posner-Schlossman syndrome)	Anterior
Trauma	Anterior, occasionally posterior in severe trauma
Malignancy (uveitis masquerade syndrome), e.g. lymphoma	Anterior or posterior
Lens rupture	Anterior
Systemic disease	
Infective disease	
Tuberculosis	Anywhere
Leprosy	Anterior
Syphilis	Anywhere
Others, e.g. leptospirosis, Lyme disease	Anywhere
Inflammatory disease	
Behçet disease	Pan uveitis
Sarcoid	Pan uveitis
Vogt–Koyanagi–Harada syndrome	Pan uveitis
Multiple sclerosis	Intermediate with some anterior 'spill over'
Autoimmune disease	
Connective tissue diseases, e.g. ankylosing spondylitis, rheumatoid arthritis, juvenile idiopathic arthritis, reactive arthritis, psoriatic arthritis	Anterior
Inflammatory bowel diseases, e.g. ulcerative colitis, Crohn's disease	Anterior

Lyme disease

Lyme disease is an infectious disease caused by *Borrelia* bacterial infection. This infection is transmitted by ticks and is more common in the Northern Hemisphere. It causes systemic symptoms including fever, headache, tiredness and a rash at the site of the tick bite. Like syphilis and leptospirosis it can cause a wide range of ocular inflammatory pictures.

Other acute bacterial infections

Commonly found environmental and eyelid bacteria such as *Staphylococci, Streptococci, Haemophilus* and *Pseudomonas,* occasionally cause intraocular infection and uveitis. They usually only enter the eye after a penetrating injury and very rarely after an intraocular operation. Very rarely, in cases of septicaemia, the bacteria may enter from the bloodstream. Unfortunately, these bacteria multiply very quickly in the aqueous and the vitreous and very soon convert the eye into a mass of pus. Systemic, topical and intravitreal antibiotic treatment should be given, but it is nearly always too late to save the eye.

Fungi and yeasts

Numerous fungi and yeasts can cause uveitis (**Figure 11.15**). Candida infection is the commonest intraocular fungus and should be especially considered in the following patient groups:

- People with immune depression such as AIDS.
- Intravenous drug users particularly if dirty /reused needles and syringes are used.
- Patients with long-term intravenous treatment lines in place, such as Hickman lines used for cancer chemotherapy.

Chronic fungal infections are often misdiagnosed as inflammatory uveitis and treated with steroids, instead of anti-fungals.

Toxoplasmosis

Toxoplasmosis retinochoroiditis is usually associated with vitritis. This may make it difficult to see the retinal lesions, which are sometimes described as looking like 'car headlight in fog'. There is sometimes mild anterior uveitis as well. Toxoplasmosis is discussed on page 351.

Herpes simplex and herpes zoster anterior uveitis

Infections with both of these viruses, e.g. herpes zoster ophthalmicus (shingles) and herpes simplex blepharitis or keratitis (see Chapter 9) can be complicated by anterior uveitis. Interestingly the primary infection can be cleared and the rash, vesicles or keratitis resolve, but the immune-mediated uveitis can continue for a long period afterwards. Therefore, steroids, which must not be used during the initial phase of the disease as they allow herpes viruses to replicate much more easily, may be required for many months or even years afterwards to control the subsequent chronic inflammation.

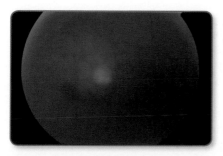

Figure 11.15 Candidal endophthalmitis. The white lesion is Candidal infection in the vitreous. The view is very hazy because there is lots of vitreous inflammation.

Herpes simplex and herpes zoster retinitis (see Chapter 20)

Herpetic infection of the retina (viral retinitis) causes a very different clinical picture to the external infection and anterior inflammation described above. Viral retinal infection provokes a vigorous posterior inflammatory response, except in patients with AIDS in whom the picture is very different, as they do not mount a normal immune response.

Parasitic worms

Parasitic worms like onchocerciasis and toxocara can cause uveitis or intra-ocular inflammation (see Chapter 16).

Inflammatory causes of uveitis

Many inflammatory conditions can cause or be associated with uveitis. Some of these are ocular inflammatory conditions, but others are systemic. It is perhaps not surprising that patients whose immune systems attack their own tissues elsewhere in the body, e.g. those with inflammatory bowel disease and rheumatoid arthritis, are also at risk of immune system inflammation in the eye.

Human leucocyte associated (HLA) – B27 associated uveitis

The HLA system is a collection of genes that code cell-surface antigen-presenting proteins that are a fundamental part of the immune system. Patients with specific variations in the HLA system have been found to be more likely to suffer from various autoimmune diseases. Patients with the HLA-B27 gene are more likely to suffer from anterior uveitis as well as from reactive arthritis and ankylosing spondylitis. A blood test can be done for HLA-B27, but the result of this blood test rarely changes the management of the patient, i.e. if the patient has anterior uveitis, they require treatment irrespective of their HLA-B27 status. HLA-B27 positivity is more common in Europeans, which may explain why anterior uveitis is more common in Europe than Africa and Asia.

Fuchs' heterochromic iridocyclitis (FHI)

FHI causes a mild to moderate non-granulomatous anterior uveitis usually in one eye only. The iris of this eye becomes depigmented and therefore the two eyes appear to be differently coloured (iris heterochromia). In time, cataract develops. The intraocular pressure often rises during episodes of inflammation and must be controlled. Steroid treatment may not help to control the inflammation in this disease, as the inflammation usually subsides without treatment.

Sympathetic ophthalmitis (Figure 11.16)

Sympathetic ophthalmitis is a rare but potentially devastating condition in which penetrating trauma in one eye provokes a granulomatous panuveitis in the other, previously healthy eye. This may occur weeks, months or even years after the initial injury. The inflammation develops gradually and is therefore often missed by the patient and eye care worker. Initially, the 'good eye' becomes painful and photophobic with gradually reducing visual acuity. Large 'mutton-fat' keratic precipitates are seen on the corneal endothelium. The disease is probably caused by an autoimmune response

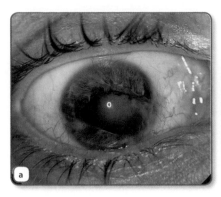
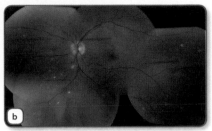

Figure 11.16 Sympathetic ophthalmitis. (a) Penetrating trauma to the right eye. This injury was caused in a knife attack. (b) Sympathetic ophthalmitis of the left eye. The patient's other eye started to develop inflammation about a year after the initial right eye injury. Note the areas of choroidal inflammation and scarring. Also, the view of the retina is slightly hazy, because of vitreous inflammation.

to the injured eye's own uveal proteins. It is very important to advise all patients who have had a penetrating eye injury of the symptoms of sympathetic ophthalmitis as urgent treatment with steroids is required to suppress the disease. Sometimes it is very hard to treat satisfactorily, and prolonged treatment with systemic steroids and other immuno-suppressive drugs may be needed. The slight risk of sympathetic ophthalmitis is removed by early surgical removal of the damaged eye, and lessened by a good early surgical repair of a damaged eye and topical steroids to suppress inflammation.

Uveitis masquerade syndrome

Uveitis is quite common in tumours of the lymphoid system. Patients with lymphomas, reticulum cell sarcomas, and Hodgkin disease may all develop signs of uveitis. It is sometimes called the uveitis masquerade (hidden or disguised) syndrome because masquerade means that the true disease is hidden or masked. Therefore, intraocular lymphoma in older patients is usually misdiagnosed as chronic diffuse uveitis. A bone marrow or lymph node biopsy may help to make the diagnosis. Inflammatory cells can also occur in other intraocular tumours such as retinoblastoma (see page 348), choroidal melanoma and metastatic tumours (see page 269).

Behçet disease

Behçet disease is a rare small-vessel systemic vasculitis. The disease is immune mediated but the environmental and genetic associations and triggers are very poorly understood. Behçet disease is diagnosed when patients have two of the following symptoms or signs: mouth and genital ulcers (**Figure 11.17**), typical skin lesions, uveitis and pathergy reaction (skin papule formation after a skin needle prick). The disease can also affect almost every other part of the body but is particularly damaging when it affects the brain (neuro-Behçet disease). In the eye, Behçet disease typically causes acute anterior uveitis, often with hypopyon (**Figure 11.18**) and inflammation around the retinal blood vessels called retinal vasculitis (**Figure 11.19**), which may

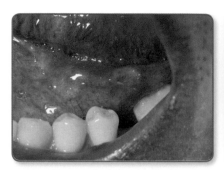

Figure 11.17 Mouth ulcers in Behçet disease.

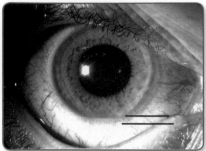

Figure 11.18 The sterile, inflammatory cells have sunk to the bottom of the anterior chamber to form a small hyopyon. This is seen as a fluid level (between red lines) and is easily missed if not specifically looked for.

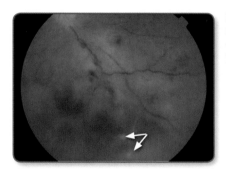

Figure 11.19 Retinal vasculitis and retinal infiltrates (white arrows) in Behçet disease. The view is hazy because of the active inflammation in the vitreous.

cause occlusions of the retinal vessels and therefore retinal ischaemia. The disease is associated with certain HLA antigens (see above), and is found especially in the eastern Mediterranean and Japan.

Vogt–Koyanagi–Harada syndrome

Vogt–Koyanagi–Harada (VKH) syndrome is a rare and poorly understood systemic disease characterised by uveitis, skin and hair depigmentation (vitiligo and poliosis). The clinical picture is very variable and in some patients the disease also affects the brain and auditory system, causing hearing loss, vertigo and inflammatory meningitis. In the eye, VKH typically causes granulomatous anterior uveitis with a variable amount of vitritis. There can also be choroidal inflammation which releases inflammatory fluid between the choroid and retina causing serous retinal detachments (**Figure 11.20**). VKH is most common in Asians, followed by African-Caribbeans.

Sarcoidosis

Sarcoidosis is a multisystem inflammatory disease. The granulomatous inflammation that it causes is similar to tuberculosis, but there is no evidence of an infectious agent and the cause of the disease is unknown. It can affect any tissue but the lungs, eyes and skin are most commonly affected.

It can cause several problems in or around the eye. Inside the eye it causes chronic granulomatous anterior and often posterior uveitis, retinal vasculitis (**Figure 11.21**) and even optic nerve inflammation. The complications of the

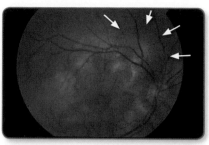

Figure 11.20 Vogt-Koyanagi-Harada syndrome. The choroidal inflammation has caused serous retinal detachment. The edge of some of the detachment has been marked with arrows, but the fluid extends under the whole macula area as well.

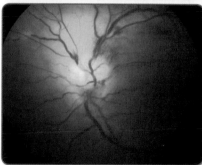

Figure 11.21 Retinitis and optic disc swelling caused by sarcoid.

inflammation, such as secondary glaucoma, cataract, retinal ischaemia and retinal neovascularisation and optic neuritis may be blinding. In the external ocular tissues, the lacrimal glands may be affected thus reducing tear production, and very rarely granulomatous inflammation of the orbit may develop and cause proptosis. It is important to distinguish between sarcoid and tuberculosis because the treatment is very different: steroids for sarcoid and anti-tuberculous drugs for tuberculosis.

Connective tissue diseases

Many connective tissue diseases, such as rheumatoid and psoriatic arthritis are associated with uveitis. These patients often have quite regular recurrences of anterior uveitis, which can usually be managed with topical steroids. Juvenile idiopathic arthritis (JIA, Still's disease) is a particular type of autoimmune arthritis that affects children. These children are at high risk of developing anterior uveitis. However, it is often completely asymptomatic, without even a red eye or photophobia. Therefore, children with a known diagnosis of JIA or with chronic joint pain should be checked regularly (every 3–6 months and more frequently in certain subtypes of the disease) for evidence of intraocular inflammation, otherwise they can slowly and quietly go blind from the complications of the inflammation.

Lens protein induced uveitis

The lens of the eye is sometimes penetrated in severe ocular trauma or inadvertently in surgical procedures and intravitreal injections or may leak from a hypermature cataract. Lens proteins are released from the lens capsule into the rest of the eye. They provoke a vigorous inflammatory response with large keratitic precipitates in the anterior chamber and endothelium and vitreous inflammation. Sometimes an inflammatory hypopyon develops.

The management and treatment of uveitis

Patients with uveitis can be difficult to look after and treat for several reasons:

- Uveitis is often chronic or recurrent and causes significant complications. In these cases, treatment and follow-up needs to be prolonged, which may be difficult in many poor and remote parts of the world.
- The treatment of uveitis with steroids and other anti-inflammatory drugs can itself have complications that may be serious. This is especially true if the treatment is systemic and if it is prolonged. Therefore, the risk of visual loss from the disease must be balanced against the risk of complications from the treatment.
- If the uveitis is caused by, or associated with, another disease then this often needs to be diagnosed and treated as well as treating the uveitis. However, this can be very difficult, even with the access to experts and 'high-tech' investigations that are available in some specialist centres.

Careful history taking and examination, both of the eye and the patient, is critical. This may reveal some important clues that help diagnose particular causes of uveitis that require specific treatment, such as toxoplasmosis, leprosy, tuberculosis, syphilis, sarcoid and intraocular lymphoma.

The basic principle of treatment for all types of uveitis is to try and identify and treat the cause and either simultaneously or subsequently use steroids to control the inflammation. If there is no apparent improvement after treatment with steroids, then consider if there is an infective (including HIV/AIDS) or malignant cause that has been missed, or if the original diagnosis was correct.

Anterior uveitis

Anterior uveitis can usually be treated topically. Acute inflammation will need steroid drops every hour until the inflammation begins to subside, and then a gradual reduction in dose over several weeks. It can be helpful to use a steroid ointment at night in the acute phase to prevent the inflammation worsening whilst the patient is asleep. The patient should also be given a mydriatic such as cyclopentolate 1% (three times/day) or atropine 1% (once/day) to prevent the iris adhering to the lens. The mydriatic usually reduces the pain a little bit. In very severe cases of inflammation or in non-compliant patients a subconjunctival injection of steroid (e.g. betnesol) and a mydriatic can be very effective. The procedure is simply to inject 1–2 mL of the mixture of steroid and mydriatic into the inferior subconjunctival space after instilling plenty of topical anaesthetic (see Chapter 4).

Chronic anterior uveitis requires longer-term steroids that are titrated to the individual patient; some patients need three or four drops per day, while others may need just a drop every other day to control the inflammation.

Some patients develop secondary glaucoma, either from the inflammation or from the steroid treatment. The treatment for this depends on how high the pressure is. Mild to moderately raised pressure can be treated with topical drops such as a beta-blocker (e.g. timolol 0.25–0.5% twice daily). More severe pressure rises may require oral acetazolamide (e.g. 250 mg slow release twice daily). If pupil block glaucoma (iris bombé) develops, mydriatic drops or subconjunctival mydriatic injection may be able to break the ring of adhesions between the iris and the lens. Otherwise an iridectomy operation is necessary.

Choroiditis

Choroiditis must be treated systemically, because topical steroid treatment does not effectively reach the choroid. High doses may be required initially and then these are tapered gradually. Systemic steroids should normally be prescribed and managed by someone with experience with these conditions as they can cause significant side effects (see page 91). Always think carefully about the diagnosis when using oral steroids. They must be used with great caution if there is a risk of any underlying infections such as tuberculosis becoming active.

In chronic uveitis other immuno-suppressive drugs, such as cyclosporin, cyclophosphamide and azathioprine may be used. These drugs can also have serious toxic side effects, and are usually given under specialist supervision. However, they may be more effective than steroids or they may allow the steroid dose to be reduced or even stopped (they are therefore often called 'steroid-sparing agents).

Uveal tumours

Primary tumours and secondary uveal tumours can occur, although both are relatively rare.

Uveal melanomas

These are the most common form of intraocular tumour, but they are very rare in black people. They usually arise in the choroid (**Figure 11.22**), but occasionally in the iris (**Figure 11.23**) or ciliary body. They mainly occur in older people. On funduscopy, they appear as a solid raised mass usually in

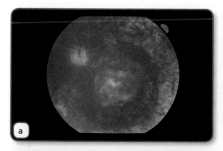
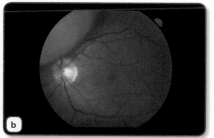
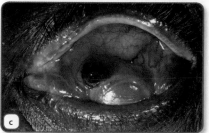

Figure 11.22 Choroidal melanoma. (a) A pigmented choroidal melanoma that has developed from a naevus. (b) A very large choroidal non-pigmented melanoma coming out of the choroid into the vitreous in the top left of the picture. (c) A choroidal melanoma that has not been treated and has grown out of the eye.

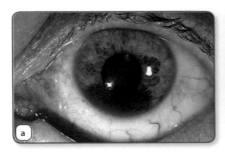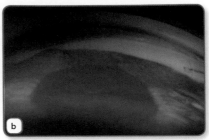

Figure 11.23 (a) An iris melanoma. (b) The same melanoma seen with a gonioscopic lens. It is growing behind the iris and lifting it up.

the peripheral fundus. They can cause retinal detachment and sometimes glaucoma. The tumour may metastasise to other parts of the body and most commonly the liver. In the early stages, it may be possible to treat the tumour with radiation therapy or an intraocular radioactive plaque, or to excise small tumours of the iris and ciliary body surgically. However, early diagnosis and very specialist facilities are required for this type of treatment. Therefore, in most cases the only treatment is to enucleate the eye.

Uveal metastases

Tumours from other parts of the body occasionally spread by metastasis to the uvea, usually the choroid. The primary sites vary but the most common is carcinoma of the breast. These secondary tumours are often multiple and may be in both eyes.

Degenerative changes

Degeneration and atrophy of the uveal tissue is common. It may occur after uveitis or glaucoma, or it may be part of the ageing process. There are also various rare primary degenerations of the uvea, which are usually hereditary.

Atrophy of the iris (**Figure 11.10**) affects both the pigment and the muscle cells. The iris appears depigmented, and the pupil is often dilated, irregular and will not react to light.

Atrophy of the ciliary body may occur. The aqueous secretion will decrease and the eye becomes soft. Atrophy of the choroid is especially common in old people, and usually involves the posterior part of the choroid around the macula. Choroidal atrophy also occurs after choroiditis (**Figure 11.13**) and onchocerciasis (see Figure 16.7). The exact pattern of the choroidal atrophy will vary, but there are usually two features:

1. *Pigment changes.* There is atrophy of the choroidal pigment, but sometimes patches of increased pigmentation. The retinal pigment epithelium may also be affected.
2. *Blood vessel changes.* The fine choroidal blood vessels (called the 'choriocapillaris') atrophy to show the outline of the larger choroidal blood vessels.

Tuberculosis

Tuberculosis (TB) remains one of the commonest infectious causes of death worldwide. Most of these deaths happen in poor countries. The ophthalmic effects of TB can be very varied and very damaging.

TB epidemiology

The WHO estimates that 9 million cases of TB were diagnosed in 2010 and there were 1.45 million deaths from the disease. The bulk of this occurs in China, India and Africa. The prevalence of multidrug resistant TB (resistant to isoniazid and rifampicin) and extremely drug-resistant TB (resistant to fluoroquinolones and at least one of three injectable drugs) is increasing. TB infection is strongly associated with HIV infection (see Chapter 20) because of the increased vulnerability to infection.

TB infection

TB is spread from person to person by inhaling the TB bacilli. The bacteria settle in the lung, which becomes the primary focus of infection. It spreads locally to the lymphatic nodes of the mediastinum, which can be seen on a chest X-ray as hilar lymphadenopathy. A few bacteria may spread around the body and lodge elsewhere but not cause symptoms. In most people the immune response keeps the infection localised and dormant ('asleep'). However it can reactivate from any of the places that it has lodged, most commonly within the first 2 years of getting the initial infection. This is called secondary disease. The most common sites for reactivation are the upper lobes of the lung, but it can occur anywhere in the body, including the eyes and brain. Occasionally, TB infection spreads rapidly and widely round the body or reactivates in lots of places at the same time. This is called miliary TB.

TB and the eye

The symptoms and signs of ocular TB

TB in the eye is not common, but it can present in many different ways. Diagnosing it correctly and starting treatment early makes a big difference, so be vigilant! The most common effect of TB in the eye is posterior uveitis and panuveitis. However, TB can affect almost any part of the eye and therefore the diagnosis of ocular TB is often missed. The diagnosis must be considered in anyone with compatible or unexplained eye signs. TB has always been an essential differential diagnosis in poor countries where the disease is common, but now must be considered in rich countries, where increased migration and the AIDS epidemic have greatly increased TB incidence. The main ocular effects of TB are listed in **Table 11.3**. Some of these are from the actual bacterium itself, such as choroidal granulomas (which has TB bacteria within it), while others are a hypersensitivity reaction to circulating tubercular protein, e.g. corneal phlycten and retinal vasculitis. Many of these are discussed in other chapters. We will discuss some of the more common manifestations below.

Table 11.3 The effects of TB in the eye arranged by anatomical location	
Location	**Effect on eye**
External	
Lacrimal gland	Dacryoadenitis
Eyelid	Ulceration and lymphadenopathy Lupus vulgaris
Orbit	Cellulitis Osteomyelitis
Anterior	
Episclera	Episcleritis*
Cornea	Peripheral ulcerative keratitis* Interstitial keratitis* Phlyctenulosis (see page 211) *
Iris	Iris granulomas
Ciliary body	Ciliary body granulomas
Sclera/uvea	
Sclera	Nodular or diffuse scleritis
Uvea	Anterior granulomatous uveitis Posterior uveitis/panuveitis
Posterior	
Choroid	Choroidal granuloma (tuberculoma) Presumed tubercular serpiginous-like choroiditis (**Figure 11.24**)
Retina	Retinitis Retinal occlusive vasculitis (Eales disease)*
Neuro-ophthalmology	
Optic nerve	Direct TB infiltration Papillitis: 'pink discs' Papilloedema from increased intracranial pressure
Cranial nerves	Diplopia can result from TB meningitis which can cause multiple cranial nerve palsies, internuclear ophthalmoplegia and gaze palsies.

*All these conditions are caused by a reaction to the tubercle protein, rather than the TB bacillus itself

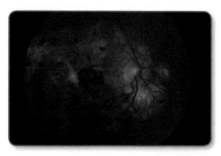

Figure 11.24 Presumed tubercular serpiginous-like choroiditis.

Interstitial keratitis (Figure 11.25)

Interstitial keratitis is inflammation of the stroma of the cornea. It is usually unilateral. The cornea is often inflamed for long periods with acute exacerbations. It is often associated with scleritis.

Uveitis

Tuberculosis may cause inflammation of any part of the uvea. Anterior uveitis is usually granulomatous with 'mutton fat' keratic precipitates and iris nodules. Posterior uveitis causes vigorous vitreous inflammation with vitreous opacities.

Patients with chronic tuberculosis can develop small nodules in the uveal tissue or rarely a large mass with an inflammatory reaction around it. Such a mass is suspicious of tuberculosis. If the disease is not treated, it may eventually spread to involve the whole eye. **Figure 11.28** shows an eye with severe uveitis and a subconjunctival tuberculoma.

Retinitis (Figure 11.26)

Retinal infection starts in the retinal vessels and can cause either extensive destructive retinitis with vigorous vitreous inflammation or form lots of small tubercles that remain localised and eventually heal (military type, or superficial exudative retinitis).

Retinal vasculitis (Figure 11.26)

Hypersensitivity to the TB protein can cause retinal vascular inflammation. This often occurs in patients who have not had symptomatic systemic TB or long after patients have been successfully treated for TB.

Choroidal tubercles

The choroid is a common place for the development of TB granulomas, because they spread there in the blood stream. They can be solitary dormant granulomas, or in miliary TB there can be multiple granulomas, which cause a vigorous posterior uveitis. (**Figure 11.27**). Tubercles can form anywhere in the body (**Figure 11.28**), but ocular ones can be very helpful in clinically confirming the diagnosis of the TB, particularly when laboratory investigations are inaccessible.

The treatment of TB

Eye-care workers sometimes make the initial diagnosis of TB when a patient presents with ocular signs. The most important part of treatment is systemic anti-tuberculous drugs. A combination of drugs will be required for 6–18 months depending on the country, the patient and the type of TB. Many ocular problems will resolve with treatment. Once the patient has received treatment for TB, steroids can be considered for the

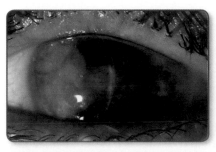

Figure 11.25 Interstitial keratitis.

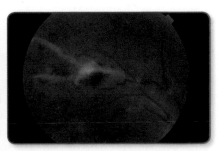

Figure 11.26 Tuberculous retinitis.

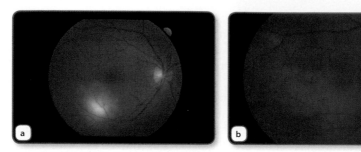

Figure 11.27 Tuberculosis affecting the choroid. (a) A choroidal tubercle in miliary tuberculosis. (b) Tuberculous choroiditis.

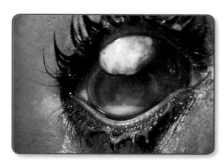

Figure 11.28 Tuberculosis of the eye. This patient has a large inflammatory granuloma under the upper lid, and a chronic uveitis with a hypopyon. Both of these are from tuberculosis, but it is unusual to see two different signs of tuberculosis in the same eye.

inflammatory complications of TB, although this should ideally be managed by an expert.

Syphilis and the eye

Syphilis is an infection caused by the spirochaete bacteria *Treponema pallidum.* Syphilis remains highly prevalent worldwide, and in recent years there has been an increase in cases, in association with the AIDS epidemic. There are three stages of syphilis:
- Primary: an infection occurs at the site of infection, usually the genitals.
- Secondary: the infection spreads through the blood stream and settles in places in the skin and mucous membranes.
- Tertiary: the infection provokes chronic inflammation and degeneration with necrosis of the cardiovascular and central nervous systems.

The eye can be affected in every stage of the infection as well as in congenital syphilis (see Chapter 22).

Ocular complications of syphilis

The main ocular complications of syphilis are described in **Table 11.4**.

Leptospirosis

Leptospirosis is another spirochaete infection. It is caught by touching soil or water that is contaminated by the urine of infected animals. Rats are the commonest source of the disease, but other animals including other rodents, dogs, pigs and even cattle can also spread it. It causes a systemic infection, which typically causes 'flu'-like symptoms, such as headache, sweats and

Table 11.4 The ocular complications of ocular syphilis			
Location	Pathology	Syphilitic stage	Comment
Eyelid	Chancre	Primary	
Conjunctiva	Conjunctivitis, nodules	Secondary	
Cornea	Interstitial/stromal keratitis	Any	Usually bilateral
Iris	Iris atrophy (**Figure 11.10**). Argyll Robertson pupil	Any Tertiary	Consequence of anterior uveitis A pupil that constricts with accommodation but not to light
Lens	Dislocation	Any	
Uvea	Anterior uveitis Chorioretinitis (**Figure 11.29**)	Any	Can occur up to 20 years after the infection. No specific identifying features, therefore diagnosis of syphilis often missed in patients with uveitis
Optic nerve	Optic atrophy (see Chapter 14)	Tertiary	

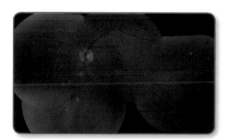

Figure 11.29 Syphilitic chorioretinitis.

chills and muscle aches. The likelihood of getting uveitis when infected with leptospirosis is unknown which is proved by small studies finding uveitis in between 2% to 92% of patients! In the eye it is typically bilateral and can cause a wide range of inflammatory pictures, including anterior or intermediate, posterior, pan-uveitis, vasculitis and optic nerve inflammation (papillitis).

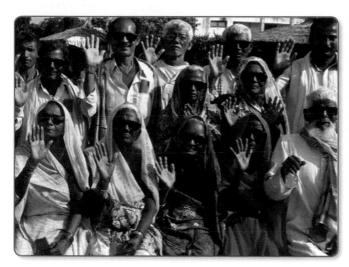

Cataract surgery with intraocular lens implantation is one of the miracles of modern medicine. These happy patients were all operated on the previous day by one surgeon.

The lens of the eye is a unique structure for several reasons:
- It is transparent, and has no blood or nerve supply.
- It has a higher protein content than any other body tissue.
- It continues to grow throughout life. New fibres form just beneath the capsule, while the older fibres are compressed towards the centre of the lens. As a person gets older, a hard nucleus is formed at the centre of the lens, with a slightly softer cortex around it and the lens becomes less transparent.

Ageing and the lens

Various degenerative and ageing changes occur in the lens, probably because of its unusual structure. These changes occur to some degree in everyone, as they grow older. The major changes that occur in the lens with age are listed in **Box 12.1** and are described in more detail below:

1. *Increase in hardness and loss of accommodation*
   The lens becomes harder. This reduces its ability to changes shape.
   The young healthy lens changes its shape during the process of

---

Box 12.1 Changes in the lens with age
1. Increase in hardness
2. Increase in density
3. Increase in size
4. Increase in opacity

accommodation when the eyes focus on a near object. It changes from being thinner to fatter every time we focus on a nearer object (**Figure 5.6**) so, with increasing age, there is increasing difficulty in focusing on near objects. This process is called '*presbyopia*' and it occurs in everyone (see page 108). Therefore, spectacles are required for close work and reading. Reading glasses are usually first needed between the ages of 35 and 50 years, and with increasing age the glasses need to be stronger.

2. *Increase in density*
    The lens becomes denser. This may change its refractive power. If the central nucleus becomes denser (called nuclear sclerosis), the refractive power of the lens increases and the eye becomes short-sighted (myopic). This is called lens-induced or index myopia. Less commonly, the outer cortex may become denser so the power of the lens decreases and the eye becomes more longsighted or hypermetropic. If the increased density is balanced throughout the entire lens, the refraction will not change.

3. *Increase in size*
    The lens becomes larger. Occasionally, a very enlarged lens pushes the iris forward so much that the drainage angle is blocked and acute glaucoma develops (see Chapter 15).

4. *Increase in opacity: cataract*
    An opacity in the lens is called a '*cataract*' (Greek: waterfall), because vision is similar to looking through a waterfall. Cataract is caused by biochemical damage to the delicate protein structure of the lens cells. Although, with age, the lens loses some of its clarity in almost everyone, it only really becomes a disease process when the patient is symptomatic from it, i.e. the patient is aware or troubled by the visual impairment. Most people over the age of 60 years have some degree of lens opacity if the eye is examined carefully, although this usually causes little or no loss of vision. These are sometimes called *early* or *immature* cataracts. As the opacity progresses, the vision becomes increasingly blurred. Eventually the lens becomes completely opaque and the vision is lost. This is sometimes called a *mature* cataract. Further degenerative changes may occur and this is often called a *hypermature* cataract. This can even involve the lens cortex becoming fluid and sometimes leaking out of the capsule. The progression of lens opacities varies greatly. Occasionally, a patient develops a mature cataract only a few months after the first signs of opacity in the lens. By contrast, early opacities may be present in the lens for many years with no obvious progression at all. However, once an opacity has formed, it does not normally disappear spontaneously.

The causes and the epidemiology of cataract

The causes of cataract are very complex. Some of the causes are clearly understood and some are not. One of the biggest problems in studying the epidemiology of cataract is to have a precise and agreed definition of exactly what is meant by cataract. The changes of cataract progress very gradually, and one observer and one study may not have exactly the same definition as another. However, the following principles are clear:

1. The biggest risk factor for cataract is age.
2. Life in tropical countries and poor countries increases the risk of developing cataract.
3. Some diseases cause or are associated with cataract.

A risk factor for cataract is something that will make it more prevalent in the community.

Cataract and age

Age is the most important cause of cataract. If we all lived long enough, we would all in the end develop cataracts, although it is not entirely clear what aspect of aging causes the lens to lose its clarity. About three quarters of normal healthy people have developed some signs of cataract by the age of 80 years, though in most cases this is not bad enough to cause serious visual loss (**Figure 12.1**).

Cataract and a tropical environment and poor countries

Cataracts are more common and occur at an earlier age in people living in hot, tropical climates. They are approximately six times more common in a typical poor, tropical country than in a rich country, with a temperate climate. It is unclear if there are differences in racial susceptibility to cataract and there are many different theories as to why cataract is so much more common in hot climates. It is probable that several or all of the factors listed below contribute to the development of cataract in the tropics.

Episodes of severe dehydration in early life

Severe dehydration caused by gastroenteritis or acute fevers can damage the lens proteins. The mechanism is called 'osmotic shock'. It is suggested that repeated episodes will eventually lead to cataract formation in later life.

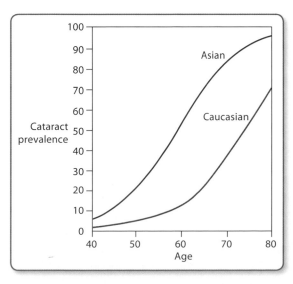

Figure 12.1 Comparing the prevalence of cataract with age in Indian immigrants and Europeans living in the same city in England and of similar economic backgrounds. All the immigrants had recently migrated to England. Cataract was defined as a visual acuity of 6/9 or worse attributed to opacification of the lens. Cataract becomes much more common with increasing age and people from a tropical environment are more likely to develop cataract at a younger age.

Solar radiation

The lens absorbs some of the sun's rays, especially in the ultraviolet wavelengths. It is thought that this causes damage to the tissue enzymes and the protein molecules, which may lead to cataract formation.

Diet

In most communities, it is found that poor people have a higher prevalence of cataract than rich people. It is possible that having a diet deficient in vitamins, especially vitamin C, may predispose to cataract formation. Furthermore high levels of vitamin C may prevent damage to the lens from solar radiation.

Heat

Heat alone may be significant, either as infra-red rays or as a rise in the ambient temperature. Glass-blowers, who work in front of very hot furnaces when making glass objects, have a greatly increased risk of cataract, probably because of the heat or infra-red rays. It seems that the prevalence of cataract is highest in those areas where seasonal temperatures become extremely high.

Cataract, and systemic and ocular disease

Many systemic diseases are associated with or cause cataract (**Table 12.1**). There are also many ocular diseases that can cause cataract. These are discussed below. Many of these systemic and ocular conditions are extremely rare. However, it is very important to conduct a thorough search for associated disease if a cataract is identified in a child or young adult. Most cataracts develop in adults but they can also be congenital. The causes of congenital cataract are somewhat different and are discussed later (see page 307).

Eye diseases and cataract

Uveitis

Both the inflammation itself and the steroids used to treat it can cause cataract (Figure 11.9)

Glaucoma

Patients with glaucoma have a higher risk of developing cataract. The likelihood of cataract increases if the patient uses pilocarpine treatment or has glaucoma (trabeculectomy) surgery.

Trauma

Eye injuries often cause cataract (**Figure 12.2**). Perforating injuries that damage the lens cause an immediate cataract. A severe non-penetrating injury will often produce cataract after a delay of some months or even years. Even simply touching the lens, which can occur in trauma or surgery will cause a localised cataract at the point of contact. This may then spread gradually throughout the lens. Intraocular surgery such as retinal detachment surgery will speed up the development of cataract even if the lens is not touched during the surgery. Most patients who have a vitrectomy will require cataract surgery within the next few years.

Table 12.1 Associations and causes of cataract

Systemic disease/risk factor	Comment/examples
Endocrine disease	
Diabetes*	Diabetics develop cataracts more frequently and at a younger age than non-diabetics
Hypothyroidism	
Other rare endocrine conditions	e.g. Galactosaemia, hypocalcaemia, hyperparathyroidism
Genetic metabolic conditions	
Wilson's disease	Disorder of copper metabolism, causing sunflower cataract
Myotonic dystrophy	Disease causing muscle wasting and causes anterior and posterior polar cataracts
Other rare metabolic conditions	
Drugs and medications	
Steroid medication*	Long term steroid use, both ocular and systemic causes cataract formation
Alcohol*	Thought to be related to rapidly maturing subcapsular cataracts
Anticholinesterase miotics, e.g. pilocarpine	
Phenothiazines	Anterior subcapsular granular opacities
Systemic infections	
Congenital viral infections*	e.g. Fetal cataracts caused by rubella and chicken pox (varicella zoster) during pregnancy
Congenital syphilis	
Congenital toxoplasmosis	
Skin Diseases	
Atopic dermatitis	Cataracts in 10% of patients with chronic disease. Typically anterior and posterior cataracts . Cataracts also occur with some other very rare skin diseases
Chromosomal disorders	
Down's syndrome*	Cataracts in 50% of patients.
Turner syndrome	
Other rare diseases	e.g. Patau syndrome, Edward syndrome
Skeletal diseases	e.g. Conradi syndrome, osteogenesis imperfecta, Pierre Robin syndrome, Rubinstein-Taybi syndrome
Syndromes that cause lens displacement	
Marfan syndrome	Autosomal dominant genetic condition
Homocystinuria	Inborn error of metabolism
Ehlers–Danlos syndrome	Inherited defect of collagen production
Syndromes that also cause pigmentary, retinal degeneration	e.g. Laurence–Moon–Biedl syndrome, Usher syndrome, Cockayne syndrome

*Common causes of cataract.

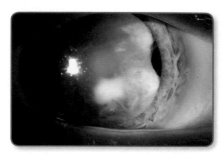

Figure 12.2 Traumatic cataract. This eye received a heavy blunt trauma damaging the zonules that hold the lens causing them to stretch and detach, and the lens to move sideways. The trauma also caused cataract to form.

Myopia

Extreme short-sightedness is associated with earlier cataract development

Radiation

Patients who have received radiotherapy to the head from any source will develop cataracts if the eyes have not been shielded.

Protective factors

At present there are no clearly identified factors that prevent cataract formation, except for avoiding risk factors such as smoking, alcohol and childhood nutritional deficiencies and diarrhoea. Periodically, people claim to have developed drops that prevent cataracts progressing. There is no evidence to support any of these, and therefore currently the only treatment for cataract is surgery.

The symptoms of cataract

Visual loss

Cataracts cause gradual loss of vision. Some cataracts, e.g. age related nuclear sclerosis, usually develops very slowly (many years) and the patient may not even notice the loss of vision. Other cataracts, such as posterior subcapsular cataract can greatly impair the vision over a few months. Eventually, when a cataract is mature, the visual acuity falls to perception of light only. Occasionally, patients present with 'sudden' loss of vision and are diagnosed with cataract in one eye and no other ocular disease. This is because although the cataract has been present for some time, they only noticed it when they closed the good eye, which had been compensating whilst the cataract was developing.

Refractive changes

Nuclear sclerosis usually causes the eye to become more myopic. This is usually up to about 4 dioptres, but can be as much as 10 dioptres! Patients who wear glasses may report that their glasses prescription needs to be changed frequently.

Dazzling

Dazzling is caused by the cataract scattering light around the eye. This is usually most troublesome in the evenings when looking at a bright light. Cortical cataracts can frequently cause very symptomatic dazzling despite hardly affecting the visual acuity. Some central cataracts can also cause dazzling as the pupil constricts in bright light, causing all light to go through the opacity, but when the light is less bright the pupil dilates, and the light can enter through the clear lens around the cataract.

Multiple images (ghosting, or polyopia)
The lens can cause variable refraction, which forms more than one image on the retina. The patient therefore sees one or more blurred 'ghost' images along with the true image. It is very important to distinguish this monocular diplopia (double vision when looking through just one eye) from binocular diplopia (double vision when both eyes are open), which is caused by conditions such as squint and neurological disease.

Haloes
These are rainbow-coloured rings around white lights that are caused by the opacities in the lens splitting the light into the colours of the spectrum. Remember that haloes are more often a symptom of corneal oedema and raised intraocular pressure from angle closure glaucoma.

Clinical examination of a cataract

The most important part of assessing a cataract is asking the patient whether they are symptomatic from it. You will be very surprised that some patients with quite mature cataracts complain very little and therefore may very reasonably decline surgery, whilst others with early cataract may complain bitterly. The examination of the cataract requires first testing the pupil light reflexes (see page 69) and then dilating the pupil. The reason for testing the light reflex is to detect other disease in the eye (and it is therefore discussed below), but this must be tested *before* dilating the pupil.

Examination of the lens

The steps of examining a patient for cataract are described in **Box 12.2**. Although a dense white cataract can easily be seen with a torch (**Figure 12.5**), the majority of cataracts required a careful examination with the pupil dilated to determine their type and density. Some types of cataract

---

Box 12.2 The steps of cataract examination
Before dilating
1. Visual acuity
2. Pupil light reflexes, including checking for a relative afferent papillary defect
3. Intraocular pressure

After dilating
4. Assess the external eye for conditions that may be connected to the cataract, e.g. trauma, atopic skin disease
5. Red reflex, using the direct ophthalmoscope
6. Slit lamp examination of cataract if available
7. Retinal and optic nerve examination

such as posterior subcapsular and those with a black nucleus will be completely missed unless a careful examination of the red reflex or slit lamp assessment is done. At this stage, it is sensible to reconsider the three different types of illumination used to examine the eye, diffuse, focal and coaxial illumination and the appearance of the normal lens. The principles of each of these are described on page 62 (Figure 3.13). Each type of illumination will give the normal healthy lens a different appearance.

Figure 12.3 shows the same eight cataractous lenses that had been removed from patients' eyes and were illuminated in two different ways. In **Figure 12.3a** they are illuminated from the front (reflected light) and in **Figure 12.3b** from behind (transilluminated light). Some are mature cataracts, and some are immature. In some the opacity is in the nucleus, which usually goes brown or black. In some the opacity is in outer cortex, which usually goes white, and this may obscure the central nucleus so it cannot be seen. Sometimes the capsule of the lens goes opaque as well, usually white. Note how the appearance varies from lens to lens, and also with different illumination. Normal lenses are usually of the same size but cataract lenses may vary considerably in size (**Figure 12.4**).

Using an ophthalmoscope

An ophthalmoscope, which uses coaxial illumination, is often the quickest and simplest way to determine if a patient has a cataract and get an idea

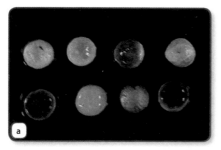
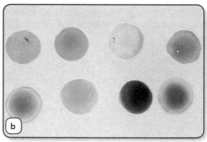

Figure. 12.3 Eight cataracts seen with different illumination. (a) The light is coming from the front of the lenses (reflected light). (b) The light is coming from underneath the lenses (transilluminated light).

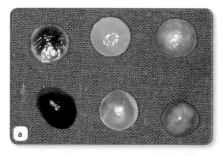
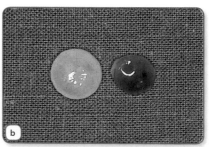

Figure 12.4 A group of cataracts against a green cloth background. (a) Variation in appearance of the cataracts. (b) Variation in size of cataracts.

about how dense this is. The +5 dioptre lens is used and the ophthalmoscope is held about 10–20 cm away from the patient's eye. In an eye without a cataract, a clear red reflex from the fundus is seen and there are no shadows or distortions interrupting this (see Figure 3.13c).

Using a slit lamp

A slit lamp is not needed for diagnosing a cataract and it is usually only specialists who have access to them. However, the focal illumination and magnification of the slit lamp give a precise view of the opacities and where they are, and make them stand out.

Type of cataract

There are three common sites within the lens where the opacity is most significant: the cortex, the nucleus and the area just in front of the posterior capsule. In the early stages, each of these different types of opacities will have a different appearance. Often in practice more than one type of opacity is present. For instance there may be changes in both the nucleus and the cortex. Eventually, the entire lens becomes completely opaque and usually appears as a white opaque mass (**Figure 12.5**).

1. **Cortical lens opacities (Figures 12.6 and 12.7)**
   These are the most common type of opacities. The opacities develop in the outer (or cortical) layers of the lens, and they appear white against the normally dark pupil. The opacities usually radiate from the centre of the eye like the spokes of a wheel. In the early stages they often do not reach the centre of the lens and the patient can see well although might report symptoms of glare. Cortical cataract has different appearances with the different types of illumination (**Figures 12.6 and 12.7**).

2. **Nucleus lens opacity: nuclear sclerosis (Figure 12.8)**
   Sclerosis actually means hardening. However, as the nucleus 'hardens', it also becomes darker in colour: first yellow, then brown, and finally black. If the lens cortex has already become white and opaque, the changes in the lens nucleus are not visible. Often, however the cortex remains transparent so the changes in the nucleus can be seen. As with cortical cataracts, the appearance of nuclear sclerotic cataract varies with the illumination (**Figure 12.8**). In cases of early nuclear sclerosis the patient may have no visual complaints except a change in their refraction. The red reflex is present but will be duller depending on how dense the cataract is.

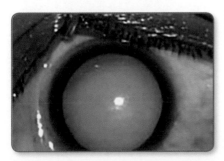

Figure 12.5 (a) A dense, mature, white cataract (vision perception of light). The pupil has been dilated with a mydriatic.

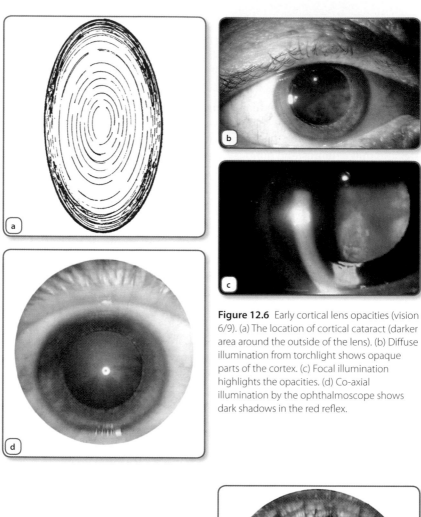

Figure 12.6 Early cortical lens opacities (vision 6/9). (a) The location of cortical cataract (darker area around the outside of the lens). (b) Diffuse illumination from torchlight shows opaque parts of the cortex. (c) Focal illumination highlights the opacities. (d) Co-axial illumination by the ophthalmoscope shows dark shadows in the red reflex.

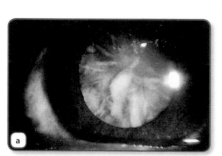

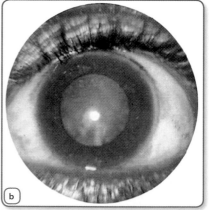

Figure 12.7 More advanced cortical lens opacities (vision 6/60). (a) With diffuse (torchlight) illumination it looks quite like a dense mature cataract. (b) With the ophthalmoscope, a partial red reflex can just be seen through the upper part of the lens.

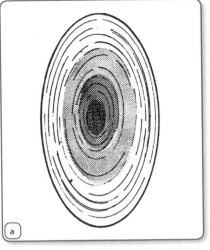

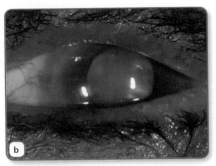

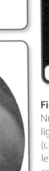

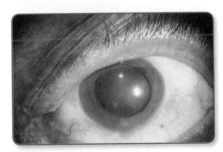

Figure 12.8 Nuclear sclerotic cataract. (a) Nuclear sclerotic cataract location. (b) Diffuse light shows the brown colour of the lens. (c) Slit lamp focal illumination shows the outer lens (cortex, red arrow) is quite clear, but the central lens (nucleus, white arrow) is yellow and opaque. (d) The red reflex is clear but slightly dull.

Figure 12.9 Dense nuclear sclerosis causing a 'black' cataract. The lens is totally opaque but appears quite similar to a normal eye when seen with diffuse illumination.

Occasionally, nuclear sclerosis progresses to a stage when the whole lens becomes black and opaque (**Figure 12.9**). These 'black' cataracts are rather unusual, and are sometimes missed because the pupil also appears black in a normal eye. However, with coaxial illumination, the red reflex is absent. The other common cause of the red reflex appearing black is a dense vitreous haemorrhage and a slit lamp may be required to distinguish them.

3. **Posterior subcapsular lens opacities**

    Overall these are less common than nuclear and cortical cataracts but are often the type of cataract that is found in younger patients. A thin, opaque layer develops just inside the posterior capsule of the lens. Because this opacity is so far back in the lens the eye appears normal with torchlight examination (diffuse illumination). With the coaxial illumination of an ophthalmoscope and the slit lamp the opacity can be clearly seen (**Figure 12.10**). Posterior subcapsular opacities have several specific clinical features:

    - They are often missed because the lens looks normal with simple torchlight examination.
    - They cause quite significant visual impairment firstly because they form quite an opaque layer and secondly they are at the back of the lens where the light rays are converging towards the retina.
    - They often cause particularly pronounced symptoms in bright light, when the pupil constricts. In dim light when the pupil enlarges the patient can often see round the edge of the opacity.

Other cataract morphologies

There are other types and appearances of cataract, especially in congenital and traumatic cataracts, but these are less common.

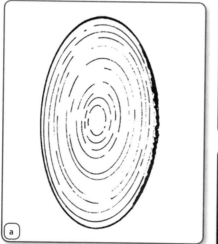

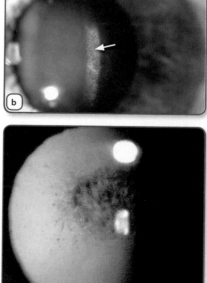

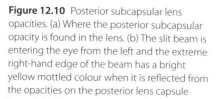

Figure 12.10 Posterior subcapsular lens opacities. (a) Where the posterior subcapsular opacity is found in the lens. (b) The slit beam is entering the eye from the left and the extreme right-hand edge of the beam has a bright yellow mottled colour when it is reflected from the opacities on the posterior lens capsule (arrow). (c) PSC cataract seen with an ophthalmoscope. The opacities stand out clearly as dark grey or black in the red reflex.

Examination of the retina

After examining the front of the eye, the pupil should be dilated with mydriatic drops so that the retina can be assessed. The retina can only be seen in patients with early cataracts, because a dense cataract obscures any view. If there is no view of the retina, then other tests should be done (as below) to try to determine if the retina and optic nerve are healthy.

The assessment of cataract in eyes with other pathology

Eyes with cataract may also have other diseases, such as retinal detachment, glaucoma and optic atrophy. It may be difficult to determine how much of the patient's visual loss is from cataract, and how much from other eye diseases. This is particularly the case in patients with glaucoma or macular degeneration, which are also common in elderly people. The following tests may be helpful.

Visual acuity

A useful guide is that if any red reflex at all is visible, the patient's vision should be 'counting fingers' or better. Therefore if some red reflex is visible, and the patient's vision is worse than 'counting fingers', some other eye disease is probably present as well.

Reading vision

If the patient is able to read, assessment of the reading vision wearing reading glasses is informative, particularly in patients who also have macular degeneration. Macular degeneration affects the vision in a different way to a cataract. A patient with early cataract alone should still be able to read moderate sized or large print even though the distance vision is getting blurred. However, if the patient also has macular degeneration, the reading vision is often much worse affected than one would expect from just the early cataract.

Pinhole vision

If the visual acuity improves with a pinhole (see page 50) it usually means that the patient needs spectacles. However, sometimes the vision improves with a pinhole but cannot be improved with spectacles. The most common reason for this is a problem in the cornea or lens that prevents the light rays from being focused clearly on the retina, which is avoided when a pinhole is used. If this situation occurs in older patients, it usually means they have a cataract, because lens opacities are so common in this age group. Visual acuity with a pinhole is also a reliable sign that the macula is healthy and that there is no macular degeneration. However, the pinhole vision will not improve in patients with dense cataract.

The pupil light reflex

This is an essential part of cataract examination and is an important way to look for serious retinal or optic nerve problems in patients in which the cataract is too dense to allow these parts of the eye to be seen. The swinging light test must be used to check for an afferent and a relative afferent pupillary defect (APD and RAPD) (see page 69). This simple test is often missed and patients with cataract and optic nerve disease therefore undergo cataract surgery unnecessarily. If the eye with the cataract also has a total APD, there must be other pathology, such as optic nerve or major retinal pathology. Therefore, cataract surgery would not be expected to improve the vision. Surgery is an unnecessary risk to the patient, provides false expectations and is a waste of precious resources as the outcome could have been predicted with this simple pre-operative test. However, if there is an RAPD cataract surgery can still be considered as some improvement may occur, but the patient must be warned about the uncertain outcome. The RAPD test is more difficult (but not impossible) to conduct in an eye that has a condition that prevents the pupil moving, such as adhesions between the iris and lens (posterior synechiae).

Projection of light

Even a mature cataract will allow some light to reach the retina. The patient should therefore be able to detect the direction the light is coming from. This is called projection of light. It is important when one sees a patient with just light perception vision to check if they have projection of light, as poor projection of light indicates serious retinal or optic nerve disease.

Intraocular pressure

If there is doubt about glaucoma the intraocular pressure should be tested. High pressure is a risk for glaucomatous optic nerve damage.

A small memory aid for the additional tests that should be conducted in patients with a cataract is: **p**in hole, **p**upil reaction, **p**rojection, **p**ressure and **p**osterior part of the eye all begin with the letter 'p'.

Complications of cataract

Phacomorphic glaucoma and phacolytic uveitis and glaucoma

A mature cataract if not removed may occasionally undergo further degenerative changes. The death and degeneration of lens cells causes the lens cortex to liquefy. These degenerate fluid proteins inside the lens capsule absorb even more fluid by osmosis so the lens swells. This is called an *intumescent or hypermature* cataract and is still sometimes referred to by its old name of Morgagnian cataract. The solid brown nucleus can sometimes be seen inside the milky-white fluid cortex (**Figure 12.11**). Intumescent

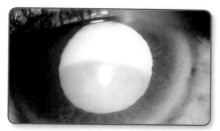

Figure 12.11 An intumescent or hypermature cataract. The brown nucleus can be seen floating inside the fluid, milky cortex.

cataracts may remain quietly in the eye for some time but there is a great risk of two serious complications developing:

1. *Phacomorphic (from the Greek for lens shape) angle closure glaucoma (**Figure 12.12 a and b**)*
   A large swollen lens pushes the iris forward and makes the anterior chamber of the eye shallower. It can cause the drainage angle to become occluded and the pressure in the eye to rise very quickly, i.e. angle closure glaucoma.

2. *Phacolytic uveitis and glaucoma (**Figure 12.13**)*
   Sometimes the lens capsule ruptures because it cannot stretch any more as the lens gets bigger. Lens protein leaks out into the anterior chamber. This causes acute inflammation in the eye (uveitis). The aqueous fluid appears milky because of the leaking lens protein. The lens protein is ingested by macrophages. The inflammation, macrophages and lens protein blocks the drainage of aqueous causing the pressure to rise in the eye.

If urgent treatment for phacomorphic glaucoma or phacolytic uveitis is not given, the eye will quickly become permanently blind from optic nerve damage. The high pressure must be controlled (usually with oral or intravenous

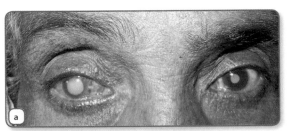
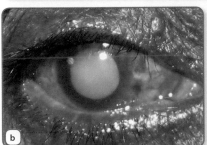

Figure 12.12 Cataract and phacomorphic glaucoma (angle closure glaucoma from a large cataract). (a) The patient has bilateral cataracts. No mydriatics have been applied to the eye but the left pupil is normal and the right is dilated and fixed. (b) A close up view of the right eye shows that it is inflamed with dilation of the ciliary vessels, and the cornea is slightly oedematous from raised intraocular pressure. Angle closure glaucoma has occurred in this eye from a swollen lens. Unfortunately, it is too late to restore the sight in this patient's right eye with surgery, but the left eye is treatable.

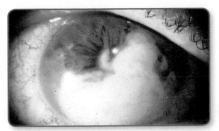

Figure 12.13 Phacolytic uveitis. The white mass is leaking lens protein and inflammatory cells. Very often this white milky mass is more evenly spread throughout the anterior chamber.

acetazolamide initially) and the lens removed as soon as possible. The inflammation is treated with intensive steroid drops before and after the surgery. If phacolytic uveitis is not treated, all the fluid lens proteins from the lens cortex will eventually leak out through the lens capsule and be absorbed. A small, solid brown nucleus inside a shrivelled capsule will be all that remains. However by this time uveitis or glaucoma have usually blinded the eye. The optic nerve damage will be detected by the tests described above, even if the retina and optic nerve cannot be seen through the opaque nucleus.

Lens subluxation and dislocation

In eyes with large, opaque, mature cataracts the suspensory ligament that supports the lens occasionally degenerates and becomes weak. The lens can sublux or dislocate (**Figure 12.14**). The signs of a subluxated or dislocated lens are described on page 311.

Aphakia and the aphakic eye

Before discussing how cataract surgery is actually done, it is helpful to consider exactly what the natural lens does in the eye, the problems of having no lens in the eye and how the function of the natural lens can be replaced.

An eye which has no lens in it is called an 'aphakic' eye (**Figure 12.15**). (Greek: 'a' = without, 'phakos' = a lens). Patients are either aphakic because

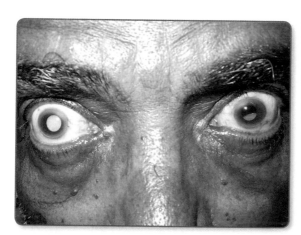

Figure 12.14 A subluxated cataractous left lens. The subluxation was only noticed after the pupil had been dilated, but careful examination would have detected iridodonesis. The right eye also has dense a cataract.

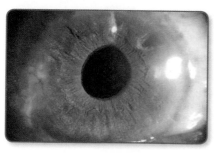

Figure 12.15 An aphakic eye following intracapsular extraction. The pupil is clear and dark and the peripheral iridectomies are visible. The pupil is very slightly distorted upwards. This may indicate that some vitreous has become adherent to the wound. There is no lens implant in this eye.

the lens has been surgically removed, or because it has dropped into the vitreous from either trauma or zonular weakness (see above). An aphakic eye has the following features:

- There is no lens to focus light rays. Although the cornea is responsible for about three quarters of light ray refraction, the lens does a further quarter. The eye becomes very hypermetropic and the patient requires a spectacle lens of at least 10 dioptres for normal distance vision (**Figure 12.16**).
- The anterior chamber is very deep, because of the loss of the lens.
- The pupil appears very black because there is no lens to reflect any of the incident light although after extracapsular extraction, some lens capsular remnants may be seen.
- The iris often wobbles when the eye moves because there is no lens to support it. This is called '*iridodonesis*'.

The optical correction of aphakia

The lens of the eye is a strong convex lens. Therefore, if the lens is removed from a normal eye (e.g. by surgery or trauma the vision will be very blurred (less than 6/60) because the eye is out of focus. There are three types of lens that can restore the focus of the lens to normal:

1. Spectacles
2. Contact lenses
3. Intraocular lenses.

Spectacles (Figure 12.17)

This is the traditional way of restoring the focusing power of the eye after cataract extraction. A pair of spectacles with a strong convex lens of about +10 dioptres will give very good visual acuity.

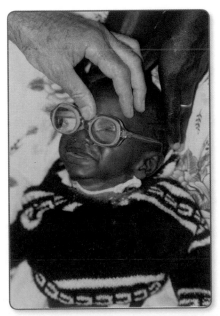

Figure 12.16 This child has had cataract surgery. A very thick 'plus' glasses lens is required to correct for the loss of the lens.

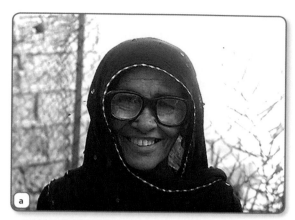

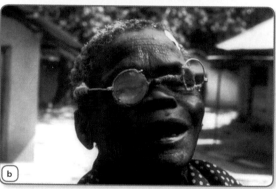

Figure 12.17 The use of spectacles. (a) A contented patient wearing aphakic spectacles. (b) The way some glasses end up looking for some people in isolated rural areas.

Advantages of aphakic spectacles
- Glasses are very cheap.
- Glasses are easy to prescribe.
- Glasses are safer than contact lenses and do not require the surgical expertise that is needed for placing an intraocular lens in the eye (see below).

Disadvantages of aphakic spectacles
- Distortion. The strong convex lens causes objects to have a different shape especially at their edges.
- Prismatic effects. Very thick lenses 'move' light. Therefore, when looking through the glasses the outside world is seen in a slightly different place to where it actually is. At first patients have some difficulty in moving around and may feel very disorientated.
- Magnification. Replacing the eye's natural lens in the eye with a spectacle lens causes magnification of the image by about 30 percent. This is not a serious problem for a patient with cataracts in both eyes, but if the other eye is fairly normal the images from the two eyes are of different sizes. This causes diplopia and prevents the patient wearing corrective glasses.
- The spectacles are heavy and uncomfortable to wear.
- Glasses are easily broken, scratched or lost (**Figure 12.17b**). In remote settings they are difficult to replace.

The optical problems of aphakic glasses were often so debilitating that in the past, patients were advised not to have cataract surgery until the cataracts were quite advanced. Also there was not much advantage in having a cataract operation in one eye if the other eye was normal. However, most people adapt to using aphakic glasses quite quickly after cataract extraction. They learn to move their head rather than their eyes to look around which helps overcome the prismatic effect and distortion at the lens edges. However, in several follow up studies after cataract operations only about half of the patients were still wearing spectacles a year after their surgery. Without aphakic spectacles the visual acuity after cataract extraction is about 3/60 so the patient remains seriously visually impaired.

Contact lenses (Figure 12.18)

A contact lens is a small corrective lens that sits on the actual cornea itself. Despite being so small it can have enough power to correct aphakia.

Advantages of contact lenses
- A contact lens is so close to the natural position of the lens, that unlike glasses it does not cause much image magnification or distortion. Therefore, it can be used to restore the vision in patients who have had cataract surgery in one eye only.

Disadvantages of contact lenses
- Contact lenses are expensive, and require expert fitting.
- Many patients find contact lenses uncomfortable and can only wear them for short periods of time.
- Many patients, particularly elderly people, find it difficult to put contact lenses in or take them out, or even to remember if they have put them in.
- The contact lenses need to be kept clean and sterilised with great care, or sight-threatening infections of the cornea can occur.

Contact lenses are therefore rarely suitable for aphakic patients in poor and tropical countries. One major use is for aphakic children, as intraocular lenses are often not used in paediatric/congenital cataract and heavy aphakic spectacles are uncomfortable and cause distortion.

Intraocular lens implants

An artificial plastic lens called an intraocular lens implant (IOL) can be placed in the eye to replace the natural, but opacified lens that is removed in cataract surgery (**Figure 12.19**). The lenses are non-irritant and non-toxic and are used in virtually all cataract extractions performed throughout the world nowadays.

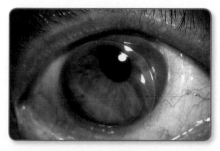

Figure 12.18 An eye with a contact lens following cataract surgery. This eye had an extensive injury which is why the pupil is updrawn and an IOL was not inserted. The green colour is from the fluorescein dye which is used to check the fitting of the contact lens.

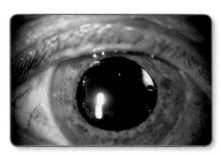

Figure 12.19 An eye with an intraocular lens implant after an extracapsular extraction. The pupil has been dilated to show the implant. The pupil is very black and there are bright reflections of light from the surface of the intraocular lens. The slightly thickened lens capsule sitting just behind the IOL can just be seen. At the edge of the IOL there is a small hole called a dialling hole. Some lenses have this hole in order to help insert the IOL into the eye.

Intraocular lenses were first used about 50 years ago but the early outcomes were not very good. Many complications occurred and many different types of lens and designs were tried. However, modern designs that are made to sit inside the lens capsule (see below) are very safe

Advantages of IOLs

- Cost: 20 years ago IOLs were very expensive and cost was considered a major disadvantage of IOLs. However, in recent years the cost has decreased remarkably; high quality lenses are available for just a few dollars, which is much cheaper than many spectacles and certainly contact lenses.
- Optical advantages: an IOL is the best way of replacing the refracting function of the natural lens because it is placed in the same place as the original lens. Therefore, there is no magnification or distortion. After measuring the length of the eye and the curvature of the cornea, the power of the lens can be chosen for an individual patient's eye in order to make the patient emmetropic (no distance glasses prescription) after the operation.
- Practical advantages: if the correct power of lens is inserted into the eye, the patient will not require any glasses except for reading. Additionally, the lens is secure inside the eye where it cannot be damaged or lost.
- Safety: modern lenses are very safe and there are few long-term complications. Unlike contact lenses, they are not an infection risk.

Disadvantages of IOLs

- Cataract surgery with an IOL requires more technical skill than simply removing the whole lens and therefore surgeons require more training and supervision. Also, IOL surgery requires an operating microscope, which may not always be available. Cataract surgery without lens placement can be done without a microscope.

The treatment of cataract

In the early stages of cataract, it may be possible to improve the vision significantly either with spectacles or by dilating the pupil. However, the main treatment for cataract is surgical removal of the lens. Cataract surgery is by far the most common eye operation and probably the second most common surgical procedure worldwide (after circumcision). Cataract surgery has been around for thousands of years; couching is a procedure in which the lens is pushed back into the vitreous and was even conducted by the ancient Egyptians. Big developments in cataract surgery were made in the second half of the 19th century with improved anaesthesia and instruments and an understanding of the importance of sterility. However, the biggest steps forward have taken place in the last 60 years, since Harold Ridley inserted the first intraocular lenses. Modern cataract surgery is a safe and straightforward operation with very few complications, although it must never be forgotten that there is always a risk of visual loss from cataract surgery.

Cataract surgery should be offered to the patient when the cataract is causing a reduction in vision or other visual symptoms such as glare, and this is significantly interfering with the patient's quality of life. Different people have different visual requirements and therefore desire cataract surgery at different levels of visual impairment. For example, a younger person who is still working in a job that requires clear vision is likely to need cataract removal at an earlier stage than an older retired person who spends most of their time at home. These days it is not the case that the cataract should be mature (or 'ripe') before it is removed and with modern surgical technique and technology the cataract can be removed at any point. If both eyes have cataract there is a lot to be gained by doing cataract surgery. However, if one eye has good vision, many people are happy with their level of vision and there is less to be gained by the removing the cataract. However, very dense cataracts in only one eye should always be removed because of the risk of hypermaturity (see above).

In modern cataract surgery there are two stages:
1. The removal of the opaque lens.
2. The insertion of an intraocular lens (IOL) implant.

In order to understand modern cataract surgery, it is easier to briefly understand the different cataract extraction procedures that have been done as the surgery has evolved.

Intra-capsular cataract extraction (ICCE)

ICCE is the removal of the whole lens, including its capsule (**Figure 12.15**). Until the latter part of the 20th century, ICCE was the most widely used cataract extraction procedure. However, as advances in technology – particular the operating microscope and intraocular lenses – have been accessible and affordable in even the poorest countries, ICCE is now rarely done.

ICCE is usually done with a cryoprobe, which adheres to the lens by forming a solid ice ball. Alternatively, a small pair of forceps may be used to grasp the lens capsule, or the lens may be expressed from the eye. After removing the lens a small piece of iris is excised, this is called an iridectomy. This is usually visible after surgery as a hole in the superior iris, or if a section of the whole iris sphincter is removed, the pupil will look 'U'-shaped and not round. It allows the aqueous to continue to circulate in the eye, because after intracapsular extraction the anterior face of the vitreous may completely occlude the pupil.

An IOL can be placed in the eye after ICCE. However, the patient does not have an intact posterior lens capsule, as occurs after extra-capsular cataract extraction (ECCE) (see below). Therefore, the lens must be placed elsewhere. The options are:

- In the anterior chamber in front of the iris (**Figure 12.20**)
- In the posterior chamber fixed to the sclera (either by sutures or tunnels to hold the IOL's 'arms') or to the back of the iris.

None of these locations are ideal and the long-term results are not as good as putting the lens in the capsular bag as is done in ECCE.

ICCE has a few advantages over more modern techniques: it is quicker and easier to teach and perform, and it does not require an operating microscope. However, the results are not as good as seen in extracapsular surgery. One common complication of an intracapsular extraction is that the capsule may rupture. Another complication is that some of the vitreous jelly may come out through the wound as well as the lens.

Extra-capsular cataract extraction with lens implantation

In the last 20 years, extracapsular extraction (**Figure 12.19**) has become the standard procedure in poor countries. This has become possible mainly because of the operating microscope, but also because of the huge reductions in price and increase in availability of IOLs. It has significant advantages over ICCE if surgeons have good training in using the technique and access to an operating microscope and IOLs.

The operating microscope

The microscope greatly magnifies and improves the view of the operation. It also provides co-axial illumination (see page 63), which is a great advantage for intraocular surgery as it creates a red reflex. Therefore, all the lens material except the posterior lens capsule can be removed, which can be seen and left intact. Without a microscope, quite large amounts of the lens cortex may be left in the eye, which cause postoperative uveitis and marked thickening of the posterior capsule. Also the posterior capsule is much more likely to be damaged during the surgery. An intact posterior capsule separates the anterior and posterior segments of the eye and keeps the vitreous and retina more stable, which lowers the risk of postoperative complications. The posterior capsule and some remaining anterior capsule, also provide a layer for an IOL to be safely and securely implanted.

Sutured and sutureless ECCE

The majority of ECCE procedures have several sutures to close the incision at the superior limbus. This is an excellent and very effective operation and

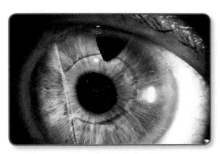

Figure 12.20 An eye after intra capsular cataract extraction with an anterior chamber IOL.

when the sutures are placed neatly and with equal tension, they are unlikely to cause problems or significant refractive changes. In recent years many ECCE surgeons have converted to a more modern type of corneal incision that is large enough to allow the above procedure to be conducted, but small enough and specially constructed for it to close and heal without requiring sutures (**Figure 12.21**).

Phacoemulsification

Phacoemulsification (phaco) means 'dissolving the lens' (**Figure 12.22**). Instead of removing the whole nucleus from the eye, the nucleus is dissolved and removed inside the eye using a very small probe. This probe produces very high frequency ultrasound which dissolves the nucleus then aspirates it. The probe fits through a very small corneal incision that is only 2–3 mm wide. An IOL is then inserted into the capsule. The IOL is folded or rolled to allow it to fit through the small corneal incision and it unfolds or unrolls in the capsule. Generally no sutures are required as the small incision seals itself.

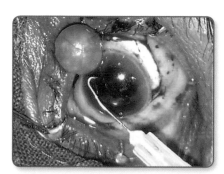

Figure 12.21 A sutureless extracapsular cataract extraction. The whole nucleus has been removed from the eye with a small 'fishhook'. This is one of several ways to remove the nucleus.

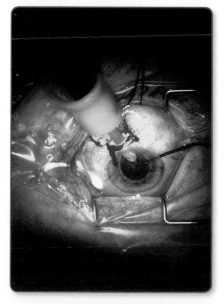

Figure 12.22 A phacoemulsification probe at work in the eye.

The main advantage of phaco is that the whole operation can be done through a very small incision without the need of any sutures. Soft, foldable intraocular lenses can be inserted through this same small incision. This is now the standard way of removing cataracts in rich countries, and is becoming popular in poor countries as well. Unfortunately, both the permanent ultrasound hardware and the consumable attachments are very expensive and the equipment requires careful management and often needs expensive repairs conducted by highly trained technicians. It is therefore not feasible in almost all poor countries except the major cities. However, as surgeons in poor countries have become very skilled at sutureless ECCE, the expensive equipment of phaco is not necessary.

Femtosecond laser cataract extraction

In the last few years a few hospitals in rich countries have been testing and using a laser to perform some parts of the cataract extraction. The Femtosecond laser can be used to cut the anterior capsular hole and to help break up the lens before it is aspirated. Currently the laser machine is extremely expensive and the surgery takes longer than conventional ECCE or phaco, without at present reducing complication rates.

Postoperative care

Nowadays with good secure wound closure with sutures or with small incision surgery, there is no need to keep patients in bed or in hospital post-operatively. Patients are usually discharged the same day. In some situations, they are seen the next day, particularly in remote places when it might be very difficult or even impossible to see them again after they return home. Patients who have had uncomplicated surgery are ideally seen 2–4 weeks after the operation.

The standard postoperative care is to apply a mixture of antibiotics, steroids and sometimes mydriatics topically to the eye for about 2–4 weeks. By then the wound should have healed and the postoperative inflammation settled.

Complications of modern cataract surgery

Complications are now uncommon during or after surgery. However, when they do occur, they can be very damaging to the vision and even blinding. The complications that may follow any intraocular operation are discussed in Chapter 4. Below are complications that are particularly important in cataract surgery.

Intraoperative complications

Posterior capsular rupture

In ECCE and phaco surgery the posterior capsule and anterior capsular rim should be left intact. If the posterior capsule is torn (sometimes called posterior capsule rupture) the following problems can or do occur:

1. The vitreous is almost inevitably disrupted and pulled into the operating area. This makes the operation much harder as the vitreous must be carefully and gently cleared (anterior vitrectomy) and it also increases the risk of retinal detachment (see below)
2. All or part of the cataract can drop through the hole in the capsule into the vitreous. Only people who have experience and expertise in doing posterior vitrectomy should retrieve lens matter from the vitreous.
3. Depending on the size of the hole, it is much harder or impossible to place the IOL in the capsular bag. Other locations have to be considered, e.g. the sulcus (in front of the anterior capsule) or the anterior chamber.
4. Increased risk of other complications that are discussed below, such as endophthalmitis, corneal oedema and post-operative inflammation.

Zonular dehiscence

The lens capsule is held in place by the zonules. If these are weak and/or are damaged and stretched by careless cataract surgery, the capsular bag will become detached in some places. This can cause two problems:
1. Vitreous may enter the anterior chamber around the side of the capsule, which will require an anterior vitrectomy (see above).
2. The capsule may not be stable enough for an IOL to be placed in it. The lens may not be well centred (**Figure 12.23**) or the whole lens and capsule may drop into the vitreous at some point after the operation.

Short-term complications

Endophthalmitis

This is perhaps the most feared complication of cataract surgery and can be disastrous for the vision. The incidence should not be more than 1 in 1000 cases (0.1%) and if it is higher than this, there may be significant sterility issues that need investigating. Acute bacterial endophthalmitis usually occurs within the first few days after surgery (some organisms, e.g. *Staphylococcus aureus* usually become evident within the first 48 hours, while others, e.g. *Staphylococcus epidermidis* are slower and may take about 5 days to become apparent). There is nearly always redness, pain, swelling and loss of vision with all the changes of acute intraocular inflammation and pus formation in the eye (**Figure 12.24**). Urgent treatment with intravitreal antibiotics is

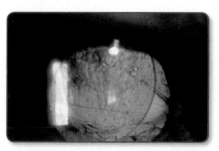

Figure 12.23 Decentration of the IOL and capsular thickening. The IOL is not centred correctly and its edge can be seen through the dilated pupil. This may be caused by zonular dehiscence or poor placement of the lens haptics. The thickening of the capsule can be seen as a dark shadow against the red reflex.

needed to save the eye (see page 85). In some situations an urgent vitrectomy is also advisable if the equipment and expertise are available.

Post-operative anterior uveitis

It is normal for intraocular surgery to provoke intraocular inflammation. This is normally controlled with post-operative steroid drops (a typical regime is dexamethasone 0.1% four times per day decreasing to once a day over 4 weeks). However, sometimes the inflammation is more intense and requires more frequent steroid or a longer period of steroid drops. If any cortical or nuclear lens matter is left in the eye during the surgery, the inflammation is often more vigorous and prolonged.

Poor wound closure

A gaping wound can allow the iris to prolapse through it or for aqueous to leak out. This prevents the anterior chamber from reforming. Poor wound closure increases the risk of endophthalmitis (see above) and intraocular haemorrhage. In the longer term a badly constructed wound may cause significant astigmatic change. Wound closure is less of a problem with well-conducted small incision ECCE and phaco surgery than with ECCE, when carefully suturing is required. Badly placed or tied sutures can become loose and cause foreign body type irritation. This can occur anytime from immediately after the surgery to months later.

Cystoid macular oedema (CMO) (Figure 12.25a and b)

CMO is a rather strange but relatively common complication in which oedema develops at the macular area after surgery. About 2–6 weeks postoperatively, the patient becomes aware that their vision is not as good as they would expect it to be. Sometimes CMO can cause the vision to be as low as 6/60. The causes of CMO are not clear, although it is more common after complicated surgery or ICCE. However, it can occur in routine, uncomplicated cataract surgery. It is treated initially with a prolonged course of topical steroid drops and non-steroidal drops. If these are ineffective, an intravitreal steroid injection (e.g. triamcinolone) often improves the vision. However, CMO can recur after the steroid effect wears off.

Corneal oedema and bullous keratopathy

Corneal oedema is quite common after cataract surgery. It occurs because the corneal endothelial cells are damaged and they are less able to pump fluid out of the cornea so it becomes oedematous (waterlogged).

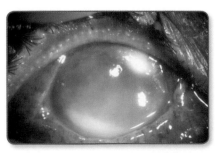

Figure 12.24 Endophthalmitis. Note the following features: inflamed (red) and swollen conjunctiva; purulent discharge on the eyelids; a very cloudy cornea that makes it impossible to see the iris clearly; an area of dense infiltrate superiorly, probably around the ECCE sutures that can be seen at the top of the eye, and a hypopyon.

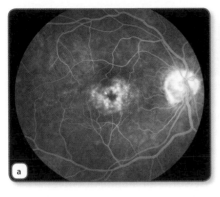

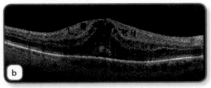

Figure 12.25 Cystoid macular oedema (CMO) after cataract surgery. (a) Fluorescein angiogram showing CMO. The oedema is the white area leaking out around the macula. (b) Ocular coherence tomogram of a cross section of the macula showing CMO. Although these two investigations will not be available in most clinics they are a helpful way of showing the CMO that occurs quite frequently after cataract surgery.

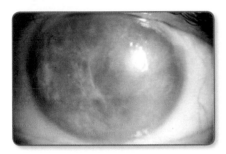

Figure 12.26 Bullous keratopathy. The cornea is swollen and hazy with fluid cysts in the corneal epithelium. Often the eye is inflamed and painful.

This usually recovers. However, sometimes it can be very severe and prolonged. This happens either when the number of endothelial cells or their function is already reduced pre-operatively, or when the corneal endothelium is damaged from long, traumatic or careless surgery. The vision becomes very blurred because the corneal stroma is thicker than normal and the eye is painful, because epithelial blisters develop (**Figure 12.26**). If it does not recover it can only be treated with a corneal graft, but symptomatically, covering the cornea with a flap of conjunctiva can relieve the pain.

Retinal detachment (Figures 13.32–13.34)

The risk of retinal detachment increases slightly after uncomplicated cataract surgery. However, it is much higher if there has been disruption of the vitreous during the surgery (see above) because it causes vitreous traction on the retina. Post-cataract surgery retinal detachment is also more common in patients who are highly myopic. The risk is of course much lower in ECCE and phaco than in ICCE in which the vitreous is always disrupted because the whole capsule is removed.

Postoperative glaucoma

The intraocular pressure often rises for a short time after any surgery. This is because the red blood cells and the plasma proteins obstruct the flow of aqueous fluid out of the eye. Persistent postoperative glaucoma can be caused by damage or obstruction to the aqueous drainage pathways.

Long-term complications

Posterior capsular opacification (PCO)

In ECCE and phaco, the posterior capsule is left intact during the surgery. It is initially transparent, but it can gradually become cloudy in the months or years after cataract surgery (**Figure 12.27**). It occurs to some degree in most people who have ECCE or phaco surgery, but may not be symptomatic in many people for many years. The opacity is caused by fibroblasts and then opaque fibrous tissue forming a thin sheet on the surface of the posterior capsule as well as new lens fibres growing on the surface of the capsule. These look like little bubbles and are called Elschnig's pearls. Very dense posterior capsular thickening can be seen with a torchlight, but in most cases it can only be detected by examining the red reflex with an ophthalmoscope or observing the shadow of the thickened capsule or using a slit lamp. Posterior capsular opacification is easily treated with a capsulotomy (making a hole in the capsule). This can be done without making another incision in the eye with a specialised type of laser (YAG laser). However, these are expensive and not available in many poor and remote areas. Alternatively it can be done under topical anaesthetic with hypodermic needle or fine capsulotomy knife. It may seem strange that during the surgery great efforts are made to keep the posterior capsule intact, but during this procedure to treat PCO a hole is deliberately made in the capsule. However, after a few months, the IOL is stable and the eye is closed. Therefore, the vitreous will not be disturbed by the capsulotomy.

Couching of cataracts

Couching has been the traditional treatment of cataract for thousands of years. It is thought to have originated in prehistoric times in India and was the only method until the arrival of modern cataract surgery. Couching still occurs in some isolated rural areas of north and central Africa and parts of Asia where there are no medical services, although it has become very rare as cataract outreach campaigns are extending out into poor and remote areas. Most couchers are uneducated, and travel from village to village, performing a few operations and then moving on. The word couching comes from the French word 'coucher', to push down, because the lens is pushed down into the vitreous using a needle or thorn. This is inserted into the eye either at the limbus, or a few millimetres behind it to rupture the suspensory

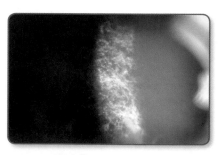

Figure 12.27 Thickened posterior capsule seen with a slit lamp.

ligament and pushes the lens back down into the vitreous. An eye often looks fairly normal after a couching operation. However, a closer examination will reveal the entry point of the needle (**Figure 12.28a**). It will also show that the lens, or fragments of the lens, is lying in the lower vitreous (**Figure 12.28b**). For the first few days after a couching operation, the patient may see a lot better. Unfortunately, complications are common, the most common of which are:

- Endophthalmitis, because many couchers do not sterilise their instruments.
- Uveitis and glaucoma. If the lens capsule ruptures, the lens matter will leak out into the vitreous and will cause severe and prolonged uveitis and secondary glaucoma.

The results of couching obviously vary according to the skill of the coucher. There are a few highly skilled couchers, who are able to totally or partially dislocate the lens into the vitreous without rupturing the capsule and who use sterilised instruments, which do not risk infection. If these patients are given spectacles to correct their aphakia, the results can be quite good. Unfortunately most couchers are less capable and severe, blinding complications are frequent.

World cataract blindness and its eradication

Cataract is by far the commonest cause of world blindness, especially in elderly people. Approximately 10 million people are blind and 57 million people have moderate or severe visual impairment from cataract. This means that about a third of all cases of blindness worldwide are caused by cataract, despite it being a completely curable disease, which can be treated with a relatively quick, cheap and highly successful operation. However, there is enormous global variation in cataract blindness; it is rarely a cause of blindness in rich countries, while in poor countries it is the commonest cause. This shows the enormous inequalities in society and the great failures of politicians and the medical profession to provide basic care to those who need it most.

Cataract surgery rates have increased rapidly in recent years, with an enormous scaling up of outreach/campaign surgery. However, with the world's

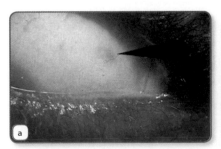 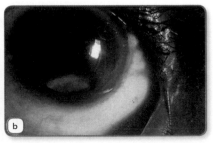

Figure 12.28 Cataract couching. (a) The dark spot in the sclera at the tip of the pointer is the place where the needle of the coucher went into the eye. (b) The same eye showing the dislocated lens in the lower vitreous, just visible through the dilated pupil.

population ageing in all but the most war-torn areas, the numbers of patients with significant cataract continues to rise quickly. Therefore, in many countries the output of cataract surgery needs to increase as much as ten times to even begin to solve the problem.

The *Vision 20/20* programme has given the eradication of cataract blindness the highest priority and some aspects of the problem have already been discussed in Chapter 1. The purpose of this section is just to summarise some of the important concepts for eradicating cataract blindness.

An effective programme to treat cataract blindness needs to treat large numbers of patients at low cost and with good results. This can be summarised in three headings: *high output, low outlay* and *good outcome.*

High output

It is obvious that with large numbers of cataract blind and very few trained surgeons available, each surgeon must achieve a high output of cases. This not only requires commitment of individuals but team-working as well, as a team of people working together can achieve so much more than an individual working alone. However, poor countries often provide very important lessons to richer countries in this respect. Some well-organised cataract centres, such as those in India, Nepal, and some outreach campaigns in Africa, have a single surgeon doing 30 or 40 procedures a day, whereas in a typical rich country cataract centre, it is rare to see a surgeon do more than 15 procedures in a day, despite enormous nursing support and expensive high-tech equipment.

Low outlay

This means that the treatment must be cheap. Obviously, the cost of treatment must be low enough so that poor people can afford it, and it should be available free of charge to those who are destitute. A high output and a low outlay work together and reinforce each other. By treating more patients, the cost of each case becomes less and as the cost becomes less, more people are able to afford the treatment, and so the output increases. There are many excellent cataract surgical programmes, which treat poor communities and are almost self-financing using the ideas of cost recovery.

When cataract surgery provision is being planned the 'indirect costs' of the patients must also be considered. These are the other costs, such as transport, food, lost earnings and child-care cover that are required simply to attend an operation, even if the operation is free. Therefore, the cost is always cheaper to the patient if it is provided closer to their home.

Good outcome

The results of cataract surgery should be very good with a low rate of complications. One of the problems of medical care in poor countries is that there is sometimes a great variation in the results of surgical treatment. In many poor countries, the very best as well as the worst surgery is available. It is quite possible to find that couching, simple cataract extraction and giving glasses, extracapsular cataract extraction with an IOL, and phacoemulsification are all carried out in the same country.

High output can sometimes lead to poor outcomes because the surgeons and the surgical team are rushing to perform as many cases as possible. Good surgical standards must be maintained at all times. It is also absolutely fundamental that high volume cataract surgery centres or campaigns in poor countries must never be used as places for training surgeons (both local and visiting surgeons) to 'practise'. The same standards of training, supervision and patient care is compulsory for all patients in all situations.

Modern cataract surgery should now either be ECCE or phaco, both with an IOL. Phacoemulsification is generally too expensive and dependent on sophisticated equipment, supplies and maintenance. It is also not suitable for some of the most mature and hypermature cataracts, which are found more commonly in poor countries.

Congenital and childhood cataract

Childhood cataract is the commonest treatable cause of childhood blindness worldwide. About 200,000 children are blind from cataracts worldwide. The majority of these are congenital (the child is born with the cataract), although it still relatively rare and is seen in about 10 out of 10,000 births. They are bilateral in about 60% of cases.

Diagnosis and examination of congenital cataract

In poor countries congenital cataract is usually detected by the parents noticing the white pupil (**Figure 12.29**). Sometimes the cataract is not noticed until it becomes clear that the child cannot see out of the eye or develops a squint because the eye is not fixating (see Chapter 18). In many rich countries, there is a routine check of the red reflex in all babies soon after they are born. A cataract is the commonest cause of an absent red reflex in a newborn baby.

One very important sign to look for when examining children with congenital cataracts is the presence or absence of nystagmus (see page 450). If nystagmus is present, macular fixation has never developed properly because of the density of the cataract in early life. Therefore, the child will not see perfectly even with successful surgery. If there is no nystagmus it is likely that the cataract was not so dense in infancy and the image on the retina was clear enough for the child to develop macular fixation. Therefore, the vision following cataract surgery is much more likely to improve.

Clinical appearance of congenital cataract

Sometimes congenital cataract may involve the whole lens, producing a dense white opacity. In other cases, only a certain layer of lens fibres may become opaque (**Figure 12.30**). This is called a 'lamellar' cataract. Sometimes the opacity may be confined to the anterior or posterior pole of the lens. These incomplete congenital lens opacities may remain static throughout life or they may progress as the child grows older.

Causes of congenital cataract

In many cases, it is not possible to discover a specific cause or associated systemic disease. A systemic disease is more commonly identified in children with bilateral cataracts (25% of cases) than in unilateral cataract (6%).

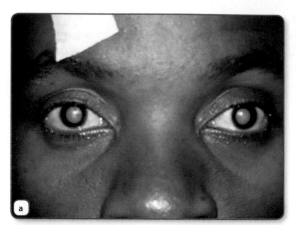

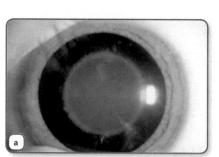

Figure 12.29 Bilateral congenital cataract (a) before and (b) after surgery.

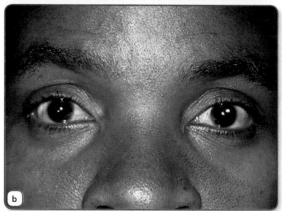

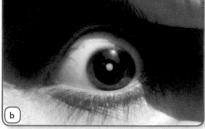

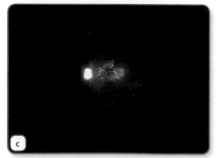

Figure 12.30 Three congenital cataracts. In all of these cataracts only one layer or area of the lens has become opaque. The rest of the lens is completely normal. If cataract surgery is performed, the whole lens has to be removed except the capsule. (a) Lamellar cataract with just one layer of the lens affected. (b) Anterior polar cataract. (c) Sutural cataract.

The major causes are:

1. Intrauterine infection, especially during early pregnancy. The major infective conditions that cause congenital cataract are shown in **Table 12.2.**
2. Anoxia or trauma to the fetus at birth or in utero before birth.
3. Metabolic disorders. These are very rare and usually require expertise and very specialised tests to diagnose.
   - Galactosaemia
   - Hypo- and hyperglycaemia
   - Hypocalcaemia

Cause of paediatric cataract

Some children are born with a clear lens but develop cataract during childhood. The commonest causes of this are:

- Trauma. When children present with cataract always consider the possibility of non-accidental injury (i.e. injury caused by the parents or other carers of the child).
- Chronic uveitis, for example in children with juvenile idiopathic arthritis (see page 267)

Management of congenital cataract

Management challenges

The management of congenital and paediatric cataract is very challenging for the following reasons:

- The eye is small and not fully developed. Therefore, surgery carries a high risk of immediate and long-term complications. If an IOL is used in

Table 12.2 The effects of common or severe intrauterine infections		
Intra-uterine Infections	Ocular complications, other than cataract	Systemic complications
Rubella (German measles)	Chorioretinitis ('salt and pepper retinopathy') Glaucoma Microphthalmos	Heart defects Deafness Learning delay Genitourinary anomalies
Toxoplasmosis	Chorioretinitis Panuveitis Microphthalmos Optic atrophy Macular scars	Cerebral calcifications, causing brain damage and epilepsy Enlarged spleen and liver
Varicella zoster	Chorioretinitis	Limb atrophy Brain damage
Herpes simplex	Keratitis Conjunctivitis Chorioretinitis	Very high fetal death rate (60%) Pneumonia Encephalitis Hepatitis
Cytomegalovirus	Chorioretinitis Optic atrophy Microphthalmos Keratitis	Enlarged liver and spleen Jaundice Brain damage

surgery, it is difficult to determine the best IOL power as it will change as the eye grows and develops.

- There is a high likelihood of the eye developing amblyopia (see Chapter 18). This is particularly likely in unilateral cataract.
- Cataract surgery will eliminate the ability of the lens to accommodate.
- The ideal management requires a team of professionals, including ophthalmologists with expertise in this subject, paediatricians to assess for other abnormalities and possibly support for the parents and the child when they go to school. This can be difficult or impossible to achieve in most poor countries.
- There is a significant possibility that the child has another ocular or systemic abnormality that may affect their general health and development.

Surgery for congenital cataract

Just as in adults, the treatment of congenital cataract is basically surgical. However, it can be a much more difficult decision whether to operate or not. The decision should be guided by two rules.

1. Is the cataract in one eye or both eyes? If the cataract is in one eye only then that eye is almost certainly amblyopic (see page 438) and there is much less to be gained by operating unless the surgery can be done very early and intensive post-operative follow-up is possible to minimise amblyopia.
2. If the cataract is bilateral, is it total lens opacity or partial lens opacity? If the cataract is total and no red reflex at all can be seen with the pupil fully dilated, then surgery should be carried out as soon as possible. If the opacity is partial and some red reflex is present with a fully dilated pupil, then it is best to delay cataract surgery until the child is old enough to have the vision tested, as vision may develop through the clear bits in the lens. Mydriatic drops may improve the vision of a child with partial or lamellar lens opacities and in some cases a peripheral iridotomy can be made to expose a clear area of the lens which may be enough for visual development.

The best technique for cataract surgery and whether to use an IOL remains controversial. If the surgery is performed before the child is 4 weeks old, there is probably a higher chance of developing glaucoma. However, the longer the cataract(s) is left, the more chance there is of developing amblyopia. There is also debate about whether to remove some of the posterior capsule and anterior vitreous at the time of surgery. Doing this reduces the development of PCO (see above), which occurs in almost every child and can be a recurrent and difficult complication in paediatric cataract surgery. However, it also increases the risk of surgical complications. The final decision on whether and how to operate will vary greatly with the facilities and skills available and how easily the child can be followed-up. However, in any event, an expert with experience of paediatric cataract surgery should perform the surgery.

Lens subluxation and dislocation

Cataract is by far the most common and important lens pathology. However, another important disorder of the lens is caused by rupture or stretching of the suspensory ligament. If the rupture is partial (lens subluxation), the lens only moves a little bit (**Figure 12.31**). It is sometimes only possible to see subluxation with a dilated pupil when the edges of the lens can be seen. Another useful sign of a displaced lens is that the iris wobbles when the eye moves (iridodonesis), because it is not resting on the lens anymore. If there is total dislocation, the lens usually drops into the vitreous. An eye with a dislocated lens appears just like an aphakic eye and needs a strong convex lens to restore the vision. A dislocated lens does not usually cause any other symptoms, but if the capsule ruptures the lens protein leaks into the vitreous and severe uveitis and glaucoma will develop. Very rarely the lens may dislocate forwards into the anterior chamber (**Figure 12.32**). This causes severe glaucoma, because the aqueous cannot circulate through the pupil. It must be treated urgently, by dilating the pupil intensively and removing the lens.

A subluxed lens usually becomes more spherical as well as moving away from the central axis. Therefore, it typically causes myopia and astigmatism.

There are several possible causes of subluxation or dislocation:

- Injury: especially a blunt, closed injury to the eye.
- Hypermature cataracts: these have a risk of dislocating or subluxating due to degeneration of the suspensory ligament.
- Congenital weakness of the suspensory ligament: this may occur as an isolated condition in otherwise normal, healthy people, or it may be part of a syndrome with changes in other parts of the body, e.g:
  - Marfan syndrome. This is a genetic condition (autosomal dominant) that affects connective tissue. Patients typically are very tall and thin with long fingers and toes, a high palate, and greatly increased risk of serious abnormalities of the aorta that can cause fatal aneurysms.

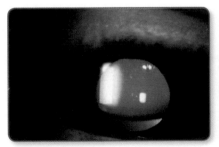

Figure 12.31 Subluxated lens. The lens is quite transparent. Its edge can just be seen when the red reflex is observed through a fully dilated pupil. This patient had myopia and astigmatism.

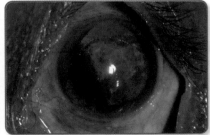

Figure 12.32 A cataractous lens that has dislocated and moved into the anterior chamber. This lens should be removed as it is likely to cause corneal endothelial damage and glaucoma, as well as obscuring the vision.

- Homocystinuria. This is a genetic condition (autosomal recessive) in which the deficiency of an enzyme causes learning delay, epilepsy, vascular disease with risk of occlusion and osteoporosis of the vertebrae.
- Weill-Marchesani syndrome. This is a rare syndrome that causes skeletal and ocular abnormalities.

The treatment of subluxed and dislocated lenses

A subluxed lens can often stay stable for many years and therefore if the patient is happy with the vision it does not require surgical removal. However, if the lens is unstable and the subluxation getting worse, it is likely that it will dislocate. Lens extraction surgery is much more difficult than normal cataract surgery and an intraocular lens cannot be placed in the capsule. The lens can be placed in the anterior chamber or supported in the posterior chamber by suturing it in place or tunnelling the lens arms (haptics) into the sclera. However it is often safer to the leave the patient aphakic and use glasses or contact lenses if available for refractive correction. Similarly, a dislocated lens can remain in the vitreous without causing symptoms or complications. Surgical removal has a high risk of complications and should only be done by someone with expertise. Therefore it is usually safer to leave the lens and use spectacles to improve the vision.

13 Diseases of the retina

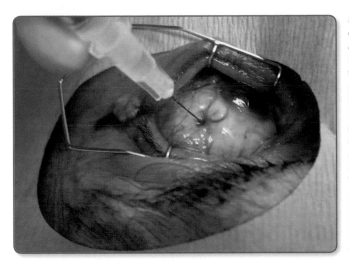

Macular degeneration and diabetic retinopathy were rare in poor countries, but increasing life expectancy and unhealthy diets mean they are now far more common. They were also untreatable, but intravitreal injections offer hope for both conditions.

When the first edition of this book was written, 'Diseases of the retina' was a small section. Many of the diseases were untreatable anywhere in the world, and particularly in poor countries. Also, most poor people were often not living long enough or eating unhealthy enough food to be affected by some of the more common retinal conditions such as age related macular degeneration (AMD) and diabetic retinopathy. Poor and tropical countries have a higher prevalence of infective diseases of the retina and choroid compared with rich countries where these diseases are rarely seen. The number of patients with these diseases in poor countries has increased dramatically over the last 30 years. However, the management of retinal conditions has greatly improved over this period for several reasons:

- There is a much greater understanding of many retinal conditions.
- Treatments exist for many more retinal conditions.
- Some of these treatments, including advanced treatments for AMD and previously complex retinal surgery are much more accessible.

A study of embryology shows that the retina is in fact a part of the central nervous system. It therefore reacts to injury and disease very much like the central nervous system and the brain.

- There are no pain fibres. Therefore, the main symptom of retinal disease is visual loss.
- The nerve cells themselves cannot regenerate after serious damage (only the supportive glial cells can). Any visual loss from retinal cell death

is therefore permanent. However, there seems to be a certain amount of reserve function. If only small or peripheral areas of the retina are damaged or destroyed, there may be no apparent loss of vision.

- The retina, like the rest of the central nervous system, has a very active metabolism, and the retinal cells need a lot of oxygen. The retinal blood vessels themselves only supply the inner layers of the retina. The outer layers – the rods, cones and bipolar cells – obtain their oxygen by diffusion from the blood vessels of the choroid. Therefore, diseases of the choroid will also affect the retina.

The commonest types of retinal disease are:

- Diseases of the retinal blood vessels called vascular retinopathies.
- Retinal and chorioretinal degenerations.
- Retinal detachments.

Less common diseases that we will consider in less detail are:

- Infective retinal disease.
- Inflammatory retinal disease.
- Retinal tumours.

Vascular retinal disease

Vascular retinopathies, like all blood vessel disorders, occur mostly in old people. They are also often associated with obesity, hypertension, diabetes and smoking. All of these used to be much less common in poor countries. However, sadly with changing diets and increasing exposure to many of the unhealthy habits of richer people, these diseases are becoming more common, particularly in urban poor people. For example, the prevalence of diabetes and therefore diabetic retinopathy is increasing in India and other Southern Asian countries faster than anywhere else in the world. In poor rural communities, where people only eat local foods such as grains and green vegetables, vascular retinal disease remains relatively uncommon.

The retina, with its high oxygen requirement and good blood supply is very susceptible to diseases of the blood vessels. The retinal capillaries are similar to the capillaries of the brain, and are less permeable than capillaries in the rest of the body. The cells that line the retinal blood vessels have 'tight junctions', which stop large molecules like proteins from passing through the walls. If protein and fluid do leak through diseased capillary walls, there is no lymphatic system to drain these exudates away from the retina. Therefore they can easily cause damage to the retinal tissues and the sight, and their effects can be seen in the retina for a long time.

The most common vascular retinal diseases are diabetic retinopathy, retinal vessel occlusions and hypertensive retinopathy. Other vascular retinopathies may be particular common in certain communities such as sickle cell retinopathy, peripheral periphlebitis (Eales disease) and Behçet disease.

Retinal examination in vascular disease

The eye is an excellent window through which the blood vessels and blood circulation in the body can be seen. The retinal circulation can be seen in great detail with the direct ophthalmoscope, which gives an image of the retina and its blood vessels about 15 times larger than their actual size. Some ophthalmoscopes also have a green filter in them. This is very useful because it makes the retinal blood vessels and any blood that has leaked in the retina much more obvious. If the retinal blood vessels show evidence of vascular disease, it is very likely that blood vessels elsewhere in the body and particularly in critical organs like the kidney and brain are similarly damaged.

The normal fundus should have no visible haemorrhages or patches of exudate and the presence of either of these suggests some underlying pathology. Vascular disease can cause haemorrhage and exudate anywhere or all over the fundus, but is often particularly concentrated around the optic disc and macula because the retinal blood supply is greatest here. Although damage to these areas causes the most visual damage, they are fortunately the easiest areas to examine with an ophthalmoscope.

Systemic examination in vascular disease

Retinal vascular disease may be the first evidence of severe systemic disease. Some retinal vascular diseases such as severe hypertensive retinopathy and arterial occlusions may indicate potentially fatal systemic disease. Therefore, it is essential to also check the patient's blood pressure and test their urine for albumin and sugar to look for kidney disease and diabetes. Other tests like a full blood count, erythrocyte sedimentation rate (ESR) and sickle cell tests are used for investigating specific diseases.

Hypertensive retinopathy

Systemic hypertension causes damage to the delicate and narrow arteries and arterioles in the retina. This ranges from mild changes that do not seem to affect retinal function or vision, to severe changes that can be blinding. There are official grades (1–4), but it is simpler to think in terms of mild, moderate and severe disease (**Table 13.1**).

Mild hypertensive retinopathy

In mild hypertension the retina itself appears normal, but there are subtle abnormalities of the retinal blood vessels. The retinal artery walls thicken, which causes the following changes that can be seen with an ophthalmoscope (**Figure 13.1**):
- The thicker artery walls reflect more light. This is called 'silver' or 'copper' wiring.
- The column of blood inside the arteries is narrower than normal.
- At places where the artery crosses a vein, the vein appears kinked or nipped.

Table 13.1 Hypertensive retinopathy		
Mild	**Moderate**	**Severe**
'Silver wiring'	Cotton wool spots	Papilloedema
Arteriovenous nipping	Hard exudates	
	Flame-shaped haemorrhages	

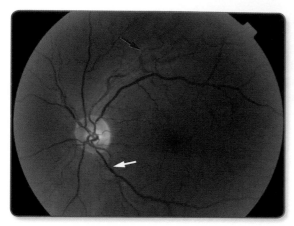

Figure 13.1 Mild hypertensive retinopathy. The following features can be seen: ① Thickening of the artery walls, with narrowing of the column of blood inside them. ② Narrowing of the vein as it is crossed by the artery (white arrow), with slight dilation on either side of the artery (AV nipping). ③ Mild tortuosity of the arteries (black arrow). ④ The arteries are just starting to develop an increase in light reflection that will gradually become more bronze-coloured ('copper wiring') and then grey coloured ('silver wiring').

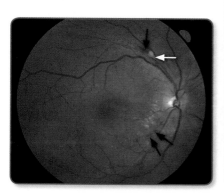

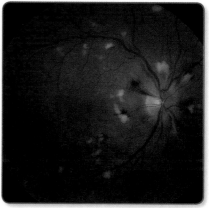

Figure 13.2 in moderate hypertensive retinopathy the arteries are very narrow and there is increased reflex (copper wiring) and AV nipping (see Figure 13.1 above for explanations). There are some haemorrhages (red arrows) and a cotton-wool spot (white arrow).

Figure 13.3 Severe hypertensive retinopathy. The cotton-wool spots and the flame-shaped haemorrhages are mainly found around the optic disc. There is also swelling of the optic disc.

Moderate hypertensive retinopathy

As the hypertension becomes worse there is leakage of protein from the blood vessels and some damage to the retinal cells (**Figure 13.2**). The same changes as described above in mild disease will be seen as well as some or all of the following changes:

Cotton wool spots

These are small round white spots with 'fluffy' edges that look a little bit like cotton wool (**Figures 13.2** and **13.3**). They are usually near the optic disc. Each spot is an area of dead or damaged axons in the nerve fibre layer of the retina with leakage of materials from the damaged nerve fibres. The nerve fibres are damaged because of blockages or narrowing of the small arterioles that supply them. Cotton wool spots come and go after a few weeks or months as the retinal macrophages 'eat-up' the damaged tissue and leaking materials. Individually they are too small to have any effect on vision, but their presence is very suggestive of a damaged and ischaemic retina, which may be affecting vision.

Hard exudates

These are denser, yellow areas, which are often found around the macula. They consist of fat and protein that is leaking from damaged blood vessels and from lipid material from the degradation of dying cells. This lipid material is contained in the macrophages where it may remain for many months, or even years. Eventually hard exudates will also disappear, although of course, new ones may continually form.

Flame-shaped haemorrhages

These haemorrhages are found in the nerve fibre layer of the retina. They occur when the superficial retinal vessels and capillaries are damaged and blood tracks between the nerves. Occasionally, a haemorrhage may spread into the vitreous (pre-retinal haemorrhage) or between the retina and vitreous (sub-hyaloid haemorrhage).

Severe hypertensive retinopathy

In severe hypertension one sees all the changes of moderate hypertension and also swelling of the optic disc. Moderate or severe hypertension usually causes fairly obvious changes in the appearance of the retina, but surprisingly little loss of vision, unless there is a lot of associated macular oedema. However, some of the complications of hypertension that may occur, such as retinal artery or vein occlusion will cause severe visual loss.

The treatment of hypertensive retinopathy

There is no specific treatment for hypertensive retinopathy itself, but the blood pressure must be treated urgently. There are two priorities:

1. Treat the blood pressure. This may be very urgent if there are severe retinal changes and very high blood pressure, as the patient is at high risk of severe medical complications such as stroke. Unfortunately, taking long-term blood pressure treatment may be very difficult, unavailable or unaffordable for many people.
2. Determine if the hypertension is being caused by an underlying disease such as kidney disease, coarctation of the aorta or some specific but rare tumours (phaeochromocytomas and paragangliomas).

Retinal vessel occlusions

Retinal vessel occlusions occur in either the arteries or the veins. A central occlusion involves the major artery or vein that enters or exits the retina, while a branch occlusion involves only a branch vessel in one area of the retina. Sometimes the occlusion is partial which causes partial obstruction of the blood flow.

Retinal artery occlusions

These occur most commonly in older people with hypertension or atherosclerosis (**Figures 13.4** and **13.4**). The most common cause is emboli that get stuck in the narrow arteries of the retina. These can come from anywhere in the body's arterial circulation, but commonly they break off from an atheromatous plaque at the origin of the internal carotid artery, or from the heart. Retinal artery occlusions usually cause a sudden and severe loss of vision because the area of retina is completely starved of oxygen. Therefore in a central retinal artery occlusion, there will be total loss of vision (unless the patient has an alternative retinal blood supply, called a cilioretinal artery). In a branch occlusion a segment of the vision will be lost. If a young, black patient has a retinal artery occlusion, sickle cell disease must be considered (see below).

On retinal examination, the arteries are very narrowed and sometimes so thin that they can hardly be seen. The area of the retina that is supplied by the blocked artery becomes white and oedematous (**Figure 13.4**). In central retinal artery occlusions, the fovea appears very red (called a 'cherry-red spot') as the healthy choroidal vasculature can be seen through this thinner area of retina. Later on, hard exudates may appear in the affected retina and the retinal vessels appear as thin, fibrotic, white streaks and many months and years later the retina is featureless, with very narrow vessels and a pale optic disc (**Figure 13.5**).

The treatment of retinal artery occlusions

The visual loss is usually permanent, although very occasionally an embolus may break up and pass on and the vision recovers. Alternatively, sometimes the pressure of blood behind the embolus forces it to move on to a smaller section of the artery allowing perfusion behind it. Therefore, if the patient is seen within the first 6 hours of the visual loss, one can try either vigorous ocular massage or paracentesis (removing aqueous from the eye to reduce the pressure). There are very occasional reports of these two measures helping

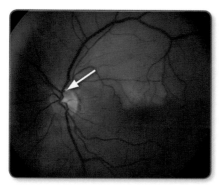

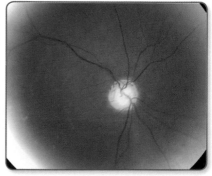

Figure 13.4 Branch retinal artery occlusion. At the top edge of the optic disc there is a yellow embolus (white arrow). The area of macula above the fovea that is supplied by this artery is pale and oedematous. The fovea looks very red because the choroidal blood supply beneath it is unaffected ('cherry red spot'). In a central retinal artery occlusion, the whole retina looks white except for the red spot at the macula.

Figure 13.5 A retina a few years after a central retinal artery occlusion. The retina is featureless, the vessels very narrow and the optic disc pale.

to move the embolus down the arterial tree and restoring the blood flow. Paracentesis is done by applying topical anaesthetic drops, then sterilising the conjunctival sac with povidone iodine 5–10% and then making a tiny incision at the limbus with a hypodermic needle (e.g. an insulin syringe) and withdrawing some aqueous. Unlike ocular massage, this procedure does carry a small risk of serious complications, such as endophthalmitis and damage to the lens of the eye. The patient should also be given aspirin to thin the blood and in some cases heparin might be considered as well.

Amaurosis fugax

'Amaurosis fugax', which means transient loss of vision, is the name given to a sudden loss of vision from temporary blockages of the retinal arterial circulation, which recover after a few minutes. Patients usually describe it as like a curtain coming down over the vision in one eye and it being all grey or black until it recovers a bit later. It is due to very small emboli blocking the retinal artery and then breaking up and dispersing. Patients with amaurosis fugax should take daily aspirin (75–150 mg), which lessens the risk of embolus formation. Ideally the patient should have a carotid Doppler scan of the neck to look for internal carotid artery thrombus, for which surgical removal could be done (carotid endarterectomy). However, this is very unlikely to be possible in most poor countries.

Retinal vein occlusions

Retinal vein occlusions are more common than artery occlusions. They usually occur in older people with hypertension and atherosclerosis. But they occasionally occur in younger people, when the commonest causes are dehydration, retinal vasculitis and some disorders of blood coagulation. A central retinal vein occlusion (CRVO) affects the whole retina, and a branch retinal vein occlusion (BRVO) affects only a segment of the retina.

The symptoms of a retinal vein occlusion are usually less severe than an artery occlusion. The visual loss is less sudden and the level of visual loss is very variable. There may also be some gradual, partial recovery of vision later. On fundus examination the retinal veins are dilated and tortuous, often with extensive haemorrhages and exudates (**Figure 13.6**) throughout the whole retina in CRVOs or in the area 'upstream' of the blockage in BRVOs (**Figure 13.7**). In severe cases there are cotton-wool spots as well because the retina is very ischaemic.

Sometimes one will see new vascular channels open, which allow blood to bypass the obstruction. These are called collaterals and form in pre-existing vasculature and must be distinguished from entirely new vessels which can be very bad for the retina (see below) (**Figure 13.8**).

The treatment of retinal vein occlusions

There is no specific treatment for retinal vein occlusions. Aspirin (150 mg daily) in the acute phase is probably beneficial if there are no contraindications. It is a good opportunity to explore the patient's risk factors, such as diet, smoking, exercise, weight, diabetes and blood pressure.

Neovascular or rubeotic glaucoma

In some cases of CRVO or BRVO the oxygen-deprived areas of retina stimulates the formation of new blood vessels (neovascularisation). Typically

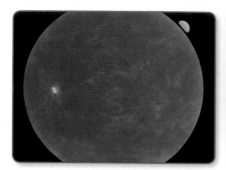

Figure 13.6 Central retinal vein occlusion. The retina and optic disc can only just be seen because of the extensive retinal haemorrhage.

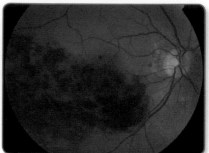

Figure 13.7 Branch retinal vein occlusion. The blood vessels in the upper half of the retina are fairly normal, although there is some 'silver wiring' change in the arteries which indicates the patient has high blood pressure. In the lower half of the retina the veins are dilated and there are haemorrhages.

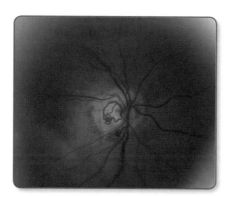

Figure 13.8 Optic disc collaterals.

this starts to occur about 3 months after the blockage. The retina has been dead for many months and the new vessels do not provide any benefit. In fact, quite the opposite; they can be very dangerous to the eye, and if possible attempts should be made to stop them growing. Otherwise, they can grow into the vitreous and bleed or into the anterior segment and drainage angle (rubeosis), causing blockage of aqueous drainage (neovascular/rubeotic glaucoma) (see Figure 15.21). Eyes with rubeotic glaucoma are usually very inflamed, painful and blind. The hazy cornea can be seen with the naked eye and the high pressure measured with a tonometer, or even just felt by palpating the eye. Rubeotic glaucoma is treated with extensive peripheral retinal laser [pan-retinal photocoagulation, (PRP)]. The PRP should be given before the rubeosis becomes extensive and the complications develop, as they cannot be reversed. The treatment works by destroying peripheral retina, which reduces the ischaemic stimulation to produce new vessels. Only a few years ago, this would have been completely impossible in almost all poor countries. However, lasers are now much more widely available and patients in some urban communities may be able to receive laser treatment.

Cryotherapy (freezing) of the retina is an alternative way of treating the isch-aemic retina. The required equipment is cheaper than lasers and it can be performed even if there is no view of the fundus (unlike when using laser). However, cryotherapy is either done 'blind' (without looking at the retina) or it requires the advanced technique of using an indirect ophthalmoscope and condensing lens at the same time as doing the cryotherapy. The treatment of blind painful eyes is discussed in more detail in Chapter 3.

Diabetic retinopathy

Diabetes mellitus (DM) is a disease of high blood sugar and disordered car-bohydrate, fat and protein metabolism. This results from either lack of in-sulin or the insulin not functioning normally. DM causes damage to blood vessels throughout the body. The small vessels of the retina are commonly affected. This causes damage to the retina itself and ultimately affects vision.

DM is a complex disease with several different causes, but in general there are two distinct types of diabetes. In type 1 DM there is autoimmune destruc-tion of the insulin secreting cells in the pancreas causing it to stop producing any insulin. Type 1 DM occurs mainly in younger people and requires insulin treatment to reduce blood sugars. Type 2 DM is more common and usually occurs in older people. It is often treated with tablets to reduce the blood sugar. In type 2 DM there is often a degree of insulin resistance as well as reduced production. Type 1 and type 2 diabetics typically have very different patterns of diabetic retinopathy.

Epidemiology

Over the last few years both diabetes and diabetic retinopathy have become increasingly common, particularly in low and middle-income countries. There are several possible reasons for this:

- *Increased prevalence of obesity*; this predisposes to type 2 diabetes.
- *Dietary changes*; many more people in low and middle income countries are now eating the unhealthy fried and processed food that was previously only available in rich countries. Sadly it is now quite common to see deep fried chicken and chips in markets throughout the world.
- *Increased life expectancy*: people are living longer in most areas of the world. There are therefore more years in which they might develop diabetes and its complications.
- *Lifestyle*. Many people are leading increasingly sedentary lifestyles. This leads to weight gain and an increased risk of type 2 diabetes.
- Racial genetic predisposition. It seems that some races, particularly South Asians, are prone to developing type 2 diabetes with changes in lifestyle.
- *Increased diagnosis*. As diabetes has become more of a problem, we are more likely to look for it and therefore diagnose cases that may have been present but never previously investigated.

Diagnosis and symptoms of diabetes

Patients with diabetes have increased urine production (polyuria), which of-ten occurs at night (nocturia), and increased thirst and water consumption (polydipsia). Eye care professionals should enquire about these signs in patients with retinas that are suspicious for diabetic retinopathy as they may be able to make the initial diagnosis of diabetes. A urine test for sugar is an excellent cheap screening tool. The diagnosis is formally confirmed by measuring the blood glucose concentration (>11.1 mmol/L random glucose, >7.0 mmol/L fasting glucose).

Classification of diabetes

There are several different systems of classification. Some of these have many grades within them that are designed for countries where there is frequent screening of diabetic patients' retinas, so that worsening can be documented. They are not particularly useful in countries where diabetic patients are seen only occasionally. In these situations the main priority is to identify patients at risk of vision impairing complications. **Table 13.2** provides a very simple classification system.

Pathological changes in diabetic retinopathy

Diabetes causes damage to large vessels (macrovascular) and small blood vessels (microvascular). Macrovascular complications make diabetics at greater risk of heart attacks, strokes and peripheral vascular disease. It is the microvascular damage that causes damage to the retina and can impair the vision. The pathological changes and the fundus abnormalities they cause, as well as the sight-threatening complications of diabetic retinopathy are summarised in **Table 13.2**. They are then described in more detail below.

Capillary closure and leakage

The capillaries become blocked. This is probably caused by the high blood sugars damaging the capillary walls and also directly affecting the blood itself and making it more 'sticky'. Capillary blockage prevents oxygen reaching the retina (ischaemia). In the early stages the retina may appear normal on fundus examination. However areas of ischaemia can be seen with fluorescein angiography (**Figure 13.11**). The damaged capillaries leak fluid (oedema) and protein (exudate) into the retina. As the disease progresses, the areas of ischaemia and leakage from vessels cause the changes described below which are visible on fundus examination.

Table 13.2 A simple classification system for diabetic retinopathy		
Type of retinopathy	**Key features**	**Treatment**
Background diabetic retinopathy	No new vessels and no severe ischaemic changes	Lifestyle changes (blood pressure, diet etc) and observation only of retina
Pre-proliferative retinopathy	Severe ischaemic changes, i.e. lots of deep haemorrhages, cotton wool spots and vessel abnormalities, but no new vessels	Consider panretinal photocoagulation, particularly if patient follow-up may be difficult
Proliferative retinopathy	New blood vessels developing at the optic disc or retina	Panretinal photocoagulation
Maculopathy	Macular oedema and exudate that is impairing the vision	Macular laser and/or intravitreal anti-VEGF agents.

Table 13.3 The microvascular changes, fundus changes and sight-threatening complications of diabetic retinopathy		
Two pathological changes	**Six clinical abnormalities seen on fundus examination**	**Four sight-threatening complications**
Capillary closure causing ischaemic areas* Capillary leakage	Microaneurysms Macular leakage – Exudate – Oedema Haemorrhages – Dot haemorrhages – Blot haemorrhages – Flame haemorrhages Changes in the veins – 'Beading' and irregularities of the veins – Venous loops – Intra-retinal microvascular abnormalities Cotton-wool spots New blood vessels	Diabetic maculopathy (macular oedema) Proliferative retinopathy (new vessels) Vitreous haemorrhage Tractional retinal detachment

*Ischaemic areas are best seen on fluorescein angiography (Figure 13.11)

Microaneurysms

Microaneurysms are small dilatations of the walls of the capillaries to form small red 'dots' around the retina (**Figures 13.9** and **13.10**) These are an early sign of diabetic retinopathy. Microaneurysms can leak blood to form haemorrhages (see below).

Intraretinal microvascular abnormalities (IRMA)

IRMA are abnormal networks of capillaries that are probably formed from the dilated remains of damaged capillaries. They are often confused with new vessels (see below), although IRMA are always flat in the retina and they are usually found right in the middle of areas of capillary occlusion, rather

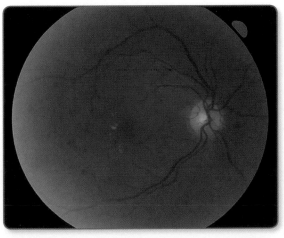

Figure 13.9 Background diabetic retinopathy and diabetic maculopathy. Note the 'dot and blot' haemorrhages and the hard exudate around the macula.

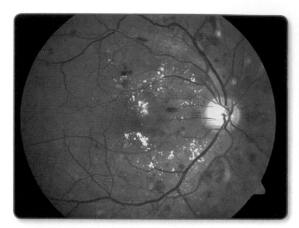

Figure 13.10 The features of more severe non-proliferative diabetic retinopathy: ① Dot and blot haemorrhages. ② Microaneurysms are the tiny red spots in the macula. ③ Cotton-wool spots are the circular white spots above the optic disc. ④ The yellowy-white areas all over the macula are macular exudate.

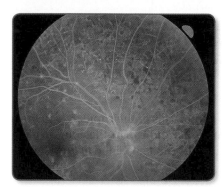

Figure 13.11 Fluorescein angiogram of diabetic retinopathy. The fluorescein is injected into the arm and travels in the bloodstream to the eye. The fluorescein dye appears white. There are lots of dark areas where no fluorescein can be seen due to capillary closure in the choroidal vascular layer. There is lots of leakage of fluorescein around the optic disc. This is coming from new blood vessels growing out of the optic disc. Some fluorescein is also leaking from other areas of the retina. There are tiny white spots, microaneurysms, scattered throughout the retina.

than on the border between healthy and ischaemic retina where neovascularisation is typically found.

Venous changes

As diabetic retinopathy progresses, the veins start to develop abnormalities. They can become 'beaded' and form strange loops in the retina.

'Dot' and 'blot' and flame haemorrhages

Weak capillaries can break down to leak blood. Bleeding in the outer plexiform layer forms small 'dot' haemorrhages. More extensive bleeding through the layers of the retina forms darker, bigger haemorrhages called 'blot' haemorrhages (**Figure 13.10**). Flame haemorrhages, are formed from blood that is tracking around nerves in the nerve fibre layer of the retina.

Cotton-wool spots (CWS)

Ischaemic infarcts of the nerve fibre layer causes CWS to form in the same way as in vein occlusions (see above).

The formation of new blood vessels (neovascularisation) – proliferative diabetic retinopathy (Figure. 13.12)

The closure of the capillaries and the areas of ischaemia in the retina stimulate new capillary vessels to grow from small veins (venules). New blood vessels always form loops so one can follow them round to see them return to where they started. They most commonly occur at the optic disc or the

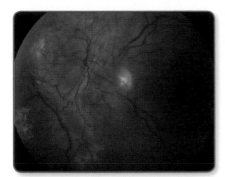

Figure 13.12 Proliferative diabetic retinopathy. The extensive new blood vessels are blocking a clear view of the optic disc

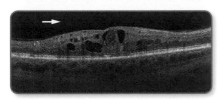

Figure 13.13 Diabetic maculopathy. An ocular coherence tomogram of the retina. This is a cross-sectional view through the retina at the macula. Note the black areas of fluid in the fovea. Although most patients and eye clinics will not have access to this modern scan, it is a helpful and clear way of showing diabetic macular oedema. The 'bubbles' of leaking fluid can be seen with careful examination with a direct ophthalmoscope or a slit lamp and condensing lens.

mid-peripheral retina. They can be small and difficult to see in the early stages, and one must specifically look for them at the optic disc and along the major vascular arcades. They can be easier to see with the green filter of the ophthalmoscope. They do not actually grow in the retinal layers, but on its surface, between the retina and the vitreous. New blood vessels are sight-threatening as they can grow and bleed into the vitreous (see below) and even to the front of the eye where they can block aqueous drainage causing severe glaucoma.

Macular oedema and hard exudate
Damaged blood vessel walls leak plasma into the surrounding retina. Although this can occur anywhere in the retina, it is worst at the macula (macular oedema) when it can greatly reduce the central vision. This is called diabetic maculopathy (**Figure 13.13**). At the edges of the fluid leakage, yellow exudates ('hard exudates') (**Figure 13.14**) appear. These consist of lipid that is being 'eaten' up by the retinal macrophages. Sometimes the fluid leaks out from microaneurysms in a circular patch with a circle of hard exudates around the outside: 'circinate exudates'. Macular oedema and exudates are more commonly seen in type 2 diabetics and is a common cause of reduced vision because the fovea becomes thick and full of fluid.

Diabetic vitreous haemorrhage and tractional retinal detachment
Vitreous haemorrhage occurs because the new vessels that are formed in proliferative retinopathy are fragile, and break easily (**Figure 13.15**). The growth of new vessels into the vitreous gel and the blood in the vitreous provokes inflammation followed by scarring. The scarring causes contraction that can pull on the blood vessels causing recurrent and increasingly persistent and

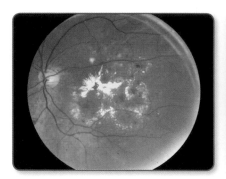

Figure 13.14 Diabetic macular exudate.

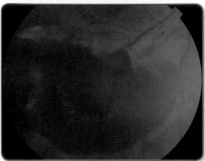

Figure 13.15 Pre-retinal haemorrhage. This bleed has come from diabetic new vessels. The blood is located between the retina and the vitreous. It is likely to spread into the vitreous.

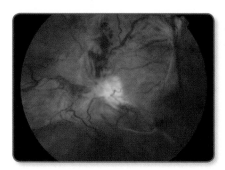

Figure 13.16 Tractional retinal detachment. The retina is being lifted away from the back of the eye by the traction in the vitreous.

severe vitreous haemorrhages. The scarring can also pull on the retina itself causing tractional retinal detachment (**Figure 13.16**). The vision is usually rapidly and irreversibly lost at this stage unless urgent and intensive surgical and laser treatment is given. This requires expertise and equipment, which is only available in very well equipped clinics. These sorts of blinding changes are more commonly seen in type 1 diabetics.

Risk factors for diabetic retinopathy

It is known that the following risk factors cause diabetic retinopathy to progress:
- Poor blood sugar control
- Increased blood pressure
- Increasing number of microaneurysms
- Duration of diabetes
- Protein and albumin in the urine
- Raised cholesterol
- Pregnancy
- Smoking

Investigation of diabetic retinopathy

Our understanding of all vascular retinopathies, and in particular diabetic retinopathy, has been greatly improved by a technique called *fluorescein angiography*. In this investigation, fluorescein dye is injected into a vein and a series of photographs taken of the retina, which show the dye travelling in the retinal vessels and capillaries. **Figure 13.11** shows a typical fluorescein angiogram of diabetic retinopathy and demonstrates the changes in the blood vessels very clearly.

Preventing blindness from diabetic retinopathy

Diabetic retinopathy is a chronic and progressive disease, which cannot be cured. However, there are ways in which it can be managed and its progress slowed. If the patient and their health-care professionals manage it well, the vision will probably be maintained for many years. However, if it is managed badly, the vision can be severely affected.

All diabetics should understand how important it is to look after their bodies and must be helped and reminded of the following:

- Keep the blood sugar controlled. Patients should be taught how to supervise their own diabetic medication to keep the blood glucose level normal throughout the day.
- Keep the blood pressure controlled: aim for less than 140/80 mmHg.
- Keep to a strict, healthy diet and avoid obesity.
- Take exercise regularly.
- Avoid smoking.

A patient's blood sugar control can be assessed by checking their HbA1c (glycosylated haemoglobin. This is the haemoglobin with glucose stuck to it and goes up if the blood sugar levels are regularly high). This test is now widely available. Ideally patients should aim for an HbA1c of 7% or lower.

Treatment of diabetic retinopathy

There are several treatments for the different stages of type 1 and type 2 diabetes. Many of these treatments are designed to stop the production of vascular endothelial growth factor (VEGF). If tissue cells do not have enough oxygen, VEGF is released.

In diabetic retinopathy, tissue cells are starved of oxygen causing the diseased retina to produce VEGF. The VEGF then stimulates the growth of new blood vessels, which leak protein and bleed. Fibroblasts invade and form fibrous tissue leading to the blinding complications seen in diabetic retinopathy.

Laser treatment

Lasers produce a focused beam of very bright light of specific wavelengths. If this light beam is shone on the retina it will burn the rods, cones and pigment epithelium, producing a scar. It can also cause small blood vessels to fibrose and close. Argon and diode lasers are the types most commonly used but others are available. A laser is not a magic treatment that can cure vascular retinopathies, but is basically an instrument of destruction, which destroys diseased and less important areas of the retina, in order to prevent complications threatening the rest of the retina.

Proliferative retinopathy: pan-retinal photocoagulation (PRP) (Figure 13.17)

PRP is the use of the laser to destroy large areas of the peripheral retina to maintain the health of the rest of the retina. This is the most effective

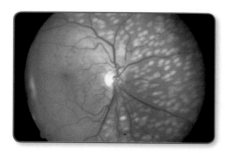

Figure 13.17 Pan-retinal photocoagulation. The retinal laser scars will become pigmented a few weeks after the laser treatment.

use of laser and can stop diabetic patients, and particularly young diabetics with long-term type 1 disease, from going blind. These patients have chronic retinal ischaemia, which stimulates the growth of new blood vessels. By destroying areas of peripheral retina, the retina's oxygen requirements are reduced, which in turn reduces the production of VEGF. This reduces the stimulus to produce the new vessels. If a thorough and timely PRP is done, the new vessels can scar and shrink and become quiet and inactive very quickly and the rest of the peripheral haemorrhages and exudate can slowly disappear. However, this must be complemented by the lifestyle changes described above. Patients must be advised that they may have visual field constriction after PRP and this can affect whether they are eligible to drive. However, good central vision can be maintained for many years.

Diabetic maculopathy: macular laser

The laser is used to destroy tiny areas of leaking vessels around the macula, or to cause mild damage in the macula, which is thought to help the retina to absorb some of the leaking fluid and exudate. This is a less effective procedure than PRP but can stabilise the central vision. The procedure is not effective if the macula is already significantly ischaemic; this can be seen on fluorescein angiography (**Figure 13.11**). The central vision will be damaged if the laser is aimed directly at the macula. Therefore laser treatment must only be carried out be well-trained eye-care professionals.

Anti-vascular endothelial growth factor (anti-VEGF) treatments

Anti-VEGF treatments inhibit new vessel formation and macular oedema. PRP is still the treatment of choice for new vessels, but the treatment of diabetic macular oedema is currently changing dramatically with intravitreal anti-VEGF injections. There is increasingly evidence that they are effective at reducing the amount of macular oedema and that they are probably more effective than macular laser. However, they need to be given regularly and remain expensive. The most widely used intravitreal anti-VEGFs are ranibizumab and bevacizumab.

Intravitreal triamcinolone

Intravitreal triamcinolone is a steroid that is also sometimes used to treat macular oedema. It can improve the vision but the macular oedema almost always returns and the vision worsens again. There is a risk of the steroid causing raised intraocular pressure.

Vitrectomy

Vitrectomy can be an essential vision saving operation in patients with persistent vitreous haemorrhage. However only ophthalmologists with considerable experience of vitrectomy surgery should carry out this procedure and it needs relatively specialised equipment that is only likely to be available in major ophthalmology units. Many haemorrhages will clear without intervention and therefore can be left several months as long as active proliferation or retinal traction are not present. It can be difficult to decide when to proceed with a vitrectomy, as there is of course some risk to any surgery. However, it is usually done in the following circumstances:

- The patient is also suspected of having active proliferative retinopathy, which cannot be seen behind the blood. Vitrectomy clears the haemorrhage so that the PRP can be done.
- The patient is suspected of having vitreous scarring and traction that is threatening to cause a retinal detachment. Vitrectomy allows the retina to be released and lasered to repair and prevent further detachment.

Cryotherapy

If laser is not available, cryotherapy can be used to destroy the peripheral retina in patients with neovascularisation. It is less effective than laser, and can do more damage to the rest of the eye. It does have the advantage that as it is done from the outside of the eye, it is possible to do the procedure without having a clear view of the retina (unlike PRP).

Cataract extraction in patients with diabetic retinopathy

It is possible that macular oedema will worsen in the short-term after cataract surgery and patients must be warned about this. However in the long-term, cataract surgery does not appear to increase the amount of macular oedema (compared to patients who do not have cataract surgery). Therefore, cataract surgery should probably not be delayed.

Diabetic screening in the community

There are large numbers of diabetics in the community and about 10% of them have diabetic retinopathy that needs treatment. There are also many people who are diabetic without even being aware of it. In such a situation, a screening service is very valuable. Even in rich countries there are many diabetics who do not receive good eye care, and diabetes is still a very common reason for blind registration. The main reason for diabetic screening is to examine the eyes of known diabetics from time to time, in order to give laser treatment as soon as it is needed. A diabetic screening clinic is also a very good opportunity for educating people about good diabetic control.

The retina should always be examined even in routine eye checks, as this is often the way that type 2 diabetes is first detected. Unfortunately in many poor countries, treatment for diabetic retinopathy may only be available in a few large cities and it may be very expensive. However, the progression can be greatly reduced simply by changing lifestyle factors, even if expensive lasers and surgical equipment and expertise are not available.

Some basic guidelines for diabetic retinopathy screening are:

- The pupil must be dilated to look at the retina properly.

- Non-doctors can be taught to screen for diabetic retinopathy.
- Young type 1 diabetics do not need to be seen very often in the first few years after their disease is diagnosed, but must be seen frequently if there is any evidence of diabetic retinopathy.
- Older type 2 diabetics should be seen once a year, and every 6 months if there are signs of background retinopathy.
- Pregnant diabetic women need to be watched very closely especially if they have any signs of retinopathy.
- All opticians should know how to recognise diabetic retinopathy.
- Retinal photography done by technicians can be a good way of screening if the equipment is available. Retinal cameras are becoming cheaper, particularly because there are now mobile phone attachments that allow high quality fundus photos to be taken (see page 78).
- Patients with background retinopathy need observation only.
- Diabetic maculopathy needs treatment and proliferative retinopathy needs urgent treatment. Vitreous haemorrhage may also require treatment.

Sickle cell disease

Sickle cell disease is a genetic disorder of the haemoglobin, which causes the red blood cells to become abnormally shaped (shaped like a sickle, or curved blade). The disease is hereditary, and is found almost exclusively in black Africans or people of African descent, especially from west Africa.

Normal haemoglobin is called haemoglobin A (HbA). Sickle haemoglobin is called haemoglobin S (HbS). Everyone has two genes for haemoglobin. Normal haemoglobin is HbAA. A person with sickle cell disease has HbSS. A person with one normal and one abnormal gene is genetically HbAS. This is called sickle cell trait (the individual is a sickle cell carrier).

All the haemoglobin in patients with HbSS is abnormal. It becomes sickle-shaped when the blood oxygen levels are low. Sickle cells are easily destroyed, causing anaemia. They also cannot flow properly through small blood vessels causing blockages and/or reduced blood supply to the tissues. This results in tissue ischaemia and infarction. Many children with sickle cell disease die young, particularly in areas where medical treatment options are limited. Those that survive often have widespread pathological changes.

Carriers with HbAS have mild or no symptoms at all. However, they may pass on the gene to their children and if the other parent does likewise, the child will have sickle cell disease. Interestingly, sickle cell trait seems to provide some degree of resistance to malaria. This natural selection in favour of the abnormal gene, probably explains why it has persisted to such an extent. In some areas of Africa up to 20% of the population have at least one sickle cell gene.

Two other genetic disorders of the haemoglobin are sometimes found together with sickle haemoglobin:

- *Haemoglobin C (HbC):* HbC is a much milder abnormality than haemoglobin S, and is also found predominantly in black Africans or people of African descent. Patients whose haemoglobin is half S and half C (genetically HbSC) are particularly prone to eye complications.

- *Thalassaemia:* This is another hereditary disorder that impairs haemoglobin manufacture. It occurs mainly in people from the Mediterranean, North Africa and East Asia.

Diagnosis

The 'solubility test' is used to show the presence of HbS (deoxygenated HbS is less soluble than normal Hb). It is a good screening test for the disease. This test cannot distinguish between sickle cell disease and trait, and therefore should be followed by quantitative haemoglobin electrophoresis, which will diagnose the exact genetic type.

Ophthalmic signs of sickle cell disease

Ophthalmic signs can occur in patients with all forms of sickle-cell disease. Surprisingly, patients with half HbS and half HbC (HbSC) have the worst sickle cell retinopathy (approximately a third will develop proliferative retinopathy), followed by patients with HbS-Thal (proliferative retinopathy in approximately one in seven patients) and the lowest prevalence of eye complications is in patients with the most severe form of the disease: HbSS (approximately one in forty patients will develop proliferative retinopathy), despite these patients having much worse systemic complications. This may be because patients with HbSS are generally quite anaemic, which helps to lower the blood viscosity, thereby reducing the risk of vascular occlusions. Mild retinal changes can be seen in patients with HbAS.

Conjunctiva

The bulbar conjunctival vessels can become very abnormal, with dilated, irregular broken sections of vessels being visible on the conjunctival surface. This probably results from infarction of conjunctival vessels.

Anterior chamber – hyphaema

Patients with sickle cell disease may develop hyphaema with minimal trauma or after ocular surgery. This can also occur with sickle cell trait. One should consider sickle cell disease/trait in all black patients with hyphaema.

Iris

White patches of iris atrophy may develop after occlusions of iris vessels (**Figure 13.18**). They are asymptomatic and the patient is not normally aware of them. Patients with proliferative retinopathy can develop iris neovascularisation (see below).

Retina

The retinal vessels become dilated and tortuous in nearly half of individuals with sickle cell disease and about a third with HbSC. It is unknown if these vascular changes have a significant impact on the retinal health.

Retinal artery occlusions can occur in patients with all types of sickle cell disease but are probably most common in HbSS patients. The symptoms and signs are described above.

The most common and often the most clinically important eye changes in sickle disease, happen in the peripheral retina. Therefore, a dilated fundal examination is essential in patients with possible sickle cell disease. The following signs may be seen:

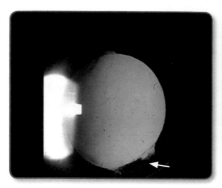

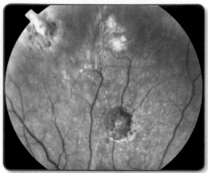

Figure 13.18 Iris atrophy in sickle cell anaemia (white arrow).

Figure 13.19 'Black sunburst' in sickle cell anaemia. This is formed from pigment being deposited in the retina after a haemorrhage.

- *Retinal haemorrhages* ('salmon patches') occur because of sudden occlusions of arterioles. They are initially bright red, but after a few days the denatured blood becomes an orange-red colour (slightly like the colour of salmon).
- *Black speculated pigmented lesions* ('black sunbursts', **Figure 13.19**). These are thought to be due to deep retina blood provoking pigment migration and deposition in the retina.
- *Retinal neovascularisation* ('sea-fans', **Figure 13.20a**): small peripheral retinal arterioles may become blocked, causing retinal ischaemia. In the same way as diabetes (see above), this causes new blood vessels to develop. These often grow into the vitreous in the shape of a 'sea-fan'. In due course these fragile vessels can bleed and ultimately cause retinal traction and detachment (**Figures 13.20b** and **13.20c**).

Although the late stages of the disease can be devastating to the vision, the early stages are often asymptomatic as they occur mainly in the peripheral retina.

Other less common or less clinically significant retinal and choroidal changes

Angioid streaks occur in approximately one in fifteen patients with sickle cell disease (**Figure 13.29**). They can of course occur in other diseases as well, including pseudoxanthoma elasticum, Paget's disease and Ehlers Danlos syndrome or be an idiopathic finding. Epiretinal membranes are seen more commonly in patients with sickle cell disease, particularly if they have retinal neovascularisation (see above).

Choroidal vessels and posterior ciliary vessels can also become occluded. This can produce visual field defects in the area of ischaemia.

The management of sickle cell disease

No treatment is given for the non-proliferative peripheral changes in sickle cell retinopathy. However, these patients need monitoring to check for proliferative disease. Destructive treatment is used to treat sea fans (areas of proliferation), e.g. laser treatment or sometimes cryotherapy. Scatter laser to

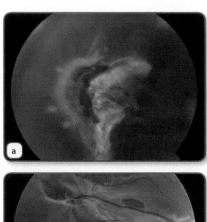

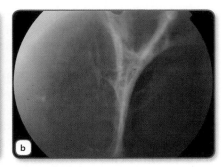

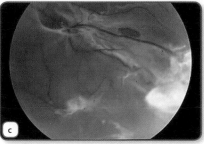

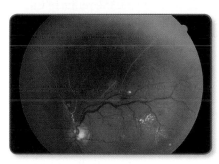

Figure 13.20 The sequence of events in proliferative retinopathy in sickle cell anaemia. (a) 'Sea fan': this is a collection of new blood vessels that develop because of the ischaemia. Note that the retina is also starting to detach in the area of the sea fan (b) Retinal traction: the retina is being lifted up because of fibrotic changes in the vitreous provoked by the new vessels. (c) Tractional retinal detachment: tears have developed in the retina and it has detached.

Figure 13.21 Retinal vasculitis. There is white sheathing of the retinal vessels above the optic disc. Some of these vessels have probably become completely occluded. There are also some haemorrhages and cotton-wool spots above the optic disc and some hard exudates around the macula. It is mainly the arteries that are occluded in this case, i.e. arteritis.

the whole area can be done or the sea fan is obliterated with intensive laser. Once traction or retinal detachment starts to develop, vitreoretinal surgery is required to try and stop the patient losing their vision.

Retinal vasculitis

Retinal vasculitis is inflammation of the retinal blood vessel walls (**Figure 13.21**). In severe cases the walls of the blood vessels may undergo necrosis (death). Vessel inflammation and damage restricts retinal blood supply, which may damage the retina. Retinal vasculitis is a complex subject for the following reasons:

- It is not a common condition, and some of its specific causes are quite rare. Therefore, many people may find it hard to recognise and diagnose. However, retinal vasculitis may be sight-threatening and some of its causes may even by life-threatening.
- Retinal vasculitis can have a very varied presentation. It may be very mild with just a few sheathed vessels or it may be severe, with extensive ischaemic changes to the retina itself.

- Retinal vasculitis may be part of a more widespread systemic disease, with blood vessels in other parts of the body also being affected. It is often difficult to determine the exact cause of the vasculitis and therefore what treatment to give.
- Treatment is possible for most of the causes of retinal vasculitis, but the treatments can be toxic and may require expertise to use. The wrong treatment can make the condition worse, or be dangerous.

In this brief description of what is a difficult disease, both to diagnose and to treat, we will firstly describe the signs and symptoms of retinal vasculitis. Then, we will discuss the more important causes and some of the difficulties with the treatment.

Signs and symptoms of retinal vasculitis

The following changes may be seen on examining the retina:

- *Sheathing of the retinal blood vessels.* This is probably caused by inflammation in the walls of the arteries and veins. It is the characteristic sign of vasculitis. Retinal vasculitis more commonly affects the veins and venules (phlebitis) but the retinal arteries and arterioles can also be affected (arteritis) in some diseases (**Figure 13.21**).
- *Vascular occlusion*: the lumen of inflamed vessels becomes narrower and the blood sticks to the wall. They block easily and the retina in this area becomes ischaemic. Cotton wool spots, retinal haemorrhages, hard exudates and neovascularisation may all develop in areas of ischaemia as described above in the section on proliferative diabetic retinopathy.
- *Vitreous haemorrhage.* New vessels are very fragile and may bleed into the vitreous.

The symptoms and severity of retinal vasculitis are very variable. Often there are initially no ocular symptoms, but the patient may have significant symptoms of systemic disease. For example, patients with tuberculosis can have severe lung disease without any ocular symptoms, but when the eye is examined peripheral vascular sheathing may be seen. When retinal vasculitis is severe it can cause visual loss because the vascular occlusion causes retinal ischaemia and vitreous haemorrhage.

It is often difficult to tell the difference between a retinal vascular occlusion caused by hypertension and arteriosclerosis, and one caused by retinal vasculitis; look for the sheathing around vessels that occurs in vasculitis and look for systemic signs of inflammatory disease. It is important to try to identify the cause of the occluded vessel, because patients with inflammatory vasculitis often respond to systemic steroid treatment, but steroids can be dangerous if the cause is infective.

Classification and causes of retinal vasculitis

The most useful classification of retinal vasculitis is to try and determine the cause. It is also sometimes classified by whether it is affecting the arteries (arteritis) or the veins (phlebitis) – or both and by whether it affects large, medium or smaller sized vessels. Both of these classifications can help point towards a particular cause of the inflammation.

The following categories of disease can cause retinal vasculitis:

- *Inflammatory/autoimmune disease*, e.g. multiple sclerosis, polyarteritis nodosa, systemic lupus erythematosus, ANCA-associate granulomatous vasculitis (formally called Wegener's granulomatosis), sarcoidosis and Behçet disease.
- *Infective disease*, e.g. tuberculosis, syphilis, viruses such as herpes simplex, herpes zoster and cytomegalovirus.
- *Cancer*: intraocular lymphoma can present with retinal vasculitis (see below).

Important causes of retinal vasculitis

Although there are numerous causes of retinal vasculitis, we will discuss a few in more detail. These diseases are either more common in poor countries or diagnosing them may save the patient's vision or even life. If retinal vasculitis is suspected, take a full medical history and make a full medical examination. If possible, a consultation with a general medical specialist may be helpful. The blood pressure must be measured and a urine sample tested. Routine blood tests, such as a full blood count, kidney and liver function and inflammatory markers (ESR and CRP) should be done, as well as tests for infection, particularly tuberculosis and HIV.

Tuberculosis (TB) (see Chapter 11)

Tuberculosis can cause retinal periphlebitis. TB testing must always be carried out in patients with retinal vasculitis in countries where TB is common or when people have visited or come from a country with TB. The vasculitis can occur in patients with active TB, but also can occur many years after the disease has been treated, and in these cases is probably an autoimmune phenomenon.

Viruses

Herpes simplex virus, herpes zoster virus and cytomegalovirus can all cause retinal infection (retinitis). Retinitis is a very different condition to retinal vasculitis. It often presents initially with vascular inflammation; in viral retinitis, the inflammation is mainly in the arteries rather than the veins.

Sarcoidosis

Sarcoidosis, which is an inflammatory disease of unknown cause, can cause a very similar clinical picture to TB. However, distinguishing between the two is very important, as TB must be treated with anti-tuberculoid drugs for a long period of time, while sarcoid is treated with steroids. If steroids are used in TB, it can mask the disease, allowing it to get much worse.

Eales disease

Eales disease mainly affects the peripheral retinal vessels. It is relatively common in South Asia and often affects young patients. It was thought to be a hypersensitivity reaction to tuberculosis, but this is not likely in many cases and there is possibly a genetic predisposition and an environmental trigger.

Behçet disease

This disease of unknown cause is much more common in people from Turkey, the Eastern Mediterranean and the Middle East. It can cause acute anterior uveitis (sometimes with a hypopyon), retinal phlebitis with occlusions and numerous systemic signs including mouth and genital ulcers. There can be some retinal infiltrates, which give an appearance of retinitis. It is discussed in more detail in Chapter 11.

Other autoimmune diseases

Numerous other autoimmune diseases can cause retinal vasculitis. For example, collagen diseases like systemic lupus erythematosus (SLE) and polyarteritis nodosa, which affect the small arteries throughout the body. It is important to try and decide if the cause of retinal vasculitis is autoimmune, as these diseases require treatment with steroids.

Tumours: lymphoma

Lymphomas can present with retinal vasculitis. They are frequently missed even by very experienced ophthalmologists and therefore sometimes called *masquerade syndromes* (disguise syndromes).

Treatment

Many of the diseases that cause retinal vasculitis are very difficult to treat even in rich countries. Great expertise and experience is required to make the diagnosis and institute treatment. However, the most important distinction is whether the cause is inflammatory or infective. Inflammatory diseases are usually treated with steroids or an alternative immune-modifying agent, while infective diseases need a suitable anti-infective agent.

Other causes of retinal vascular disease

Other haematological diseases, such as anaemia and leukaemia may cause retinal haemorrhages and exudates. It is therefore important to always check the full blood count and inflammatory markers (ESR and CRP) if retinal haemorrhages are seen, but the diagnosis is unknown.

Retinal artery macroaneurysms (**Figure 13.22**) are 'sac-like' areas of widening retinal arteries. They are associated with raised blood pressure and athersclerotic vascular disease. They can leak exudate or blood, which may affect vision if they are in or near the macula and laser treatment may be considered. Away from the macula they usually do not require treatment.

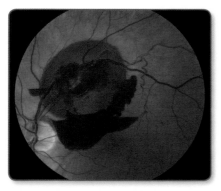

Figure 13.22 Retinal macroaneurysm, which has burst and bled into the retina and vitreous.

Retinal degenerative disease

Age-related macular degeneration (AMD)

AMD is the pathological changes that occur in the macula of the retina in people over the age of 55 years. AMD is only diagnosed when there is no other disease process, i.e. it is simply associated with aging. It is the commonest cause of severe visual impairment in older people in rich countries. It is less common in poor countries, which have a younger population, lower life expectancy and many other more important diseases. However, life expectancy is increasing throughout the world and therefore AMD is becoming much more common. Also there are now treatments for some forms of AMD. Some of these treatments are relatively cheap and easy to administer and therefore will be increasingly available. AMD is divided into two distinct types: 'wet' (exudative or neovascular) and 'dry' (geographic atrophy).

Pre-AMD changes

Before the development of obvious wet or dry AMD there is an accumulation of lipid material beneath the retinal pigment epithelium (RPE). This forms clumps of pale yellow deposits under the retina, which are called drusen (**Figure 13.23**). Larger, 'softer' (more fluffy edges) drusen are more likely to develop into AMD than smaller, 'harder' drusen. The retina in the macular area also starts to become atrophic which is seen as areas of hyper- and hypopigmentation. These changes can look very dramatic but do not usually greatly impair the vision.

Wet AMD

In 'wet' AMD clumps of new blood vessels that come from the choroid (choroidal neovascularisation) invade through defects and cause damage in the membrane between the retina and the choroid (Bruch's membrane) and into the subretinal area. The vessels leak fluid, exudate (lipid and protein) and blood under (subretinal) and into (intraretinal) the macula. Therefore, the macula is described as being 'wet'. The neovascularisation and exudation severely damage the retina and RPE. A fibrovascular mass of scar tissue is formed between the retina and choroid, which impairs the retinal function.

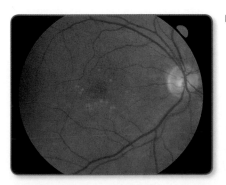

Figure 13.23 Drusen.

Clinical appearance

In the early stages, small areas of the macula are raised from the leaking fluid (**Figure 13.24**). In the later stages, there is a mass of dense pale scar tissue in the macular area, and often some hard exudates from lipid deposits in the macrophages and haemorrhages (**Figure 13.25**). This type of degeneration is sometimes called 'disciform macular degeneration' because of the disc like shape of the white scar under the macula.

Symptoms

In the early stages there is often some kinking or distortion of objects or straight lines, although this is often missed by the patient if the other eye is healthy. Patients at risk of macular degeneration can be given a piece of paper with squares on (Amsler grid) in order to test each eye for distortion. The distortion is usually followed by quite rapid loss of central vision over the course of a few days or weeks. Ultimately, the central vision usually ends up being 6/60 or worse. However, the peripheral vision remains intact.

Treatment

A diagnosis of wet AMD used to be very bad news, as the central vision would fall to 6/60 or even count fingers relatively quickly. However in recent

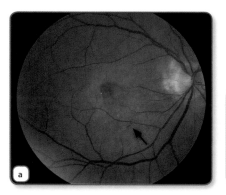
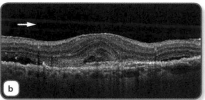

Figure 13.24 (a) Wet macular degeneration. The slightly paler appearance around the fovea is caused by fluid leakage into and under the macula from the choroidal neovascular membrane. There is a small haemorrhage inferior to the fovea. (b) The fluid leakage can be seen in this ocular coherence tomogram which shows a cross section of the macula (red arrow).

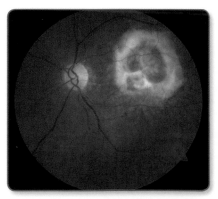

Figure 13.25 Macular disciform scar from wet age related macular degeneration.

years there has been a revolution in the treatment of wet AMD. Intravitreal injections of anti-vascular endothelial growth factor (anti-VEGF) can stop the disease progressing. This can stop the vision worsening and in about a quarter of patients, the vision improves a bit. However, treatment is needed soon after the leakage of fluid, before there is too much scarring, as late treatment will not make much difference. The treatment involves an initial course of three injections given over 3 months. If there is continued exudation of fluid in or under the retina, further injections need to be given. Some patients may end up receiving as many as fifty injections in order to keep the disease from progressing. At present two main anti-VEGF agents are widely used (although others are becoming available). Ranibizumab (Lucentis) was designed as an AMD treatment. Bevacizumab (Avastin) was designed for systemic chemotherapy, and therefore the vials have much more drug in them. Each vial of bevacizumab can be divided into several intravitreal injections. It is therefore much cheaper. Two large randomised trials have shown that ranibizumab and bevacizumab have similar efficacy. At present ranibizumab is far too expensive for many people. Bevacizumab is more affordable, but does require suitably equipped and skilled manufacturing pharmacies to divide the vials.

Dry AMD

Dry AMD is a gradual atrophic process of the RPE and the choriocapillaris. There are no new or leaking vessels. There is no treatment for dry AMD, although it is possible that a very healthy diet with many green vegetables, may slightly slow down the progress of the condition. Smoking can make AMD progress more quickly.

Clinical appearance

In 'dry' AMD there are well-demarcated areas of pigment loss where there is atrophy of the RPE (**Figure 13.26**). Sometimes the normal, large choroidal vessels are seen through the atrophic RPE (a 'window defect').

Symptoms

Patients describe distortion and reduction of vision and particularly the reading vision. The visual loss is very much more gradual and usually less severe than in untreated wet AMD. Many patients are not aware of the gradual change, particularly if it is unilateral.

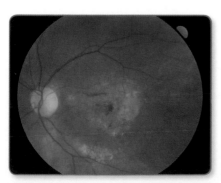

Figure 13.26 Dry age related macular degeneration. The appearance of a mixture of pigmented and pale areas in the macula is often called 'geographic atrophy'.

Other conditions associated with choroidal neovascularisation

Myopic retinal degeneration

Very myopic eyes are very large. The axial length of the eye is sometimes over 30 mm, compared to the normal eye of about 24 mm. In these myopic eyes, the RPE, choroid and retina become very stretched and thin. There is often degeneration and atrophy around the optic disc, and especially around the macula (**Figure 13.27**) Defects can develop in the choroid and RPE ('lacquer cracks'). Similarly to wet AMD, choroidal neovascularisation (CNV) can develop in these cracks (**Figure 13.28**).

Angioid streaks (Figure 13.29)

Angioid streaks are cracks in Bruch's membrane, which occur in a variety of diseases including sickle cell anaemia (see above) and pseudoxanthoma elasticum. The vision is usually normal unless the streak goes straight through the fovea. However, CNV can develop in these cracks and the exudate and haemorrhage and subsequent scarring can severely reduce the vision.

Treatment

These CNVs that occur in myopic degeneration and angioid streaks can sometimes be prevented from progressing with intravitreal anti-VEGF injections.

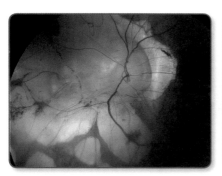

Figure 13.27 Severe myopic chorioretinal degeneration.

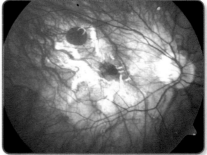

Figure 13.28 Myopic lacquer cracks. The white lines are breaks in Bruch's membrane and therefore the underlying choroid and sclera can be seen.

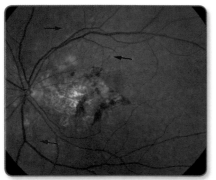

Figure 13.29 Angioid streaks. The arrows point to the streaks radiating away from the optic disc. This patient also has extensive macular atrophy and scarring, probably because they developed a CNV from their angioid streaks.

Hereditary chorioretinal disease

Many genetic disorders cause choroidoretinal degenerations, and the symptoms usually appear in childhood or teenage years. The incidence of these genetic disorders varies in different parts of the world, but is likely to be higher in isolated communities or areas where consanguinity (children born to parents who are close relatives) is more common. The two most common disorders are retinitis pigmentosa and albinism.

Retinitis pigmentosa (RP)

RP is the characteristic retinal appearance that is caused by a huge and wide-ranging group of inherited diseases. The majority of these diseases only affect the retina, but others are systemic disorders of which the retinal disease is one small part of the whole syndrome. RP can have autosomal dominant, recessive and sex linked inheritance. Even some mitochondrially inherited diseases can cause RP.

Clinical appearance (Figure 13.30)

RP particularly affects the peripheral retina. Sharply defined patches of retinal pigmentation are seen along the small peripheral retinal arterioles ('bone spicules'). The retinal arteries and arterioles become narrowed and eventually are completely absent in the peripheral retina. RP is common in east Asia, especially among those communities in which cousins marry each other.

Symptoms

Patients with RP usually report poor vision at night, dawn and dusk. Although they have gross constriction of their visual field, they are often not aware of this. However, they may be aware that they bump into things quite frequently. For example, one of our patients with RP was unaware that he had the disease but stopped cycling as he kept hitting things with his handlebars. Eventually central visual reduction or loss develops, usually between the age of about 50 and 80 years.

Treatment

There is no established treatment for RP yet, although gene therapy (injecting viruses into the eye to alter genes of the retina) trials are showing some

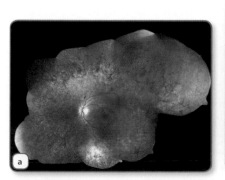
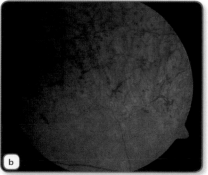

Figure 13.30 Retinitis pigmentosa. (a) Widespread stippled pigmentation across the whole fundus. Narrowed arteries disappear completely in the periphery. (b) A highly magnified view through an ophthalmoscope shows the pigmentation.

promise for a few genetic subtypes of the disease. It will be many years before these are widely available. Patients with RP are more likely to develop premature cataract and surgery can give surprisingly useful improvements in vision. Patients with RP need strong support from their family and community.

Albinism

Albinism is a failure to produce the melanin pigment in the skin and the eye. Both the skin and the fundus therefore look pale. The visual acuity is diminished because there is poor macular fixation, and there is often nystagmus. There are partial forms of the disease where some pigment is produced. These children may be very blond with pale blue eyes, but may not look particularly different to other white children and have good vision.

Albinism is untreatable, but patients are likely to be very photosensitive and at risk of sunburn and skin cancer. Therefore, sunglasses and covering their skin with clothes or sun cream is important. The vision in albinism does not usually deteriorate. It is very important therefore, that these children are taught in schools for sighted children using low visual aids and not in blind schools using Braille.

Juvenile macular dystrophies

There are several rare diseases that affect the macula of young people causing poor visual acuity. Most of them are genetically inherited although in some cases the symptoms do not appear until adolescence or early adult life.

Onchocerciasis

In certain areas, onchocerciasis is an important cause of choroidoretinal degeneration (see Figure 16.8).

Retinal detachments

The normal retina lies in close contact with the underlying retinal pigment epithelium (RPE). When a retinal detachment occurs, the retina separates from the RPE, and protein-rich fluid fills the space in between. Retinal detachments are not a very common cause of blindness. However, it is one major retinal disease that can be treated and early surgery, if successful, will preserve and in some cases restore the sight. Unfortunately, if surgical treatment is delayed, secondary changes will occur, which eventually make the retinal detachment untreatable. Therefore, it is important to be able to recognise a retinal detachment in the early stages.

Posterior vitreous detachment and asteroid hyalosis

A posterior vitreous detachment (PVD) is a normal ageing change, but it is important to discuss it here, as the symptoms of a PVD can be very similar to a retinal tear, and distinguishing between the two is critical. As the vitreous ages it becomes less viscous and more liquid. The aging vitreous detaches from the retina, typically in patients over the age of 50 although often earlier in myopes. This is a normal aging process. It is can be accompanied by some flashing lights caused by the traction on the retina and some new floaters caused by the change in structure of the vitreous. There is a small risk of the traction causing a retinal tear, which is typically 'U' shaped (**Figures 13.31 and 13.33**). If this occurs there is a significant risk of developing a retinal detachment (see below).

Asteroid hyalosis is the developing presence of small white, shimmering opacities in the vitreous. For unknown reasons, they are usually unilateral. Although their appearance can be dramatic, they are usually asymptomatic other than sometimes causing some 'floaters'.

Causes of retinal detachment

The retina may detach either because there is vitreous traction pulling it away from the RPE or because there is fluid leakage between the two layers, which separates them (Figure 13.31).

1. **Rhegmatogenous retinal detachment**

   This means a retinal detachment caused by a hole or break in the retina. This is the commonest cause of retinal detachment. Fluid leaks through the hole and separates the retina from the RPE (**Figures 13.32–13.34**). There are two common types of breaks in the retina:

   - 'U' shaped tear: these are created by vitreous traction and occur suddenly. They usually occur during the natural posterior vitreous detachment (see above).
   - Atrophic holes in the peripheral retina: these are usually round and in the thin peripheral retina, particularly in myopic people. They my be present for some years without causing any symptoms. If this edge become lifted up then fluid will pass beneath the retina causing detachment.

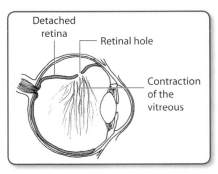

Figure 13.31 Illustration of how a retinal hole causes retinal detachment.

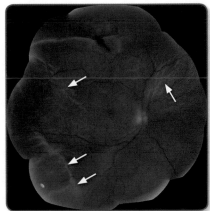

Figure 13.32 Complete retinal detachment. There is a large tear in the superior retina (red arrow). The wrinkled retina (white arrows) shows that the whole retina has detached. The macula is also detached and therefore vision will be very poor (compare with **Figure 13.33**). Vision may improve after successful retinal detachment surgery, but it is unlikely to recover fully.

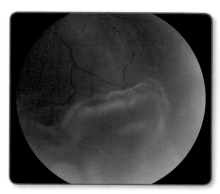

Figure 13.33 Inferior rhegmatogenous retinal detachment. This retinal detachment has been caused by a small peripheral tear in the retina. This photograph is of the inferior retina. The superior vision will be affected. But, as the macula has not detached, the central vision will not be reduced (compare with **Figure 13.32**).

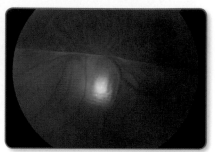

Figure 13.34 This retinal detachment has been caused by a very large (giant) retinal tear. The whole of the upper half of the retina has detached and folded over. If the upper half of the retina is detached, it is the lower half of the vision that will be affected.

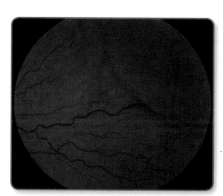

Figure 13.35 Serous retinal detachment. The retina is detaching because of fluid underneath. In this patient, the fluid has been caused by an underlying tumour.

Rhegmatogenous retinal detachments are usually very raised and the folds of retina can almost be seen to 'float' around in the vitreous like bits of material.

2. **Fluid leakage: serous retinal detachment (Figure 13.35)**
   Several pathological processes can cause fluid to leak into the subretinal space. These include inflammatory diseases of the choroid or sclera such as scleritis and primary and secondary tumours of the retina. Serous detachments are often more dome shaped, solid and less mobile than rhegmatogenous detachments.

3. **Tractional retinal detachment (Figure 13.16)**
   In conditions that cause retinal neovascularisation, such as diabetes and sickle cell anaemia, the new blood vessels can grow into the vitreous causing inflammation and scarring. This pulls ('traction') on the retina detaching it from the RPE. This is discussed in more detail above.

Risk factors for retinal detachment

Retinal holes and vitreous degenerations may occur in otherwise normal eyes. However, they are more common in the following conditions.

1. **Myopia**

   Myopic eyes have a thinner more stretched retina that frequently has peripheral atrophic holes in it (**Figure 13.36**). Moreover this thin retina is more likely to tear during vitreous detachment causing a 'U' shaped tear.

2. **Following intraocular surgery**

   There is a slightly higher risk of retinal detachment after cataract surgery, even if there are no surgical complications. However, the risk is much higher after any cataract surgery in which the posterior lens capsule is torn or after intracapsular cataract extraction. This disturbs the anterior face of the vitreous, which can put traction on the posterior face and the retina and may cause a tear to develop.

3. **Blunt ocular trauma**

   Significant blunt trauma can cause great disturbance in the vitreous. This can create a retinal tear. It can also cause the very peripheral retina to separate from the peripheral RPE at the ora serrata (the edge of the retina). This is called a retinal dialysis (**Figure 13.37**). These can be difficult to see as they are very peripheral.

4. **Hereditary conditions**

   Several retinal conditions predispose to retinal detachment either because the retina is thin and very poorly adherent to the RPE or because the vitreous is abnormal. For example, Stickler syndrome and connective tissue disorders such as Marfan syndrome and Ehlers-Danlos syndrome.

Symptoms and natural history of a retinal detachment

Patients with new 'U' shaped retinal tears usually present with flashing lights (photopsia) and floaters. Patients with a retinal detachment also have visual

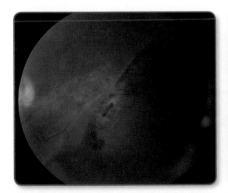

Figure 13.36 Lattice degeneration and peripheral retinal holes. These are more common in myopic people.

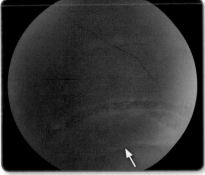

Figure 13.37 Retinal dialysis. This peripheral detachment occurred after blunt ocular trauma. The line of pigment at the end of the dialysis indicates that it has been present for a long time and may have stopped progressing at this boundary. The edge of the dialysis where the retina has torn away from the ora serrata is marked with an arrow.

field loss, which is often described as being like a curtain covering the peripheral vision. The three F's to remember are: floaters, flashing lights and visual field loss.

Floaters

Floaters are specks in the vision that move around the eye with eye movement, but with a characteristic delay from inertia. They are caused by opacities in the vitreous jelly or the posterior vitreous face that cast a shadow on the retina. They are particularly noticeable in bright light. They are a common symptom in normal, healthy eyes and are caused by bits of vitreous debris. Typically, normal floaters are seen as grey or translucent. Floaters from a retinal tear or detachment are more commonly described as dark or black. They are caused by pigment that has been released from the retina around the tear, or blood from tearing a small retinal vessel.

Flashing lights

Vitreous traction causes flashing lights in some people. This is probably from the traction causing electrical discharges from the retina. They are often described as being in the temporal peripheral visual field. Bilateral flashing lights are usually not caused by ocular changes, and more likely to be caused by migraine or anxiety.

Visual field loss

Visual field loss in a patient with flashes and floaters is very suggestive of a retinal detachment. The vision is lost in the area corresponding to the area of retina that has detached. Remember this is reversed, i.e. an upper half retinal detachment will cause a lower half loss of the visual field and vice versa. As the retinal detachment spreads, the visual field defect will enlarge accordingly. This is often described as being like a curtain coming across the vision. If the detachment spreads to the macula, the visual acuity will be greatly reduced.

Natural history

Retinal detachments progress at very different rates. The retina may begin to detach almost immediately after a tear. Sometimes, however, a hole or tear may be present for months or even years without progressing to a detachment. Similarly, a detachment may spread to involve the whole retina within a few hours, or remain localised to part of the retina only. Retinal detachments caused by retinal holes or tears usually progress much more quickly in the upper than the lower part of the retina.

Examination of retinal tears and detachment

Retinal holes and vitreous degenerative changes can be very difficult to detect, as the peripheral retina can be difficult to examine thoroughly. It is essential to dilate the pupil. An indirect ophthalmoscope, a slit lamp with a 90 dioptre or a three mirror gonioscope lens, are better tools for examining a retinal detachment than a direct ophthalmoscope. These instruments enable more peripheral retina to be viewed and they give a three-dimensional view, which means the tear or detachment can be seen lifting away from the retina. With more experience one can learn to indent (pressing on the eye as posteriorly as possible with something like a cotton bud) the retina in order to view the most peripheral areas, whilst examining with an indirect ophthalmoscope. When a retinal hole occurs there are often some pigment cells released into the vitreous. If a slit lamp is available, these orange pigment cells may be seen floating around in the vitreous just behind the lens. If vitreous pigment cells are seen in an eye that hasn't previously had significant trauma or surgery, there is a very high likelihood of a tear being present. The characteristic examination features (**Figure 13.32–13.34**) of a retinal detachment are:

- The retina is displaced forwards. It will therefore be necessary to use positive lenses with a direct ophthalmoscope to bring it into focus.
- The surface of the retina is irregular and wavy.
- The retinal vessels also appear slightly darker than normal, because less light is reflected from the choroid.
- The background pattern of the choroidal vessels and pigment is no longer clearly visible, because more light is reflected from the detached retina.
- If it is a relatively recent rhegmatogenous detachment the retina may appear to wave around as the eye moves.

The other eye must also be examined very carefully. Retinal degenerations and holes are often bilateral. Therefore, prophylactic treatment of the other eye may be necessary. This is especially important if the first eye has already become blind from a retinal detachment.

Treatment of retinal holes, tears and rhegmatogenous retinal detachment

When the retina first becomes detached, it is quite mobile and can be reattached. However, after some weeks, fibroblasts grow over the surface of the retina. These probably come from the pigment epithelium, and pass through the retinal hole. They form a membrane on the surface of the retina, making it much more rigid and it cannot easily be re-attached. In a long-standing detachment, secondary uveitis and a secondary cataract may also develop and phthisis can even occur.

Retinal holes and tears

Retinal holes or tears (where the retina has not yet detached) should be treated by scarring the area around them to prevent fluid (or more fluid) entering into the subretinal space and causing a retinal detachment. The technique is either to photocoagulate the retina with a laser, or to freeze the surface of the sclera with a cryoprobe.

Retinal detachment

Once the retina has become detached more extensive surgery is needed. The principle of treatment is to remove the subretinal fluid and get the retina to stick to the retinal pigment epithelium and to scar around any holes or tears (as described above). Two methods used by retinal surgeons are:

1. An operation inside the eye to remove the vitreous and replace it with a substance (gas, heavy liquid or oil) that pushes the retina back against the RPE.

2. An operation outside the eye to indent the overlying sclera so that the choroid is pushed up against the retina (**Figure 13.38**). This indent is usually held in place with something like a silicone rubber sponge that is sewn onto the surface of the eye. If the retina has been completely detached for a long time, and is no longer mobile, it will not become reattached with this type of operation. Instead complex intravitreal surgery inside the eye is required.

Both surgical methods require highly trained surgeons and specialist equipment that will usually only be available in eye units in larger cities.

Results of surgery

Patients who have their retinal detachments surgically treated before the macula is detached have a very high chance (approximately 80% or greater in good surgical centres) of maintaining their normal vision. Patients who have surgery after the macula has detached but before the retina has become rigid have a good chance of maintaining some vision, but may not regain good central vision. Patients who have surgery on long-standing retinal detachments with scarred, rigid retinas have a very low likelihood of regaining useful vision and the best one can hope for is 'counting fingers' vision.

Patients who have had their retinal detachments repaired with intraocular surgery (vitrectomy), which has become by far the more common method, are likely to develop a cataract within the first year or two after surgery.

Retinoblastoma

Retinoblastoma is a highly malignant tumour of the retina that occurs in infants. It is the commonest intraocular tumour in children, although fortunately it is still very rare. Retinoblastoma can be an inherited tumour in 5–10% of cases (the abnormal tumour suppressor gene is inherited from one of the parents). These cases are frequently bilateral.

The tumour grows between the retina and the choroid and also into the vitreous, forming a white mass in the posterior part of the eye. It may then burst through the sclera or cornea to form a progressively enlarging fungating mass in the orbit. Alternatively, it may spread down the optic nerve into the brain. It may even spread to the lymph nodes, bones and liver. In the advanced stages of the disease, the diagnosis is usually obvious. A tumour

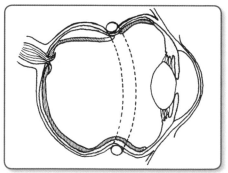

Figure 13.38 Surgical treatment of a retinal detachment. The retinal hole is sealed off by indenting the outside of the eye. An elastic silicone band has been placed around the equator of the eye.

which is still confined to the eye is much more difficult to diagnose. However, it is essential to make the diagnosis in the early stages before the tumour has spread beyond the eye, because in the early stages the child's life can be saved. Once the tumour has spread beyond the eye the child will probably die from the tumour. Retinoblastoma used to be a death sentence in poor countries. However, treatment programmes involving complex regimens of chemotherapy, radiotherapy and surgery are starting to be set up, with amazing and life saving results.

Symptoms and signs of retinoblastoma

Retinoblastoma can present in different ways:

1. **A white mass inside the eye (Figure 13.39)**
   The retinoblastoma obstructs the light from reaching the retina. Therefore the normal red reflex (see Chapter 3) is lost and instead there is a white reflex from the tumour. The pupil response is usually absent which helps distinguish it from other the other causes of a white reflex (see below).

2. **A squint**
   If a child cannot see out of one eye a squint will develop relatively quickly. This may be the first sign of retinoblastoma.

3. **A painful inflamed eye**
   The tumour may become partly necrotic causing uveitis, or it may close off the drainage angle of the anterior chamber causing acute glaucoma. In both cases, the child will present with a painful, blind and inflamed eye.

4. **Proptosis**
   The tumour may spread backwards into the orbit and push the eye forward.

5. **A fungating mass (Figure 13.39b)**
   This occurs when the tumour bursts through the cornea and may be the first presentation of the tumour.

Other causes of an absent red reflex in children

1. Congenital cataract (see Chapter 12). This is more anterior in the eye and the pupil response is normal. This is the commonest cause of a white reflex. The rest of the pathological causes below are very rare.

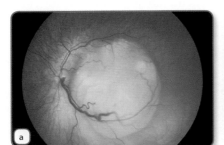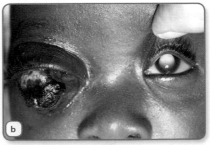

Figure 13.39 Retinoblastoma. (a) An early retinoblastoma. (b) Advanced, bilateral retinoblastoma. In the right eye, the retinoblastoma has taken over the whole eyeball. In the left eye the white mass behind the pupil looks rather like a cataract but is more posterior than a cataract and the pupil does not react to light.

2. Parasitic granuloma. Typically this is caused by toxocara, which is a nematode worm.
3. Tuberculosis or other causes of severe exudative uveitis.
4. Persistent foetal vasculature. This is the remnants of the foetal intraocular vascular system which should disappear just before birth but occasionally persists.
5. Retinopathy of prematurity.
6. Coats disease. This is a rare telangiectatic and exudative disease that typically occurs in one eye of young boys (**Figure 13.40**).
7. Camera flash angle. The widespread usage of digital cameras throughout the world has meant that millions more photos are taken than ever before. At certain angles it is possible for the flash to cause a white reflex in one eye. Ophthalmic examination must be done to exclude pathology and because the parents may be very anxious if they are aware of the possible causes of a white reflex. The retinal examination will obviously be normal with a clear view of the retina.

Treatment of retinoblastoma

The treatment of retinoblastoma has changed dramatically in recent years. Enucleation used to be the only option, but now highly specialised treatments which mainly use chemotherapy are used. These advanced treatments are even being used for some of the poorest patients in the world. For example, there are now successful programmes in South Asia and Africa. However, in many other poor countries, immediate enucleation remains the only available treatment for tumours that are still confined to the eye. If this is performed, the optic nerve should be cut back as far as possible. As long as the tumour is confined to the eye, the prognosis is good. The unaffected eye must be very carefully examined under anaesthetic with a fully dilated pupil as there is a risk of early retinoblastoma lesions in that eye. If these are detected at an early stage they can be treated and destroyed with laser photocoagulation or cryotherapy and thus preserve the eye.

If the tumour has spread beyond the eye the prognosis is very poor. Palliation with radiotherapy and cytotoxic drugs may help and occasionally may save the child's life. Exenteration (removal of the entire contents of the orbit) is still occasionally necessary, when chemotherapy is not available, as it may make the child more comfortable by reducing the secondary infection, discharge and smell until death occurs.

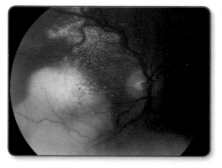

Figure 13.40 Coats disease.

Retinal infections

Retinitis

Retinitis actually means 'inflammation of the retina'. However, primary retinitis is almost always caused by infection. The retina can also become secondarily inflamed, because of severe disease in neighbouring tissues, such as the sclera (scleritis) and the intraocular contents (e.g. endophthalmitis). Retinal infection is very rare, although it has become much more common with the AIDS epidemic, particularly in areas of the world where many patients have HIV and are not receiving antiretroviral drugs. This is discussed in more detail in Chapter 20.

Toxoplasmosis

Toxoplasmosis is caused by a protozoan parasite, *Toxoplasma gondii*, and is an important cause of chorioretinitis. Infection with the organism is widespread throughout the world (it is thought that over one third of the entire world population is infected, but of course asymptomatic). A particularly high prevalence of infection and ophthalmic manifestations is seen in Latin America, some parts of northern Europe, South East Asia and Africa and may relate to eating less cooked meat. The disease is particularly severe in congenital infections and in immune-compromised individuals.

Life cycle

The organism has a complex life cycle of which some details are uncertain but the main host is thought to be the cat. Cysts are found in cats' faeces. If the secondary host, which is either man or other animals, eats these cysts they will transform into active infective protozoa. They invade the tissues and bloodstream and multiply, then again forming tiny cysts. The life cycle is completed when the cat is again infected, by eating meat that contains cysts. Therefore, humans can become infected, either from eating food contaminated by cat's faeces or by eating meat that contains cysts which has not been properly cooked. It also appears that these cysts (oocysts) can contaminate water supplies and this may be a significant route of infection.

Congenital infection

Congenital toxoplasmosis is relatively rare despite the high prevalence of toxoplasm gondii. It probably does not usually cross the placenta and cause foetal infection. However, infants who do suffer from congenital toxoplasmosis can have severe ocular and cerebral complications, including hydrocephalus, brain calcification and blinding chorioretinitis. As many as 80% of congenitally infected infants will have some chorioretinal lesions (**Figure 13.41**).

Some years later the cysts may become active again and the organism starts multiplying to produce inflammation in the retina and the choroid. Blood tests show that a majority of people have had some infection but in most cases this does not cause any disease at all. However in a few people, probably those who are infected as a fetus, there may be quite severe and recurrent chorioretinitis in later life. Toxoplasmosis is particularly common in west Africa. However, there are not many domestic cats in west Africa and the infection may live in some other host to complete its life cycle.

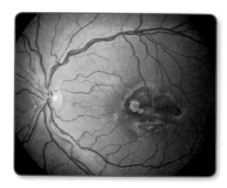

Figure 13.41 Congenital toxoplasmosis macular chorioretinal scarring.

Symptoms and signs

The eye is the main focus of symptoms and signs of toxoplasmosis. Over 80% of patients with the disease have eye involvement without significant systemic disease, although some people do get 'flu like symptoms with lymphadenopathy when they get infected. The immune reaction to the infection is thought to be the main cause of the destructive effects of the disease.

Toxoplasmic chorioretinitis has a characteristic retinal appearance with irregular focal patches of necrotising granulomatous retinitis, associated with granulomatous choroiditis, vitritis and sometimes anterior uveitis (**Figure 13.42**). When the disease is inactive there are just pigmented and atrophic scars on the retina and the choroid (**Figure. 13.43**). Occasional inactive toxoplasmosis scars are extremely common and almost the norm in some countries.

Once an individual has a primary infection, reactivations may occur at any time causing a new phase of ophthalmic complications, but is particularly likely in immune-compromised individuals.

Diagnosis

The diagnosis of toxoplasmosis is usually determined by the clinical appearance. Many people who have positive serological tests have no symptoms or signs at all, so these tests are not always very helpful. They are also very expensive. However, negative tests are useful; the absence of anti *T. gondii* IgG and IgM virtually excludes the diagnosis. The diagnosis can be confirmed with a very specialised test of the aqueous [polymerase chain reaction (PCR) testing], but this test is not available in most poor countries.

Treatment

Multiple treatments have been and are used for treatment. This of course indicates that none of them is particularly good. There are two important questions:

1. Does the episode of active toxoplasmosis need treatment? It is often a self-limiting condition. Therefore, if the macula is not threatened and the immune response is not too severe the episode can be carefully monitored without treatment. However, if the episode is severe, the central vision in danger or the patient known to be immunocompromised, treatment is likely to be required.

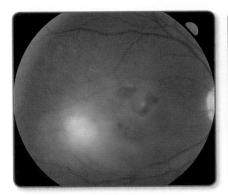

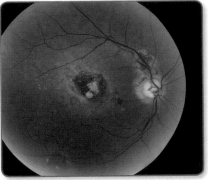

Figure 13.42 Active toxoplasmosis chorioretinitis. The active area has the appearance of a 'headlight in the fog'. The fog is the vitreous inflammation. The blood vessels in the area of the active lesion are not regular, as they are inflamed.

Figure 13.43 Old choroiditis from toxoplasmosis. There are several patches of pigmented scarring of the choroid and retina from previous episodes of toxoplasmosis. The lesions have distinct edges.

2. What is the best treatment? Active toxoplamosis is treated with antbiotics for the infection and steroids for the inflammation. The best antibiotic choice is unknown. The 'classical' antibiotic treatment is sulfadiazine, pyrimethamine and folinic acid, but this carries a risk of toxicity. Other antibiotics, including azithromycin, and clindamycin and a combination of sulfamethoxazole and trimethoprim, may be as effective. There is also some doubt about how well any drugs reach the retina where the organism is found, and whether they are active against the cysts. Sight-threatening disease should be managed by a specialist if at all possible, particular as some of the treatments can have toxic side effects.

Prevention must not be forgotten. In most situations it will not be possible to test pregnant woman to see if they are seronegative (and therefore at risk of primary infection during pregnancy). Therefore, it is sensible to advise all pregnant women to avoid undercooked or raw meat, to drink well filtered or boiled water and to avoid contact with cat faeces.

Toxic retinopathy

Most systemic drugs and chemicals do not harm the retina. However, a few can either slowly damage the retina if they are taken for a long period of time, or rapidly damage it if taken in large doses.

Chloroquine retinopathy

Excessive doses of chloroquine and its derivatives can damage the macula. Chloroquine was a very effective drug against malaria, although there is now widespread resistance. It is cheaply and easily available in many parts of Africa and therefore is frequently over-used. The initial changes are irregular pigmentation around the macula and fine deposits in the cornea. Both these early changes are very slight and are very difficult to detect, but the loss of visual acuity is often quite severe. Eventually, further pigmentary changes around the macula produce the appearance of a target or 'bull's eye' (**Figure 13.44**). The loss of central vision is permanent. Therefore, chloroquine should only be taken under medical supervision. Patients, particularly in Africa, with an unexplained loss of central vision should be specifically asked about their consumption of chloroquine, as they may not think to mention it, and the vision will continue to deteriorate if the diagnosis is not made and they continue to take it every time they have a cold or fever.

Other drugs

Other drugs that are becoming increasingly available in poor countries that can cause toxic retinopathies are listed in **Table 13.4**. These drugs tend to only cause retinal pathology if they are either taken in excessive doses or taken for very long periods of time.

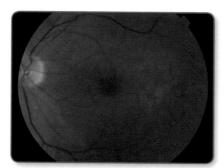

Figure 13.44 Chloroquine retinopathy showing a circular pattern of abnormal pigmentation.

Table 13.4 Systemic medications with ocular effects			
Drug	**Clinical use**	**Effect on retina and vision**	**Reversible with stopping treatment?**
Sildenafil (Viagra)	Erectile dysfunction	Visual cell excitation causing blue tinge in vision, light hypersensitivity and hazy vision	Yes
Vigabatrin	Epilepsy	Peripheral visual field loss (pathology unknown)	Usually no
Tamoxifen	Breast cancer chemotherapy	Macular crystals: reduced central vision	Usually no
Phenothiazines	Psychiatric disorders	Reduced central vision. Variable mechanisms depending on specific drug	Variable

14 Diseases of the optic nerve and visual pathways

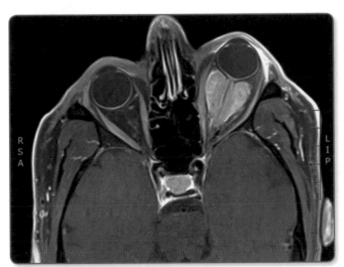

When we look at the optic nerve we are looking at part of the brain. This tumour coming from the optic nerve sheath causes blindness and may gradually grow to follow the optic nerve back to the brain.

The optic nerve and visual pathways connect the eye to the brain (see Figure 2.5). The optic nerve is in fact a part of the central nervous system. Therefore, when you are looking at the optic nerve in the eye, you are looking at an extension of the brain; it is surrounded by a meningeal sheath and cerebrospinal fluid. Some diseases of the brain will be visible by the effects they have on the optic nerve.

Diseases of the optic nerve

The optic nerve contains the axons from the retinal ganglion cells passing backwards to the brain. As it is susceptible to many kinds of damage, diseases of the optic nerve are very common. The damage may be in one or both eyes. However, any optic nerve disease will always cause some loss of vision and some loss of the pupil light reflex. There are a number of different clinical terms used to describe optic nerve damage, which can be confusing. We will go through them now as they are so important for understanding and diagnosing optic nerve disease:

- *Optic neuropathy:* this is a general name for any damage to the optic nerve.
- *Optic neuritis*: this is a general name for inflammation of the optic nerve. This is an active process.

- *Optic disc swelling:* a swollen appearance of the optic disc on funduscopy from any cause.
- *Papilloedema* refers to the specific situation of optic disc swelling caused by raised cerebrospinal fluid pressure in the brain (see **Box 14.1**).
- *Optic atrophy:* loss of optic nerve fibres, which causes the whole optic disc or areas of it to appear pale on funduscopy. This is the outcome of previous disease, e.g. the end result of optic neuritis is usually optic atrophy.

Optic neuritis

Inflammation of the optic nerve can occur anywhere along its path from the eye to the optic chiasm. At any location, it usually causes considerable visual loss, and also a reduction of the pupil light reflex. There are two forms of optic neuritis: *papillitis* and *retrobulbar neuritis*.

Papillitis

This is the name for optic neuritis in the anterior part of the nerve inside the eye, including the optic disc (see **Box 14.1**). It gets its name from the papilla, which is another word for the optic disc. A fundus examination shows slight oedema of the optic disc, and blurring of its margins (see Figure 16.8).

Retrobulbar neuritis

This is the name for optic neuritis in the posterior part of the nerve behind the eye. Therefore, the optic nerve head, which you can see on fundus examination, looks completely normal. Often, the patient complains of some pain behind the eye especially on looking upwards. This occurs, because the dural sheath that surrounds the optic nerve is attached to the same fibrous ring that the extraocular muscles originate from at the apex of the orbit. Therefore, moving the eyes also pulls on the inflamed optic nerve. There is a common saying about optic neuritis: 'The patient sees nothing, and the doctor sees nothing', i.e. the patient's vision is greatly reduced but the eye and optic nerve look normal, or only slightly swollen if the patient has papillitis (**Figure 14.1a and b**).

Disease course

Patients with optic neuritis usually present with rapid loss of vision and an aching eye that is worse with eye movements. The colour vision is impaired. This can easily be checked by holding up a red object and covering each

---

> **Box 14.1 Distinguishing papilloedema and papillitis**
> Papilloedema is often confused with papillitis. However, in papilloedema there is obvious swelling of the optic disc, but little change in vision. In papillitis, the opposite occurs: the changes in the optic disc are slight, but there is considerable loss of vision. Papilloedema is usually bilateral, while papillitis is usually unilateral.

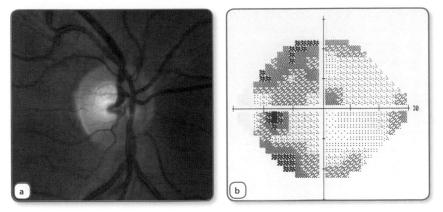

Figure 14.1 Retrobulbar neuritis. (a) A normal looking optic disc. (b) The visual field test of the same patient shows quite widespread areas of field loss.

eye in turn. A patient with optic neuritis typically describes the red as much less bright or much less 'red' in the affected eye. A relative afferent pupillary defect is present (see page 69). During the next week or so, the vision often recovers significantly, as the inflammation and oedema settles. However, there is nearly always some permanent visual loss, because of dead nerve fibres, which cannot regenerate.

Treatment of optic neuritis

Intravenous steroids (e.g. methylprednisolone 500 mg–1 g/day for 3 days) sometimes speeds up the improvement in vision, although does not alter the final visual outcome or affect the risk of further recurrences. They only need to be given in the short-term. Also, they should be administered by an expert as there is a small risk of serious side effects from large doses of steroids. Oral steroids are also sometimes used to speed up the recovery, but it is possible that this treatment causes more frequent recurrent episodes than if intravenous steroids or no treatment at all is used. The reason for this is unknown.

Optic disc swelling and papilloedema

Numerous conditions can cause the optic disc(s) to swell (**Table 14.1**). Many of these are very rare, and it is beyond the scope of this book to describe them all. However, you must try to identify serious and possibly life-threatening causes of optic disc swelling. First, decide if the swelling is in one or both eyes. If the optic nerve of only one eye is swollen, it may be caused by inflammation (see above), pressure on the nerve behind the eye such as from a tumour, or vascular problems, such as a central retinal vein occlusion. However, if both optic nerves are swollen, there are two possible, very serious and acutely life-threatening causes: papilloedema (**Figure 14.2 and 14.3**) and severe hypertension (see Figure 13.3).

Papilloedema

Optic disc swelling from raised intracranial pressure (papilloedema) is almost always bilateral although one disc may be more swollen than the other

Table 14.1 Causes of a swollen disc

Raised intracranial pressure (papilloedema) ►

Cerebral tumour

Idiopathic intracranial hypertension

Encephalitis and meningitis

Retinal and optic nerve vascular disease

Very high blood pressure ('malignant hypertension) ►

Retinal vein occlusion

Arteritic anterior ischaemic optic neuropathy (temporal/giant cell arteritis) ►

Non-arteritic anterior ischaemic optic neuropathy

Diabetic papillitis

Inflammatory eye disease

Uveitis

Optic neuritis (papillitis)

Scleritis

Neuroretinitis

Optic nerve tumours

Glioma

Meningioma

Lymphoma

Metastasis

Orbital tissue swelling

Thyroid eye disease ►

Orbital inflammatory diseases

Pseudo swelling, i.e. the disc is raised but is not actually swollen (oedematous)

Optic disc drusen

High hypermetropia

► There are many more very rare causes, but we have included the ones that are either common or very serious. The conditions marked with a red flag are potentially fatal or rapidly blinding if they are not treated urgently.

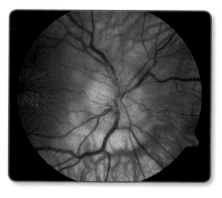

Figure 14.2 Papilloedema. There is swelling of the optic disc and the retina surrounding it including the macula where there is a 'macular star' (left of picture).

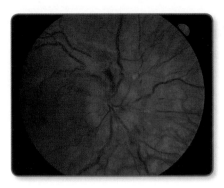

Figure 14.3 Very severe papilloedema. The optic disc is very swollen and there are haemorrhages around it.

(**Figure 14.2**). At first, the optic disc is swollen with fluid (oedema), but there is little or no loss of vision. Eventually, however, the optic nerve degenerates and the vision starts to fail. In long-standing cases, small, dilated blood vessels are present on the surface of the disc. If papilloedema is diagnosed, it is essential to discover the cause and give treatment as soon as possible. The raised intracranial pressure can be caused by numerous diseases, but the two most common are: brain tumours and idiopathic intracranial hypertension, which is a condition in which the cerebrospinal fluid pressure is increased for unknown reasons.

Severe (malignant) hypertension

Very raised blood pressure can cause the optic discs to swell dramatically (see Figure 13.3). It also causes haemorrhages in the retina. It is sometimes called malignant hypertension to indicate how serious the condition is, as the high blood pressure is not just causing damage to the eye, but also to other important organs such as the brain and kidneys, and therefore there is a significant risk of death unless the blood pressure is treated. It is discussed in more detail in Chapter 13.

Optic atrophy

Optic atrophy simply describes an optic disc that has lost a significant number of nerve fibres. This can be caused by any condition that affects the retinal ganglion fibres or optic nerve (**Box 14.2**). There is always some loss of vision, usually with reduced visual acuity, and the pupil light reflex is either diminished or absent. The exact pattern of the visual loss depends upon the cause of the atrophy, and upon which fibres have degenerated in the optic nerve. In mild cases, there may only be a loss of brightness or colour discrimination. However, a careful visual field test will reveal small defects, usually between the blind spot and the centre of fixation (called central and paracentral visual field defects). In severe cases, there may be total blindness in one or both eyes.

The exact appearance of the optic disc will vary according to the cause and the stage of the optic atrophy. In the first few weeks after any optic nerve damage, the disc appears normal. After that the disc appears pale and white because the optic nerve fibres and the small blood vessels nourishing them

> **Box 14.2 Causes of optic atrophy**
> 1. Optic nerve damage
>   - Glaucoma
>   - Inflammation: optic neuritis (and multiple sclerosis)
>   - Toxic chemicals, e.g. lead, arsenic, excessive alcohol, methanol, pipe tobacco, cassava
>   - Drugs, e.g. quinine/chloroquine, ethambutol
>   - Nutritional deficiency, e.g. vitamin B deficiency, generalised malnutrition
>   - Tumours, e.g. glioma, meningioma, optic chiasm tumours
>   - Distant pressure on the optic nerve, e.g. papilloedema
>   - Trauma
>   - Infection, e.g. syphilis, tuberculosis, measles, onchocerciasis, typhoid
>   - Optic nerve vascular disease, e.g. ischaemic optic neuropathy (including giant cell arteritis), diabetes
>   - Hereditary diseases, e.g. Leber hereditary optic neuropathy
> 2. Severe retinal damage, e.g. retinitis pigmentosa, retinal artery occlusion

both atrophy. Sometimes just one side of the disc (usually temporal) is pale (**Figure 14.4a**) and sometimes the whole disc is pale (**Figure 14.2b**). If the optic atrophy follows papillitis or papilloedema, the disc is pale but there is often fibrous tissue or pigmentation around the disc (see Figure 16.9). If the optic atrophy is caused by severe retinal changes (e.g. retinitis pigmentosa or retinal artery occlusion) these will also be seen on fundus examination. If the optic atrophy is caused by glaucoma, the disc is cupped as well as pale (see Figures 15.7–15.9). The optic nerve cannot regenerate, and so visual loss from any form of optic atrophy is permanent.

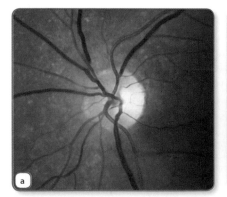 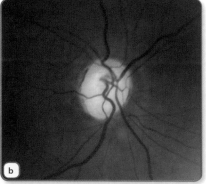

Figure 14.4 Optic atrophy. (a) Temporal pallor, i.e. only the lateral side of the disc is pale. (b) The whole disc is pale.

Causes of optic neuropathy, optic neuritis and optic atrophy

There are many causes of optic neuropathy and optic atrophy. Because they all produce a similar clinical picture, it can be difficult to find a specific cause. In patients with optic nerve disease of unknown cause it is important to take a very good history, as you may identify a cause that can either be treated or a causative agent that can be stopped. Some causes of optic neuritis and optic atrophy are especially important in the tropics and poor communities:

Malnutrition

Malnutrition is more likely to damage the optic nerve than most other parts of the nervous system. The precise relationship between malnutrition and optic neuropathy is not clear, as malnutrition by itself is not a common cause of optic atrophy. However, optic nerve damage is much more common when there is malnutrition (particularly of vitamin B) in combination with infections such as measles and tuberculosis or toxins such as excessive alcohol and some types of tobacco (see below). Vitamin B deficiency has been identified as the specific cause of optic atrophy in certain situations, such as amongst chronically malnourished prisoners of war. The disease was found only in those camps where the diet was deficient in vitamin B, and including yeast extract or other sources of vitamin B in the diet could prevent it.

Toxins

These can also damage the optic nerve, especially if the patient is also malnourished. The three best-known examples are tobacco (particularly pipe tobacco), cassava and methyl alcohol. Pipe tobacco contains cyanide. Cyanide binds to vitamin B in the blood stream. The body is normally able to detoxify cyanide in small quantities, but excessive pipe smoking may produce an excess of cyanide, which therefore reduces the level of vitamin B available to the body. However, the exact relationship between tobacco and optic neuropathy remains controversial as many of these patients have other risk factors, such as vitamin B malnutrition, cassava rich diets (see below) or excessive alcohol usage as well. Therefore, although this condition used to be referred as tobacco-alcohol-amblyopia, it is probably part of the nutritional/toxic optic neuropathy spectrum.

Methyl alcohol or methanol is particularly likely to cause optic neuropathy. Methanol is sometimes present in home brewing and illegally brewed alcohols. During digestion, methyl alcohol is metabolised into formaldehyde or formic acid. It is probably these metabolic products that cause serious damage to the optic nerve and the ganglion cells of the retina. At first, the patient is prostrate with headache, nausea and delirium. When they recover, they are either blind or have severe visual loss. Urgent treatment is required, ideally by an expert as the patient may have severe metabolic acidosis that requires correcting. One part of the acute treatment, surprisingly involves giving ethyl alcohol as this delays the metabolism of the methanol. Unfortunately, patients usually present much too late for this treatment and all that can be done is to determine the cause of the optic atrophy. There are occasional reports of tragic consequences of wedding parties and social events when methanol or methylated spirits are added to communal drinks containers, causing many of the guests to become severely visually affected and even blinded.

Cassava is a cheap staple food in many tropical countries. It also contains high levels of cyanide and must be prepared very carefully to make it safe to eat. Poor people, who may already be generally malnourished, may also eat badly prepared cassava, further increasing the risk of optic neuropathy. Cassava neuropathy also causes damage to the long tracts in the spinal cord, which makes walking difficult. In some reports of cassava neuropathy, the visual field defects have been in the periphery rather than the centre of the vision.

Treatment of nutritional, tobacco, alcohol and cassava optic neuropathies

If malnutrition is suspected, it is necessary to give nutritional advice. It may also help to give vitamin B supplements, such as yeast or multivitamin tablets tablets. If tobacco or alcohol are also being used excessively, the patient must be encouraged to stop these immediately and large doses of vitamin B complex given. If poorly cooked cassava is being eaten hydroxycobalamin injections can be given. However, it is unclear exactly how useful this treatment is.

Drugs

Many drugs can be toxic to the optic nerve. The most important of these are:
- *Ethambutol*, which is used against tuberculosis.
- *Quinine*, which is used to treat malaria, and sometimes to produce an abortion. Patients in many malaria endemic countries can easily buy quinine at pharmacies. Some patients take quinine every time they have any fever or illness and risk causing optic neuropathy from excessive consumption.
- *Arsenical drugs*, which were once used against trypanosomiasis.

Infections

Infection is particularly likely to damage the optic nerve in debilitated or malnourished patients. This may be an acute, generalised infection such as measles or typhoid, or a more localised optic nerve infiltration as can occur with tuberculosis. All forms of meningitis can damage the optic nerve. Two important chronic infections that must be considered when you see a patient with optic neuropathy are syphilis (see page 275) and onchocerciasis (see Chapter 16). Although syphilis can damage the eyes in many ways, the most serious and common complication of syphilis in the eye is probably optic neuritis followed by optic atrophy. This may occur in congenital, secondary, and all forms of tertiary syphilis, especially in tabes dorsalis.

Vascular diseases

The optic nerve requires a healthy blood supply. Therefore, diseases that damage its blood supply will cause optic nerve damage. Anterior ischaemic optic neuropathy (AION) is the most common and important vascular optic nerve disease. It can be divided into arteritic anterior ischaemic optic neuropathy (AAION), when there is an inflammatory cause of vessel narrowing and non-arteritic anterior ischaemic optic neuropathy (NAAION) when no inflammatory cause is identified.

Artertitic anterior ischaemic optic neuropathy: giant cell arteritis (temporal arteritis, cranial arteritis)

Giant cell arteritis (GCA) is an inflammatory disease of large and medium-sized arteries. In all of ophthalmology, GCA is perhaps one of the most important diagnoses to make quickly and to treat quickly, as it can rapidly cause bilateral irreversible blindness and can even cause strokes and heart attacks. GCA typically occurs in people over the age of 60 years. It presents with headache centred over the temporal artery in the forehead, and pressure on the temporal artery itself may be particularly painful. Patients often also describe pain on combing their hair, pain on chewing, shoulder and neck ache and night sweats, fever or generally feeling unwell. As it progresses, patients may start to develop fluctuating visual loss and blurred vision and then finally complete visual loss as the optic nerve becomes severely ischaemic. When you examine the patient you might find specific tenderness over the temporal artery and it may feel firm and nodular. The optic disc may be swollen (**Figure 14.5a** and **b**) GCA also causes both the blood sedimentation rate and the serum viscosity to rise. A biopsy can be taken of the superficial temporal artery in the forehead, if there are facilities available to examine it. A positive biopsy confirms GCA is present; however, a negative biopsy does not exclude the disease and treatment should still be given if there is reasonable clinical concern. If you suspect GCA it is essential to start oral or intravenous steroids immediately (e.g. oral prednisolone 1–1.5 mg/kg once daily). The steroids must often continue for a long time. For example, 1–2 years, with the dose being adjusted according to the patient's symptoms and inflammatory blood markers.

Non-arteritic anterior ischaemic optic neuropathy

NAAION is a condition that usually occurs in old people. The precise cause is not known, but it appears that there is interruption of the blood flow in

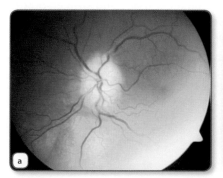 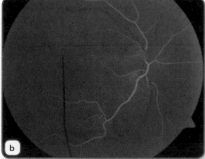

Figure 14.5 (a) Optic disc swelling from giant cell arteritis. Emergency steroids are required to try and save the vision in both eyes of a patient like this. (b) Fluorescein angiogram in giant cell arteritis. Normally, a fluorescein angiogram is quite bright because of fluorescein dye passing into the choroidal circulation. In this case, the background is very dark because the blood supply to the choroidal vessels has closed off from the arteritis.

the short posterior ciliary arteries, which supply the optic nerve, causing optic neuropathy (**Figure 14.6**) and then optic atrophy. It is more common in people with atherosclerosis and diabetes. It usually causes sudden loss of vision, sometimes of just one half (superior or inferior) of the vision. There is no known treatment for it. Diabetic patients can suffer from a similar optic neuropathy called diabetic papillitis. This is probably a variant of NAAION.

Head injuries

Severe blunt injuries especially on the temple can cause optic nerve damage. They probably do this by rupturing small blood vessels in the optic foramen or by causing compressive swelling of the optic nerve.

Demyelinating diseases

These are diseases of the central nervous system, which cause the myelin sheath surrounding the nerve fibres to degenerate. The most common demyelinating disease is multiple sclerosis. Multiple sclerosis involves the optic nerve more than any other part of the central nervous system. It is an important cause of optic neuritis and optic atrophy all over the world. However, it is more common in cold and temperate climates than in the tropics, but the reason for this is not known. In multiple sclerosis, the nerve fibres lose their myelin sheath. This causes a fairly sudden loss of function, usually followed by gradual and partial recovery. Optic neuritis is described in more detail above. With each attack, the residual disability increases. Although demyelinating disease is much less common in hot climates, when it does occur it seems to be more severe and there is often less recovery.

Tumours or other space-occupying intraorbital or intracranial lesions

These may press on the optic nerve and damage it. There are three locations/mechanisms by which this can happen:

Orbital lesions

Any orbital mass, such as tumours, inflammatory tissue and swollen orbital tissue from thyroid eye disease can press on the optic nerve and damage its blood supply, leading to optic atrophy. These usually cause proptosis as well.

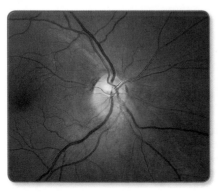

Figure 14.6 Non-arteritic anterior ischaemic optic neuropathy. The lower half of the optic nerve is swollen. This would cause visual loss in the upper half of the visual field.

Chiasmal lesions

Lesions of the optic chiasm are an important cause of optic nerve damage. At the optic chiasm the nasal fibres from each retina cross over to the other side, and these fibres are usually the first to be damaged by any chiasmal lesion (see Figure 2.5). These nasal retinal fibres are responsible for the vision in the temporal visual field. Therefore, chiasmal lesions cause temporal visual field defects, although sometimes other more complex visual field defects occur. The optic disc usually looks normal because the optic chiasm is such a long way behind the optic disc. Patients are often not aware of the temporal visual field because the nasal visual field in the other eye compensates for it. Therefore, chiasmal lesions are often not diagnosed until they are quite advanced. The most common chiasmal lesions are pituitary tumours, but meningiomas, craniopharyngiomas and metastases can also occur. Most chiasmal lesions can be excised by neurosurgeons.

Raised intracranial pressure

Any intracranial tumour can cause raised intracranial pressure. This, in turn, causes bilateral papilloedema, which may eventually lead to optic atrophy.

Retinal disease

Any disease causing extensive destruction of the retinal ganglion cells such as retinitis pigmentosa or retinal vascular occlusions will cause optic atrophy, as the whole length of the ganglion cell will atrophy including the section in the optic nerve.

Inherited optic atrophy

There are certain rare causes of optic atrophy that are inherited genetically, although the disease often does not appear until teenage years or even later. The most common is called Leber hereditary optic neuropathy, which nearly always affects young men, and may have quite a sudden onset and occur in one eye first and then the other eye.

Glaucoma

Glaucoma is the most common cause of optic atrophy, although the appearance of the atrophic optic disc is different from the other causes of optic atrophy. It is so common that there is a whole chapter about it in this book (see Chapter 15).

Diagnosis of optic nerve disease

Optic nerve disease is not always easy to recognise because the changes in the appearance of the optic disc are often not obvious especially in the early stages. Loss of vision is usually the only symptom of optic nerve disease, although in some forms of optic neuritis there may be some pain. The onset may be gradual or sudden, according to the cause. Optic nerve disease should always be suspected in patients with visual loss without any obvious cause for it. Two fairly simple tests will usually confirm a suspected diagnosis of optic atrophy: the pupil light reaction and the visual field.

- The pupil light reaction is always reduced or absent in optic nerve disease. If the disease is unilateral then an afferent defect on the affected side will be very obvious (see page 70). If the disease is bilateral then the pupil abnormalities are much more difficult to detect, although you may see that both react more slowly than a normal pupil. Other causes of visual loss such as refractive error, amblyopia, macular disease, functional visual loss (non-organic visual loss, i.e. the patient has better vision than they are telling the health practitioner) do not affect the pupil light reflexes.
- The visual field. Specialised equipment is needed for a complete visual field examination but a black screen and a white spot can be used. Optic nerve disease always causes visual field defects and sometimes the type or shape of defect will lead to the diagnosis (**Figure 14.7**). Defects with a horizontal edge (e.g. the superior or inferior half of the vision is lost) are usually from the blood supply to the front of the optic nerve (e.g. ischaemic optic neuropathy). Defects with a vertical edge are usually from lesions in the chiasmal region or behind the chiasm. Defects in the central part of the visual field are usually from toxic causes or optic neuritis.

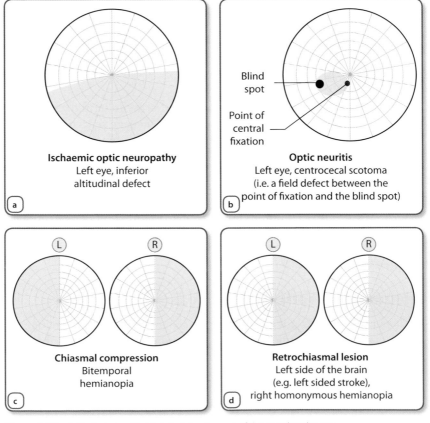

Figure 14.7a-d Typical visual field defects in diseases of the visual pathways.

It is often difficult or even impossible to find a specific cause for many cases of optic atrophy. It may help to ask about the patient's diet, habits, general health and any drugs they are be taking. A neurological history and examination may also be advisable. Three tests may be useful if there is still no explanation for optic atrophy. These are:

1. A serological test for syphilis.
2. A 'skin snip' test, in areas where onchocerciasis is endemic.
3. A radiological examination of the pituitary region in cases of suspected pituitary tumour. A CT scan will show all pituitary lesions but even a plain lateral X-ray of the skull will show most of them.

Always remember that glaucoma is the most common cause of optic atrophy and that sometimes glaucoma can develop in an eye with normal intraocular pressure.

Urgent treatment of optic nerve damage

Most optic nerve damage is irreversible, and so there is very little treatment for patients with advanced optic atrophy. However, some causes of optic nerve damage can be treated - and in particular giant cell arteritis – if urgent treatment is given. This can stop the progress of the disease or even reverse some damage in some conditions. Therefore, it is important to try and determine the cause. The specific treatments for the individual causes of optic nerve disease are discussed above.

Congenital abnormalities of the optic disc

The optic disc is quite a common site for congenital abnormalities.

Optic nerve hypoplasia

In optic nerve hypoplasia, the nerve and the disc are small and poorly developed. This usually causes some generalised loss of vision.

Coloboma

A coloboma is a developmental defect in one segment of the optic disc and sometimes of the retina (**Figure 14.8**) and iris as well. It is usually of the lower part of the optic disc. These patients will have a visual field defect in the upper half of their vision.

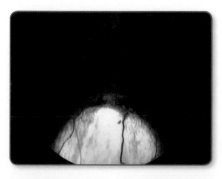

Figure 14.8 Retinal coloboma.

Optic disc pit

An optic nerve pit is a defect in the centre of the disc (**Figure 14.9**). It may cause oedema of the macula, and therefore blurring of the vision.

Persistent fetal vasculature of the optic disc

Embryonic blood vessels, which grow into the vitreous and normally disappear by birth may persist into adult life, leaving small vascular loops or spots (sometimes called Bergmeister papilla) coming from the optic disc. They do not cause any symptoms.

Diseases of the posterior visual pathways and cortical blindness

The visual pathway continues onwards behind the optic chiasm, initially as the optic tract, which goes to the lateral geniculate body. It then spreads out into a much wider area called the optic radiations. Finally, the afferent pathway (the part of the pathway going to the brain) ends up in the occipital cortex.

Any disorder of the visual pathways behind the chiasm will affect exactly the same part of the visual field in each eye. This is called a 'homonymous defect' (**Figure 14.7**). Disorders of the left side of the brain produce defects in the right visual field of each eye, and vice versa. The most common defect is the loss of one complete half of the visual field in each eye. This is called a 'homonymous hemianopia'. Sometimes, however, only a quadrant or a small sector of the visual field is lost in each eye (quadrantinopia). The 'edge' of these visual field defects is always well-defined and distinct, rather than gradual. Damage to the visual pathways behind the chiasm is usually the result of a cerebrovascular accident (stroke), but occasionally, and particularly in younger patients the field defect may be caused by a tumour in the cerebral cortex. Occipital lobe strokes also cause a hemianopia, although depending on the location of the stroke there is sometimes macular sparing. Occasionally, bilateral occipital strokes can occur, causing blindness (cortical blindness). However, there is often recovery of at least some vision. Very occasionally patients with cortical visual impairment or blindness are not aware of the visual loss and may keep bumping into things. Complete cortical blindness may also occur in young children after an attack of encephalitis. A typical patient with cortical blindness cannot see and yet the pupil light reflexes are normal and the eyes look normal on examination.

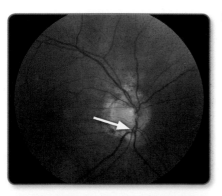

Figure 14.9 Optic disc pit (arrow).

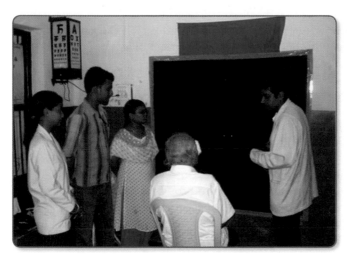

A simple visual field test can detect glaucoma. It can then be treated to prevent irreversible bilateral blindness.

Glaucoma is the second commonest cause of world blindness after cataract. Despite being very common, glaucoma is a difficult disease to define. However, the best way to think about it is as a disease in which the optic nerve gets damaged at the point where it enters the eye, and the damage is usually caused by the pressure in the eye [intra-ocular pressure (IOP)] being higher than normal. There are many different types of glaucoma (**see Table 15.1**)

Table 15.1 The main types of glaucoma
Primary open angle glaucoma
Primary closed angle glaucoma
Acute angle closure
Chronic angle closure (peripheral anterior synechiae often present which obstruct drainage)
Secondary open angle glaucoma. The drainage can be obstructed by:
Blood (traumatic glaucoma)
Inflammatory cells (uveitic glaucoma)
Lens cells (phacolytic glaucoma)
Blood vessels (rubeotic/neovascular glaucoma)
Pigment cells (pigment dispersion glaucoma)
Lens capsule particles (pseudoexfoliation glaucoma)
Steroid treatment (topical or systemic)
Secondary closed angle glaucoma. The obstruction can be caused by
A swollen/enlarged lens (phacomorphic glaucoma)
Aqueous misdirection into the vitreous (malignant glaucoma)
Ciliary body rotation (plateau iris)
Congenital glaucoma

but the most common are primary open angle glaucoma and primary closed angle glaucoma. The secretion and drainage of aqueous is described on page 34; re-reading this will help you to understand glaucoma. It is also important to remember that the disease is only defined as 'glaucoma' if there is damage to the optic nerve, i.e. simply having raised IOP does not mean that a patient has glaucoma, but of course they are at significant risk of developing optic nerve damage.

Primary open angle glaucoma (chronic simple glaucoma)

This is the most common type of glaucoma in most countries and ethnicities. In primary open angle glaucoma (POAG), the aqueous fluid is produced and circulates normally in the eye. However, for reasons that are not clear, the aqueous does not drain properly through the trabecular meshwork and into the canal of Schlemm. This causes the pressure to be persistently slightly raised above the normal level. About 1% of the world's population suffers from POAG.

Risk factors

Anybody can be affected by POAG, but there are three well-known risk factors:

Age

The prevalence of glaucoma rises with age and the older a person is the more likely it is that they will have glaucoma. It is uncommon under the age of 30 years but quite common over the age of 60 years. About 10% of people over the age of 80 years have glaucoma to some degree although often it is not severe, and frequently does not cause any significant visual impairment during the person's lifetime.

Families

The disease tends to run in families. If a patient has glaucoma their immediate relatives are about ten times more likely than others to have it or develop it in the future. Therefore, the close relatives of a patient with glaucoma should always be examined. However, there seem to be many different genes that determine if an individual will get it, and therefore many relatives of patients with glaucoma never develop the disease.

Race

Black people are about five times more likely to develop POAG than those of other races. They tend to develop it at a younger age and the disease is often more severe. In west Africa there seems to be a particularly severe form, which can affect teenagers and young adults. African patients from poor countries are further disadvantaged as they often present much later with much more advanced, and often end-stage, disease.

The signs and symptoms of open angle glaucoma

POAG is often undiagnosed because it does not usually cause any symptoms until it is very advanced. The rise in intraocular pressure (IOP) is not high enough or quick enough to cause any pain or inflammation in the eye. The first and most important structure to be affected is the optic nerve where it enters the eye (the optic disc) and this will affect the vision. There are three characteristic clinical features of the disease:

1. Gradual loss of vision: often the patient will not be aware of this until it is very advanced. It can be detected much earlier by automated (e.g. Goldman or Humphrey) visual field testing if this is available.
2. Changes in the appearance of the optic disc.
3. Increased IOP.

In some cases of advanced POAG, changes in the pupil reactions to light and the pupil diameter may be seen.

Gradual loss of the field of vision

This is the only symptom caused by the optic nerve damage in POAG. This visual loss from glaucoma progresses slowly and in a characteristic pattern. The normal visual field is shown in **Figure 15.1**. In a nasal, superior and inferior direction it stretches to approximately 60° from the point of fixation. On the temporal side the field of vision is larger: about 90° from the fixation point. The blind spot is the area where the optic nerve enters the eye and so has no retinal photoreceptors. In the visual field, the blind spot is found 15° to the temporal side of central fixation (remember, the optic disc is *nasal* to the fovea, but images are reversed).

An area of visual field loss is called a scotoma (from the Greek word for a dark patch). The typical glaucomatous visual field loss is an arcuate-shaped scotomas spreading from the blind spot either above or below fixation. **Figure 15.2** shows a large arcuate scotoma below fixation. A similar scotoma will usually develop above fixation (they can develop in either order or at the same time) and they will gradually enlarge as the glaucoma progresses until the only vision left is in the macular area and the extreme temporal periphery (**Figure 15.3**). Therefore, advanced glaucoma is one cause of 'tunnel vision' (**Box 15.1**), i.e. the peripheral vision is lost causing the patient to feel like they are looking down a tunnel. Eventually, even this central vision is lost. However, the visual field loss is usually a slow process taking many years or decades.

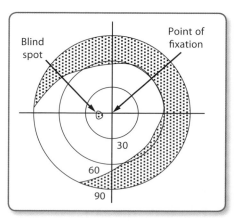

Figure 15.1 The normal visual field of the left eye. The white area is where the patient can see and the shaded area is outside the normal visual field.

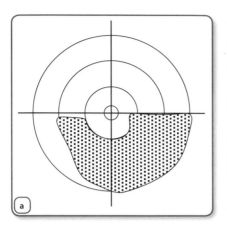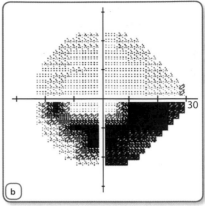

a

b

Figure 15.2 (a) A typical visual field defect in early glaucoma. There is a large lower arcuate scotoma. This visual field loss indicates that there is damage to the superior fibres of the optic nerve. (b) Automated visual field analysers are widely used for testing visual field defects and would produce a print out like this.

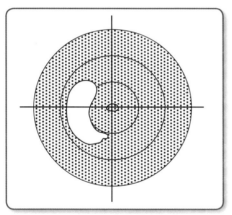

Figure 15.3 A typical visual field defect in advanced glaucoma. Only a small area of visual field around the macula and a patch of vision in the temporal field remains (the white crescent).

Box 15.1 The major causes of tunnel vision

- Optic nerve damage
  — Glaucoma
  — Atypical presentations of optic neuritis
- Retinal disease
  — Retinitis pigmentosa
  — Widespread peripheral chorioretinitis
- Cerebral lesions
  — Migraine
  — Bilateral macular sparing occipital lobe stroke
- Hysteria (also known as functional or malingering, i.e. there is no organic cause for the visual loss)

Defects in the visual field need careful examination with special apparatus to detect them at the early stages. They also need an alert and co-operative patient. Reasonably cheap and portable screening tests for glaucoma field defect are now available (**Figure 15.4**). The Bjerrum screen (see page 55) is still a cheap and excellent test but requires patience.

Open angle glaucoma may be very far advanced by the time it is first discovered for the following reasons:

- The visual field defects start in the peripheral visual field, where they are not noticed.
- Small central blind spots are often not noticed – most of us are unaware of our own blindspot. The human brain and the other eye fill in gaps in the visual field.
- The progression of visual field loss is usually very slow. Therefore, patients adapt to it and the other eye compensates without being aware of it.
- Patients in the poorest areas do not have regular visits to optometrists, which is where early glaucoma is frequently discovered in richer countries.
- There is no pain or inflammation.

Changes in the appearances of the optic disc

The optic nerve is damaged by raised IOP. It is not known exactly how this damage occurs but it is possible that the raised IOP impairs the blood supply to the optic nerve head. It is also not known why some people's optic nerves are not damaged by quite high pressure and other people's are damaged by slightly raised or even 'normal' pressure.

There are about 1.2 million nerve fibres (called axons) in the optic nerve passing from the retinal ganglion cells to the brain. They run in the nerve fibre layer of the retina and join at the optic disc before piercing the sclera at a place called the lamina cribrosa (where the retinal artery and vein also enter/exit the eye) to form the optic nerve. There is considerable variation in the size of the normal optic disc. In some people it is larger than average, and in others it is smaller. There is also some variation in the number of axons, with larger optic nerves having on average more axons than smaller nerves.

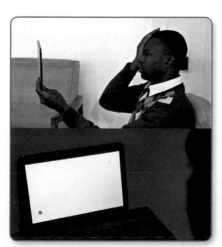

Figure 15.4 This simple visual field screening test, to check for the early field defects of glaucoma, is being done with a tablet/smart phone/laptop application (app). These portable devices and their apps allow quick testing to be conducted by field workers in remote places.

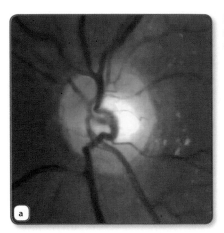

Figure 15.5 (a) A normal optic disc with an orange-pink neural rim and the white optic cup. (b) A diagram of the normal optic disc.

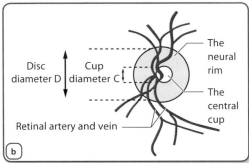

The normal optic disc has two parts: an outer part that is pale orange-pink in colour and a central part that is white and hollowed out (**Figure 15.5a and b**). The outer part, called the neural rim, is made up of all the axons in the nerve. The orange-pink colour comes from the fine capillaries which form the blood supply to the nerve and their supporting cells called glial cells, as the axons themselves are transparent. The central white part, called the 'cup' because of its shape, contains no nerve fibres. The white is the lamina cribrosa of the sclera at the bottom of the cup. It can be difficult to understand what the cup and the rim are. If you imagine many hundreds of bits of string going down a funnel, then the rim is made up of all the bits of string and the cup in the middle is where there is no string so you can look straight down the funnel and see a layer of tissue half way down the funnel, which is the lamina cribrosa.

If the optic disc is large there is plenty of room for all the nerve fibres at the edge and still leave a large cup in the centre. If the optic disc is small there may be no central white cup area at all (in our analogy above, this means that the whole funnel is full of bits of string), as all the nerve fibres have to be squeezed into a smaller space. **Figure 15.6a and b** shows a diagram of a small and a large optic disc; both are normal. The normal cup in a healthy eye is sometimes called the 'physiological cup'.

As glaucoma damages the optic nerve, nerve fibres die off. Therefore, the neural rim gets thinner. This means that more of the cribriform plate becomes visible, i.e. the cup becomes larger (**Figures 15.7 and 15.8**). You should try to measure the vertical diameter of the whole optic disc and the

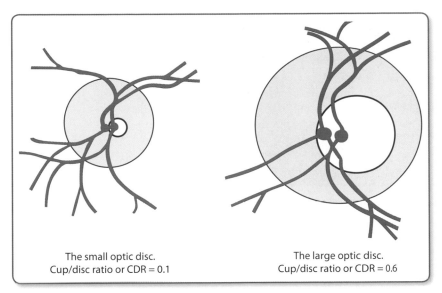

The small optic disc.
Cup/disc ratio or CDR = 0.1

The large optic disc.
Cup/disc ratio or CDR = 0.6

Figure 15.6 A normal small and a large optic disc.

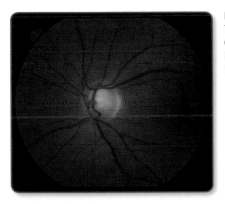

Figure 15.7 Early glaucomatous optic atrophy. The cup is oblong and the cup:disc ratio equals 0.7 (vertically). There is the beginning of a notch in the superotemporal part of the disc. The inferotemporal neural rim is quite thin.

vertical diameter of the optic cup. The cup diameter divided by the disc diameter is called cup/disc ratio or CDR. The larger this is, the more likely it is that the patient has glaucoma. As a guide, a CDR of less than 0.5 is probably normal and CDR of more than 0.5 is probably abnormal. However, it also greatly depends on the overall size of the disc; a big disc may have a CDR of more than 0.5 and still be normal and a small disc a CDR of less than 0.5 and yet be damaged by glaucoma. As glaucoma progresses, eventually the entire neural rim atrophies and disappears causing the whole disc to be white and hollow. The retinal vessels can be seen diving over the edge of the disc (because they have no neuroretinal rim to rest on) and reappearing out of focus at the bottom of the cup. At this stage the eye is blind because there are no surviving axons in the optic nerve (**Figure 15.9**).

Apart from enlargement of the optic cup, there are other slightly more subtle changes in the optic disc that are often seen in early glaucoma (**Box 15.2**). Although they are not so obvious, these changes are important because they help to diagnose glaucoma in its early stages before the patient has gone blind:

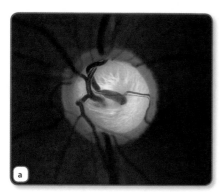

Figure 15.8 (a) The optic nerve in advanced glaucoma. (b) Features of the optic nerve in advanced glaucoma.

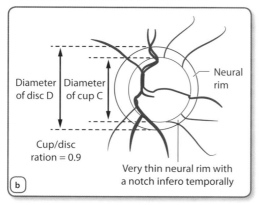

Diameter of disc D | Diameter of cup C

Neural rim

Cup/disc ration = 0.9

Very thin neural rim with a notch infero temporally

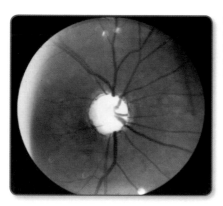

Figure 15.9 Complete (end-stage) glaucomatous optic atrophy. There is no neural rim at all. The retinal vessels dive over the edge of the disc and appear out of focus deep in the bottom of the optic cup.

Box 15.2 Summary of the optic disc changes in early glaucoma
- Vertical cup to disc ratio (CDR) more than 0.5
- Vertical diameter of cup larger than horizontal
- Retinal vessels pushed to the nasal side of the disc
- Unequal CDR in the two eyes
- Thinning of the neuroretinal rim especially on the temporal side
- Notch in the neural rim
- Tiny haemorrhage at the disc margin

- Vertical enlargement of the cup: the nerve fibres at the top and bottom of the disc are most sensitive to damage from glaucoma. Therefore, a cup that is vertically enlarged (i.e. oblong like Figure 15.7) is particularly suspicious for early glaucoma.
- *Neuroretinal rim notch*: sometimes glaucoma causes the loss of one small segment of nerve fibres which causes a localised notch in the neuroretinal rim.
- *Asymmetry of the cup/disc ratio*: If the two eyes have a different cup/disc ratio the eye with the larger cup may have glaucoma.
- *Disc margin haemorrhage*: for unknown reasons a small disc margin haemorrhage is sometimes seen in patients with glaucoma and can be an early sign that glaucoma is developing (**Figure 15.10**).
- *Displacement of the retinal vessels*: in the glaucomatous disc they are often displaced towards the nasal side of the disc as the cup enlarges.

The visual field changes should match the optic disc changes. For instance, a notch in the bottom of the disc should have a visual field defect in the top of the visual field, because the image is upside down on the retina.

All these optic disc changes can be seen with a direct ophthalmoscope. Dilating the pupil makes the disc easier to see, but the disc can be seen through an undilated pupil. The very best way of examining the disc is through a dilated pupil with a slit lamp and a 90 or 78 dioptre condensing lens or a contact lens. This gives a three-dimensional view of the disc, which makes it much easier to assess the cup size.

Increased intraocular pressure

The normal IOP is 10–20 mmHg. There is some variation during the day. Measurement of the IOP is essential for glaucoma assessment. Well-maintained equipment is required for accurate pressure measurement. The methods of measuring the IOP are described on page 75. The higher the IOP is, the more likely that the optic nerve will be damaged. However, there is considerable variation as to how sensitive different people's eyes are to raised IOP. If the pressure is consistently over 30 mmHg then the patient is highly likely to either already have or to develop glaucoma. Between 20 and 30 mmHg the eye may remain normal or may have/develop glaucoma. If the pressure is raised but the optic nerve and visual field are healthy the

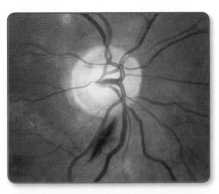

Figure 15.10 A small disc margin haemorrhage, which is sometimes a sign of glaucoma. The optic disc cup is slightly enlarged suggestive of early glaucoma.

patient is described as having 'ocular hypertension'. Some people develop the changes of glaucoma even though the pressure is below 20 mmHg. This is called 'normal tension' glaucoma. It seems that the black people have more glaucoma partly because their eyes are more sensitive to raised IOP.

Other changes

Changes in the pupil responses

As glaucoma affects the optic nerve, the pupil motor fibres in the optic nerve are damaged. Glaucoma therefore causes a diminished pupil light response due to an afferent defect in the pupil light reflex. Glaucoma usually affects both eyes but often one eye is more affected than the other, in which case a relative afferent pupil defect will be seen in the worse affected eye (see page 69). This can be a very useful screening test for glaucoma because the only equipment required is a torch. Glaucoma is the most common cause of optic nerve atrophy, and therefore a relative afferent pupil defect is always suspicious of glaucoma.

Changes of advanced glaucoma

Advanced glaucoma causes more extensive damage to the eye. The sphincter muscle of the iris atrophies, causing the pupil to become dilated and non-reactive. Glaucoma comes from the Greek word for dark blue, possibly because the early Greek scientists thought that the inside of the eye looked dark blue through the damaged dilated pupil. If the pressure in the eye is consistently very high, the corneal endothelial cells may be unable to keep the cornea dehydrated. The cornea will then look hazy from oedema although this is much more common in acute closed angle glaucoma and secondary causes of open angle glaucoma. At this advanced stage, there may be some discomfort in the eye.

Pigment dispersion syndrome and pseudoexfoliation

Pigment dispersion syndrome (PDS) and pseudoexfoliation (PXF) can be considered variants of primary open angle glaucoma. However, in these two conditions there are other changes in the anterior segment of the eye, which contribute to the raised pressure. These changes should be looked for as it will help confirm the diagnosis.

Pseudoexfoliation

PXF is the deposition of white fluffy material around the anterior segment of the eye. The white material is most visible on the lens capsule (**Figure 15.11**) and on the iris at the pupil margin. The fluffy material probably originates from the suspensory ligament of the lens and patients with PXF are at a much greater risk of glaucoma, perhaps because the fluffy material impedes aqueous drainage. It is important to recognise PXF prior to cataract surgery because the abnormal zonules in these patients increases the risk of a zonular dehiscence (see page 301) or of the whole lens dropping into the vitreous during the cataract surgery. Interestingly the name *pseudo*exfoliation was created to distinguish it from *true* exfoliation in which layers of the lens capsule split off (rather than deposition of material on the lens), which often happens in people such as glass blowers who are exposed to high levels of infra-red radiation.

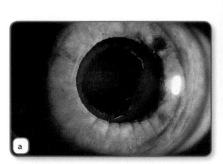 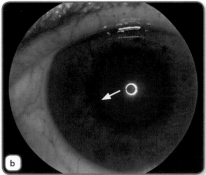

Figure 15.11 Pseudoexfoliation of the lens capsule. (a) Focal illumination from the slit lamp shows the abnormal material at the edge of the lens. There is also some white material present on the pupil margin. (b) The abnormal material can also be seen against the red reflex using the direct ophthalmoscope (white arrow).

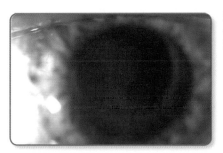

Figure 15.12 Pigment on the corneal endothelium in pigment dispersion syndrome (Krukenberg spindle).

Pigment dispersion syndrome

In PDS pigment cells are shed from the iris. They are deposited on the endothelial surface and in the drainage angle. Therefore, the following three signs are usually seen:

1. Iris transillumination: the iris transmits some light when the slit lamp beam is shone straight into the eye.
2. Krukenberg spindle (**Figure 15.12**): this is vertical strip of pigment cells on the inner (endothelial) surface of the cornea.
3. Drainage angle pigmentation: the drainage angle can be seen with a slit lamp and a gonioscopy lens. The drainage angle in patients with PDS is often very heavily pigmented. This probably restricts aqueous outflow, and therefore these patients are at a higher risk of developing glaucoma.

The diagnosis of open angle glaucoma

Glaucoma is a progressive disease and any visual loss is permanent, and therefore it is important to try and diagnose it as early as possible. The signs can be easily detected when they are very advanced, but are much harder to spot in the early stages, especially with the limited diagnostic equipment and expertise that is available in many parts of the world. If there is uncertainty about the diagnosis of glaucoma, the examination should be repeated again after 6 months or a year, or else the patient should be referred to some-one with more advanced diagnostic equipment. *It is a mistake to miss a case of early glaucoma, but it is equally a mistake to start patients on a lifetime of treatment when they may not even have glaucoma at all.*

Management principles for open angle glaucoma

There are two aims in managing open angle glaucoma:
1. *Early detection*: to identify and diagnose the disease before the patient has lost a significant amount of vision.
2. *Effective treatment*: to give treatment that prevents any further sight loss.

It might be helpful to consider the vision throughout the lifetime of three imaginary patients to explain in detail the importance of both early detection and effective treatment. **Figure 15.13** is a graph that plots the loss of optic nerve fibres either from glaucoma or just from ageing on the vertical axis against the age of the patient on the horizontal axis. The lines across the graph show that quite a lot of nerve fibres can be lost before even the most expensive and sophisticated test can detect any loss of vision. When about one-third of the nerve fibres have been lost, then sophisticated tests with visual field analysers will demonstrate the beginning of a visual field loss. When about two-thirds of the nerve fibres have been lost, the patients them-selves will begin to notice that there is something wrong with their sight. When over 90% of the nerve fibres have been lost the patient will have a seri-ous visual handicap, although they will still have a small amount of residual vision.

In **Figure 15.13**, the blue line represents the first imaginary patient who is in fact normal and does not have glaucoma. Note that with in-creasing age, there is some slight loss of function of the optic nerve fibres. This indeed happens in everyone and is part of growing old. However, it is not until the age of over 80 years that any visual field defect at all can be detected and obviously this person would die of old age before reach-

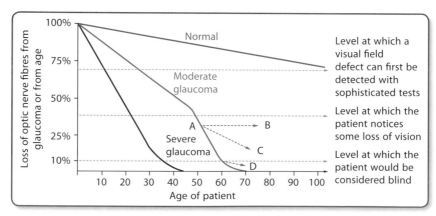

Figure 15.13 The loss of optic nerve fibres with age in glaucoma. The y axis shows the percentage of normal nerve fibres. The x axis shows the age of the patient.

ing the level at which any loss of vision from nerve fibre loss would be experienced.

The solid green line represents a patient with moderate glaucoma. At the age of 40 years the visual field defects can be detected with sophisticated visual field tests. At the age of 50 years they start experiencing some loss of vision and at the age of 60 years, they are almost blind. At the age of 70 years, their vision is reduced to no perception of light. Now, let's imagine that their glaucoma is diagnosed at the age of 50 years and treatment is commenced at position A on the graph. If the treatment is entirely successful, the patient follows dotted green line to B, i.e. there is only very slight further loss of vision due to increasing age. If the treatment is only partly successful, the patient follows dotted line C, i.e. the vision will continue to deteriorate but not quite so fast. If the treatment is started much later, at position D, when the patient is almost blind, it may not make much difference whether it is successful or not, as it may just slightly postpone the inevitable complete loss of vision.

The red line represents an imaginary patient with severe glaucoma, who develops a visual field defect at the age of 20 years, experiences loss of vision at the age of 30 years and is blind by 40 years. For this patient, any intervention needs to be both early and effective.

The management of glaucoma clearly demonstrates the relationship between preventive medicine based in the community and treatment that is based in a hospital or clinic. Both are essential to prevent blindness from glaucoma. There is no point in having excellent treatment facilities for glaucoma, if the disease is not detected until the patients are almost blind. There is also no point in having a good programme of early detection of glaucoma, if no treatment is available for those patients who are discovered by the community health programme.

Treatment of open angle glaucoma

The aim of treatment is to reduce the IOP to normal levels. This usually prevents further damage to the optic nerve. The lost vision will never recover. There is no purpose in treating eyes that are already blind with no perception of light unless they are causing pain. It wastes the patient's time and money and only creates false hopes.

Open angle glaucoma nearly always affects both eyes, but one eye is often more damaged than the other. One eye may be blind, while the other still has some useful vision. The IOP can be lowered either medically or surgically.

Medical treatment

Table 15.2 summarises the different possible medications used in open angle glaucoma. Chapter 4 (see page 92) describes the drugs used in medical treatment. The usual plan of treatment is to start with one type of drop and review the patient after a month. The first choice of drop depends upon availability, expense, age of the patient (e.g. it is best to avoid pilocarpine in young patients) and other health problems of the patient (e.g. beta-blockers must be avoided in patients with asthma or a slow heart rate). Until recently a beta-blocker has been the first drug to be used in poor countries. However, latanoprost is now 'off patent' and is therefore sold very cheaply throughout

Table 15.2 The medical treatment of open angle glaucoma		
Drug category	**Advantages**	**Disadvantages**
Topical beta-blocker, e.g. timolol, levobunolol, betaxolol	Cheap, effective	Systemic side effects, therefore must be used if asthma, obstructive airway disease, very slow heart rate or abnormal rhythms
Pilocarpine 1-4%	Cheap, easy to prepare	Frequent instillation required (3–4 times/day), side effects of accommodation and miosis (i.e. vision darker) and 'ice-cream' headache
Prostaglandin agonist, e.g. latanoprost, travoprost, bimatoprost	Once/day, latanoprost cheap as patent expired, few side-effects	Some are very expensive, increased periocular pigmentation and eyelash growth
Topical carbonic anhydrase inhibitors, e.g. dorzolamide, brinzolamide	Few systemic side-effects	Local irritation
α agonist, e.g. brimonidine	Few systemic side-effects	Local irritation
Adrenaline 1%	Few systemic side-effects	Localised redness and irritation, not widely available or used now
Acetazolamide tablets (e.g. slow release 250 mg twice daily)	No local side-effects	Side-effects common, e.g. nausea. Serious systemic effects possible particularly long-term, e.g. nausea, dizziness, abdominal pain

The drugs below the grey dividing line are either less effective or have more side effects - and are therefore mainly used as second line treatment

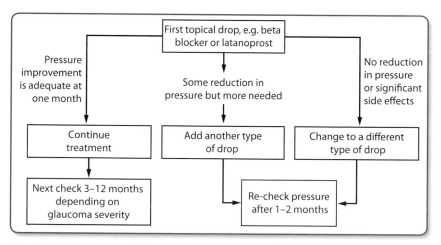

Figure 15.14 Glaucoma medical treatment strategy.

the world. It has the advantage of usually having less side effects and only needing to be used once a day.

Figure 15.14 shows a general strategy for treatment. Different drops will be available in different parts of the world. However, this strategy should be possible in any place where more than one type of drop is available. Acetazolamide tablets can also be given but they have many long-term complications and are usually avoided for long-term control of glaucoma.

Once the pressure has been controlled, then medical treatment for open angle glaucoma must continue for the rest of the patient's life. There should also be regular supervision to make sure that the IOP remains under control, and that there has been no further loss of vision. The visual field, the optic disc and the IOP should be checked at least once a year in stable patients and ideally every 6 months if there is any cause for concern. *It is not acceptable to give the patient some drops and send them away and forget about them.* The expansion of available drops in the last few decades has meant that where medical services are good, most cases of mild and moderate glaucoma can now be controlled satisfactorily with drops.

Medical treatment in poor countries

Unfortunately, there are many reasons why long-term medical treatment is not usually recommended or even possible in poor countries. These include:

- *Expense*: patients cannot usually afford treatment for the rest of their life.
- *Compliance*: the patient may not be able to use the drops properly, or apply them regularly.
- *Availability*: many drops are not available in poor countries
- *Follow-up*: regular follow-up visits may not be possible due to cost or accessibility. Therefore, high pressure or glaucoma that is progressing may be missed.
- *Side effects*: if a treatment causes significant side effects, there may be no other drops available to use instead.
- *Education*: glaucoma does not cause symptoms until patients are almost blind. It can be very difficult to educate patients to take their treatment despite the lack of symptoms.
- *Drop storage*: some drops are supposed to be kept either in the fridge or somewhere cool, which is not possible in the climates of many poor countries.

Even in ideal circumstances medical treatment may not control the glaucoma. Therefore, for most low income patients it is not usually recommended. Surgical treatment is recommended instead.

Surgical treatment

The aim of surgery is to improve the flow or drainage of aqueous fluid from the eye. These operations are sometimes called drainage operations. The aqueous fluid can then pass straight into the subconjunctival space, where it is slowly absorbed. The most widely used operation is called a trabeculectomy because an area of the deeper part of the limbal sclera containing the trabecular meshwork is removed whilst preserving the superficial sclera (**Figure 15.15a and b**). The remaining sclera acts as a partial barrier to the flow of aqueous fluid from the eye. There is therefore less danger that the aqueous fluid will drain away too quickly causing very low pressure and of course the eye remains 'sealed' which minimises the risk of intraocular infection.

When surgery works well it can keep the pressure well controlled permanently and prevent further visual loss. The effects of successful surgery should last for many years and usually the patient's lifetime. Unfortunately, there are several problems with surgical treatment. These include:

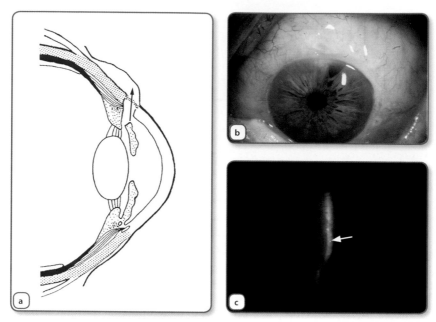

Figure 15.15 Glaucoma drainage surgery: trabeculectomy. (a) The passage of aqueous fluid after a trabeculectomy operation for glaucoma. (b) Trabeculectomy surgery seen with torchlight. This is a very large bleb that may be overdraining aqueous. A normal bleb is usually flatter than this, but much harder to see in a photograph. (c) Trabeculectomy seen with a slit lamp to show the raised area of conjunctiva (the 'bleb', arrow) where the aqueous is coming out from the anterior chamber.

The psychology of surgery

The biggest problem in the surgery of glaucoma is possibly the psychological one. The operation does not restore vision; it only prevents future sight loss. Therefore, the patient will undergo a fairly major eye operation without any immediate benefit. In fact, if any complications arise they will actually see less well, and even if the surgery is uncomplicated the vision may be temporarily a bit worse and the eye uncomfortable. Many patients with glaucoma are already blind in one eye and only have partial vision in the other. They are obviously anxious about having any operation and may resist or refuse surgery. It is also a difficult situation for the surgeon who cannot make the patient better and risks making them worse.

Technical skill of the surgery

Glaucoma surgery requires a high level of technical skill and good equipment. Careful attention to small details is essential for successful glaucoma surgery.

Careful short-term postoperative care

The eyes must be carefully watched for a few weeks after glaucoma surgery and postoperative medication is essential. This is in contrast to cataract surgery where much less postoperative care is needed.

Uncomplicated glaucoma drainage surgery

After a trabeculectomy operation, the IOP may be low for a few days, but usually the pressure stabilises at a normal level. As the aqueous fluid leaves the eye, it forms a small blister (bleb) under the conjunctiva at the operation site. Most of the aqueous fluid is eventually absorbed by the subconjunctival veins or lymphatics, or passes slowly through the conjunctiva into the tears. Some may pass directly into the canal of Schlemm or into the suprachoroidal space.

Complications of drainage operations

All the usual short-term complications of any intraocular surgery can occur after glaucoma surgery, such as infection and inflammation. There are also four important complications that may occur in the short or long-term after glaucoma drainage operations:

1. *Blockage of the drainage outflow pathway*
   Fibrosis and scarring sometimes block the aqueous drainage pathway in the first few months after surgery. The pressure then rises and the patient is again at risk of damage to the optic nerve. This complication is commoner in black people, perhaps because they are more likely to form scars. Topical steroid treatment for up to 3 months after the operation helps to prevent this fibrosis and scarring. Topical cytotoxic drugs, such as 5 fluorouracil and mitomycin C, are now frequently used at the time of surgery to reduce fibrosis.

2. *Low pressure (hypotony)*
   Sometimes aqueous drains too well and the pressure in the eye goes too low. This can cause choroidal effusions and macular oedema both of which can greatly reduce the vision.

3. *Endophthalmitis and blebitis*
   Bacteria can enter the eye from the conjunctiva and through the drainage pathway. Initially the drainage bleb becomes infected, red and inflamed ('blebitis') (**Figure 15.16**) which then spreads into the eye (endophthalmitis). This is a rare but very serious complication.

4. *Cataract*
   All intraocular surgery, including glaucoma surgery, promotes the formation of cataract. The precise reason for this is not known.

The overall long-term success rate for glaucoma surgery is about 80%. Most of the failures are due to the drainage bleb not working. If the patient does

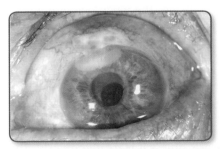

Figure 15.16 Infection of the trabeculectomy drainage bleb ('blebitis'). The fluoroscein dye is staining an area of corneal epithelial defect and infection in the area of the bleb infection.

have worse vision than preoperatively, it is often due to poor surgical technique or postoperative care, although of course rare and serious complications can happen to even the most careful surgeons.

Glaucoma surgery follow-up

Ideally, one should follow up all patients who have had a glaucoma operation for the rest of their lives, because the drainage pathway may become blocked. However, this is just as difficult as following up patients on medical treatment. Fortunately, a glaucoma drainage operation that functions successfully for the first few months usually continues to function successfully for many more years.

Other surgical procedures

Non-penetrating glaucoma surgery (deep sclerectomy and visco-canalostomy)

The principle of a deep sclerectomy is to dissect out a section of the trabecular meshwork but to leave a very thin piece of tissue so that the anterior chamber is not entered. In a visco-canalostomy, the canal of Schlemm is identified and dilated. There is less research into the long-term outcomes of these procedures, but it appears that they reduce pressure less than conventional trabeculectomy, but that they have less complications.

Drainage tubes/valves

In these procedures a small plastic tube that joins the anterior chamber to the subconjunctival space is sewn into the eye. Aqueous drains down the tube. These devices are usually recommended for patients with glaucoma in which a trabeculectomy has already failed or there is a high risk of it failing, e.g. secondary neovascular glaucoma and uveitic glaucoma.

Laser treatment of POAG

Argon laser trabeculoplasty (ALT) and selective laser trabeculoplasty (SLT)

Both ALT and SLT are procedures in which a laser is used to make about 10–20 small burns on the trabecular meshwork. This often produces a significant fall in the IOP. Although this procedure is safer than surgery, the pressure drop is often less than with surgery, and after several years the pressure may rise again. It can be repeated once or twice, but after this, further repeat treatments are ineffective.

Ciliary body destructive procedures

It is possible to lower the production of aqueous fluid from the ciliary processes, rather than by improving the drainage. The usual technique is to apply a diode laser, diathermy or cryotherapy superficially to the sclera overlying the ciliary body. Unfortunately, the results are unpredictable, with the pressure dropping dramatically in some patients and very little in others.

Angle closure glaucoma

Angle closure glaucoma usually comes on suddenly and with severe symptoms. It can be a rapidly blinding disease, unless it is treated quickly. The

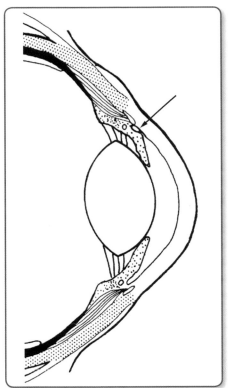

Figure 15.17 An eye with a shallow anterior chamber. The arrow shows where the periphery of the iris has come forward to touch the back of the cornea causing angle closure.

disease mechanism and clinical presentation are very different to open angle glaucoma. The only similarity is that high pressure causes damage to the optic nerve.

The process starts when the iris bows forward causing the peripheral part of the iris to touch the back of the cornea (**Figure 15.17**). This closes the drainage angle of the anterior chamber and prevents the aqueous reaching the trabecular meshwork. Therefore, the IOP suddenly rises. As the pressure rises the peripheral iris gets pushed forward even more, further closing the anterior chamber angle. This is a vicious cycle, i.e. the more the angle closes, the more the pressure rises and the more the iris is pushed forward to keep the angle closed. Modern classification systems advise that the disease should not be called angle closure *glaucoma* until there is damage to the optic nerve, i.e. if an acute attack is treated quickly and successfully, then the optic nerve may be undamaged and therefore, the patient does not have glaucoma. Therefore, some people prefer to call this *primary angle closure*.

The risk factors for angle closure

Angle closure glaucoma only occurs in eyes with a shallow anterior chamber. In these eyes, the peripheral iris lies close to the back of the cornea and the drainage angle is already smaller than 'normal' eyes. The depth of the anterior chamber varies from person to person.

General risk factors

The major risk factors for having a shallow drainage angle are:

- *Hypermetropia*: these eyes are smaller than emmetropic or myopic eyes. Therefore everything in the eye, including the drainage angle is more compressed.
- *Age*: the drainage angle becomes narrower with age because the natural lens gets larger throughout life, pushing the iris forward. Occasionally a very swollen cataractous lens is entirely responsible for the angle closure glaucoma even in a patient who previously had a normally sized anterior chamber and drainage angle (see page 290).
- *Ethnicity*: some races are more likely to suffer from angle closure glaucoma, e.g. the Chinese and Mongolians and the indigenous Indians of North and South America. It is rare in Africans.
- *Gender*: angle closure glaucoma is slightly more common in women than men

Risk factors for precipitating an acute attack

Many people have eyes that are at risk of suffering from acute angle closure glaucoma, because they have a shallow anterior chamber. These people are at risk when the pupil is mid-dilated causing the iris to bunch up and close off the angle. The factors that are often responsible for precipitating an attack in people who are at risk include:

- Watching something in dim lighting conditions. It was often said that elderly patients would develop acute glaucoma whilst in church because the poor light caused the mid-dilated pupil.
- Excitement, as the pupil dilates.
- Mydriatic drops
- Medicines with an atropine-like action, e.g. some antidepressants and gastrointestinal sedatives. Acute angle glaucoma sometimes occurs after a change of medication.

Examination of the anterior chamber

A shallow anterior chamber with a narrow drainage angle is the defining characteristic of eyes that are either at risk of developing AACG or in an attack of angle closure glaucoma. It is very important to be able to recognise a shallow anterior chamber, because these eyes can often be treated before they suffer AACG (see below). The following methods can be used to examine the anterior chamber:

- *Slit lamp and gonioscopic mirror*: this is the best way to examine the anterior chamber. The mirror allows the drainage angle to be seen in detail and with practice it becomes possible to assess if the drainage angle is narrow and at risk of closing.
- *Slit lamp alone*: a thin light beam should be shone into the eye at the edge of the cornea. The slit beam will clearly show the distance between the back of the cornea and the iris. This is the basis of the Van Herrick test, in which the thickness of the peripheral anterior chamber is compared to the thickness of the peripheral cornea.
- *Torch alone*: it is more difficult to assess the anterior chamber with only a torch. However, a reasonable assessment can be made by shining a

bright torchlight from the side of the eye. If the anterior chamber is deep the whole surface of the iris will be illuminated. If the anterior chamber is shallow then the iris will bow forwards, which will cause half of the iris on the side of the light to be illuminated and the other half to be in shadow (**Figure 15.18**).

The signs and symptoms of acute angle closure glaucoma

Symptoms

In a typical case the following symptoms occur:
- *Rapid reduction of vision*, typically over 1–2 days. This is usually in one eye, but AACG can occur in both eyes simultaneously especially if it has been precipitated by a change in systemic medication.
- *Severe pain in the eye*, although patients often describe this as headache on the same side of the head as the affected eye. If the patient has bilateral acute glaucoma, the patients often do not localise the pain to the eyes and instead report a severe headache.
- *Nausea and vomiting*: this can be so pronounced that patients have undergone abdominal investigations and treatments and even surgery because it has wrongly been assumed that the symptoms must have been caused by abdominal problems.

Signs

In a typical case, the following signs are seen (**Figure 15.19**):
- A *shallow anterior chamber*. Although the anterior chamber in the affected eye may not be visible because of corneal oedema, the other

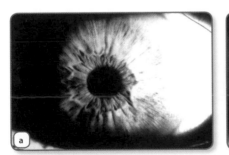
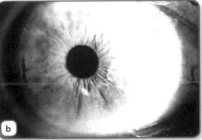

Figure 15.18 Shallow anterior chamber seen with torchlight shone from the side. (a) If the anterior chamber is shallow, some of the iris is in shadow. (b) If the anterior chamber is of normal depth, there is no shadow on the iris. The iris on the left hand side of (a) is not well illuminated.

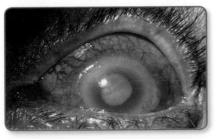

Figure 15.19 Acute angle closure glaucoma. The cornea is hazy, the pupil is half dilated and slightly irregular, and there is ciliary vasodilation. There is also quite dense cataract, which makes an attack of acute glaucoma more likely.

eye must be examined and is very likely to have a similarly shallow anterior chamber.

- *A red eye*, but with more marked redness around the limbus because of ciliary blood vessel dilatation.
- *Corneal haziness*, caused by oedema
- Non-reactive, mid-dilated pupil. It is often slightly vertically oval in shape.
- *Very high intra-ocular pressure*. This can be felt by pressing on the eye, which will feel stony hard and acutely tender.
- *Reduced vision*. This is caused both by the corneal oedema and from the acute rise in IOP shutting off the blood supply to the optic nerve.

Self-resolving episodes of angle closure

In some patients there may be 'minor' attacks of angle closure with spontaneous recovery. These episodes involve shallowing of the anterior chamber with closure of the drainage angle and an intra-ocular pressure rise, but somehow the vicious cycle is broken, perhaps by pupillary constriction and the angle re-opening before the damage has become permanent. During an episode the patient typically has eye pain, blurred vision, nausea and sees haloes or rainbow coloured rings around bright lights. The haloes or rainbows are caused by corneal oedema. The symptoms resolve after a few hours, although the severity of these episodes varies greatly from patient to patient. Patients who are having a non-resolving attack of AACG often recall these attacks in the past, but as they got better spontaneously they did not seek help. Sometimes untreated attacks cause a segment of the iris to atrophy, which distorts the pupil. Self-resolving attacks also leave pigment staining in the angle from the iris coming forward; this can be seen with the gonioscopy lens.

The treatment of AACG

With immediate treatment, there is a high chance of partial or complete recovery of sight. Without treatment, the poor blood supply to the optic nerve rapidly progresses to permanent damage and blindness especially in old people.

The first aim of treatment in acute glaucoma is to lower the IOP. This is usually done medically, but it can be done even if medicines are not available.

Medical treatment for acute angle closure glaucoma

Medical treatment must be started immediately (**Box 15.3**). The different medications that should be used are:

- *Pilocarpine* 2–4%: this should be given to both eyes frequently (e.g. four times daily) until successful iridotomies have been done on both eyes. Pilocarpine constricts the pupil and makes the iris taut, which helps to pull it away from the back of the cornea, and opens up the angle of the anterior chamber. There is a view that the pilocarpine does not penetrate an eye with very high pressure, but we would still recommend it is given to both eyes, as some may penetrate.
- *Acetazolamide* 500 mg (orally or intravenously) reduces the production of aqueous. The effect is quicker if it is given intravenously.

> **Box 15.3: The emergency treatment of acute angle closure glaucoma**
>
> **Immediate treatment**
> 1. Keep the patient lying on their back as much as possible
> 2. Pilocarpine 2–4% to both eyes
> 3. Acetazolamide 500 mg iv or orally
> 4. Dexamethasone 0.1% to the affected eye
> 5. Topical glaucoma drops can be given, e.g. beta blockers or alpha agonists, but adrenaline should not be used
>
> **Treatment options if intra-ocular pressure not reducing**
> 1. Mannitol infusion 1.5–2 g/kg (e.g. approx 80–100 g for average weight person) intravenously over 30–60 minutes
> 2. Glycerol 1–1.8 g/kg as 50% solution
> 3. Corneal indentation
>
> **Continuing treatment after intra-ocular pressure reduced until iridotomy done**
> 1. Pilocarpine 2–4% q.d.s.
> 2. Acetazolamide 250 mg q.d.s. (or the slow release formulation b.d.)
>
> **Iridectomy or iridotomy**
> A surgical iridectomy or laser iridotomy must be done in both eyes as soon as the view of the iris is clear enough to do this safely.

Acetazolamide must not be used in patients with sickle cell anaemia and must be used with great caution if there is kidney or liver disease, when a reduced dose may be appropriate. Acetazolamide can then continue to be given every 6 hours to keep the pressure reduced.

- *Dexamethasone* 0.1% is given to the affected eye because an eye with high pressure can become very inflamed.
- *Other glaucoma drops*: beta-blockers, such as timolol or α agonists such as apraclonidine or brimonidine can be used to help reduce the pressure.
- *Mannitol or glycerol* can be used if acetazolamide is not effective. These are both hyperosmotic agents, which work by reducing the vitreous volume. They should be avoided in patients with kidney problems and significant heart disease.

Treatment with corneal indentation

Corneal indentation can be a very effective way of ending an attack of acute angle glaucoma, even if no medicines are available. The technique is to press very firmly on the central or inferior cornea with something like a cotton bud or squint hook. Even the round end of a large paper-clip could be used if it is carefully cleaned first. Firm pressure that indents the cornea should be maintained for 30 seconds and repeated 4–6 times. It is very painful for the patient and often causes a corneal abrasion, but the pressure can push the iris back, allowing aqueous to enter the anterior chamber and break the cycle.

Iridectomy/iridotomy

The permanent treatment for acute angle closure is to make a small hole in the iris to permanently allow aqueous to move between the posterior and anterior chambers, which prevents the iris bowing forward and blocking the drainage angle (**Figure 15.20**). The iris hole can be made surgically (iridectomy) or with a YAG laser (iridotomy), although lasers are usually only available in the major cities of many poor countries. An iridectomy is a fairly simple operation with a good success rate and few complications. A segment of peripheral iris is excised through a small limbal incision. After a successful iridectomy, there is no risk that acute angle closure will occur again.

An iridectomy/iridotomy must be performed on both the affected and the unaffected eye as soon as the IOP has returned to normal, and the ocular inflammation has subsided, as there is a high-risk of the other eye developing acute glaucoma later.

If a YAG laser is available, it can be used to perform an iridotomy as soon as the view of the iris is clear enough. The great advantage of this procedure over a surgical iridectomy is that it does not require surgical entry into the eye, which is particularly appealing to the patient when treating the healthy eye.

However, in some eyes that have had acute glaucoma the iris does not 'unstick' from the back of the cornea and allow the drainage angle to function again. In these eyes, the surgical iridectomy may not be effective. Even though aqueous can drain freely through the iridectomy to the anterior chamber, it cannot drain into the trabecular meshwork. Therefore, the pressure will rise when the medical treatment is stopped. If there is still vision to preserve, these eyes will need either cataract surgery with freeing up of the drainage angle (goniosynechialysis) and/or a trabeculectomy to reduce the pressure.

In some patients the primary cause of the acute angle closure is a swollen, hypermature cataract. In these patients the cataract should be removed. In fact, an increasing number of eye surgeons feel that it is a good idea to remove a cataract relatively early in patients with narrow angles as this eliminates the risk of angle closure glaucoma.

If an episode does not settle and is not treated, eventually, the pain and inflammation subside. However, the features of end-stage glaucoma remain: a hard eye with a dilated pupil, atrophy of the iris and total atrophy of the optic nerve.

Chronic angle closure glaucoma

Some patients with narrow drainage angles do not develop acute angle closure. Instead the narrow angle causes a chronic restriction to aqueous

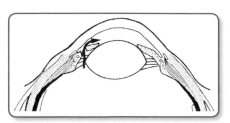

Figure 15.20 The flow of aqueous fluid after an iridectomy operation.

drainage. The pressure rise is more chronic and less severe and there are no symptoms. They develop very gradual visual field loss similar to that of open angle glaucoma.

Secondary glaucoma

Sometimes complications of other eye diseases cause a rise in the IOP. This is called secondary glaucoma.

Neovascular glaucoma

Neovascular glaucoma is the growth of new blood vessels on the iris surface and into the drainage angle (**Figure 15.21**). These blood vessels obstruct the drainage of the aqueous, and produce a very severe type of glaucoma, with a very high IOP. It is also known as rubeotic or thrombotic glaucoma. Iris neovascularisation is almost always a complication of vascular disorders of the retina that cause marked retinal ischaemia such a retinal vein occlusion and diabetic retinopathy. These conditions also cause new blood vessels to grow on the retina and into the vitreous as a response to the retina being starved of oxygen. Most of these eyes are already blind from the retinal disease, and the aim of treatment is only to relieve pain in an inflamed, hard eye. Topical steroids and mydriatic drops may do this, but an injection of dilute phenol, alcohol or chlorpromazine into the retrobulbar space is often a cheaper and more permanent method of pain relief in a blind eye (see page 100).

Glaucoma secondary to intraocular inflammation

A rise in IOP is quite common with anterior uveitis (see Chapter 11). The drainage angle may be blocked by inflammatory cells or occasionally the pupil margin may become adherent to the lens causing *pupil block glaucoma*.

Glaucoma secondary to trauma

Trauma may cause bleeding in the anterior chamber. The red blood cells can obstruct aqueous drainage at the drainage angle. Trauma and intraocular surgery can also cause the iris to be pushed backwards. Although the angle looks wider and more open on gonioscopy (angle recession), it is actually damaged and torn by the trauma and aqueous drainage is reduced.

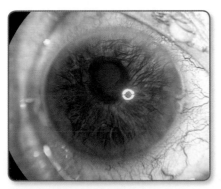

Figure 15.21 Neovascular glaucoma. The blood vessels are spreading all over the iris.

Ghost cell glaucoma

Sometimes degenerated blood cells get into the anterior chamber, from vitreous bleeds or from trauma. This can block aqueous drainage causing glaucoma. This is sometimes called 'ghost cell' glaucoma because the cells are very difficult to see, like a ghost.

Malignant glaucoma (ciliary block glaucoma)

Malignant glaucoma is a rare complication of any intraocular surgery. The aqueous fluid does not pass into the anterior chamber, but instead collects either behind the vitreous body or behind the iris and lens. The iris is pushed forward against the back of the cornea and so blocks the aqueous drainage pathway. Treatment involves initially mydriatic drops, and then urgent and often complex surgery, usually to remove the vitreous.

Steroid induced glaucoma

In some patients the IOP rises with steroid treatment. These patients are called *steroid responders*. The pressure usually returns to normal when the treatment stops. Steroid induced glaucoma can be a particular problem when intraocular injections of steroid are used. These are used increasingly frequently for conditions such as post-operative and diabetic macular oedema.

Paediatric glaucoma

Paediatric glaucoma is raised intraocular pressure causing optic nerve damage in children. It is rare, but often seriously damages the vision for the following reasons:

- Children with glaucoma are likely to have the disease for the rest of their life, i.e. they are at risk of high pressure and optic nerve damage for many years.
- Paediatric glaucoma is often associated with other abnormalities of the eye. These can be either congenital abnormalities such as cataract and abnormal eyeball size or shape, or other conditions that develop in childhood such as uveitis. These other conditions may also impair the vision or make the glaucoma more difficult to manage.
- Paediatric glaucoma is often very difficult to manage, requiring intensive treatment and technically very difficult surgery with regular follow-up.

Paediatric glaucoma can be divided into primary congenital glaucoma, which exists at birth (or even before birth) and the high pressure is caused by drainage obstruction alone, and secondary glaucoma in which the drainage obstruction results from another ocular or systemic condition.

Primary congenital glaucoma

Congenital glaucoma is a rare condition, in which the angle of the anterior chamber does not develop normally in the embryo. The exact cause is not known, but one theory is that a mesodermal membrane covers the trabecular meshwork. This prevents the drainage of aqueous fluid causing the IOP to rise. Congenital glaucoma is usually bilateral, but one eye is often more diseased than the other.

Symptoms and signs

- *Photophobia and eye watering*, which are probably caused by the corneal oedema and the high pressure. Although paediatric glaucoma is rare, the diagnosis must be considered when parents describe their child as having increased light sensitivity and watering.
- *Enlarged cornea* (buphthalmos, from the Greek for ox-eye) (**Figure 15.22**): the cornea and sclera of the fetus and neonate is less rigid than in an adult and therefore it stretches in response to the pressure.
- *White lines on the cornea* (Haab's striae): as the cornea stretches, it causes splits in Descemet's membrane, which are seen as horizontal, faint, white lines on the cornea.
- *Corneal oedema*: the cornea is hazy or oedematous because of the high pressure

If congenital glaucoma is suspected, the infant should be examined under a general anaesthetic both to measure the IOP and the diameter of the cornea and to exclude other diseases like retinoblastoma. The treatment is surgical but it is usual to give drops (e.g. latanoprost, or timolol, although timolol should not be used in neonates) and acetazolamide first to try to lower the IOP. The standard operation is called 'goniotomy'. It involves incising along the trabecular meshwork in the angle of the anterior chamber.

Congenital or juvenile glaucoma needs surgical treatment and if successful this will preserve the sight for the rest of the child's life. However, glaucoma surgery in a child is much harder than in an adult, and these patients should if possible be referred to an expert.

Secondary childhood glaucoma

Secondary glaucomas usually develop in early childhood. They can be associated with other congenital eye and systemic conditions or with conditions that develop later in childhood. The causative or associated conditions include:

- Congenital conditions:
  - Iris and trabecular meshwork dysgenesis, e.g. Rieger, Axenfeld and Peter anomalies
  - Aniridia
  - Coloboma
- Acquired conditions:
  - Aphakia
  - Uveitis
  - Trauma

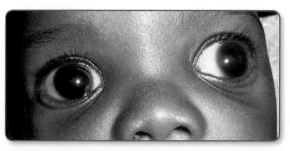

Figure 15.22 Congenital glaucoma, buphthalmos. The corneas are very large and a squint has developed because of the poor vision in one or both eyes.

- Steroid usage
- Retinoblastoma

The management of secondary childhood glaucomas requires treatment for both high pressure and any underlying disease. Similar surgical procedures are used as those used for primary congenital glaucoma.

The prevention of blindness from glaucoma

If a patient is diagnosed as having advanced glaucoma in one eye and the other eye is fairly normal, every attempt must be made to try to find the exact cause. This determines the management for the other eye, which is now the patient's only seeing eye. If the affected eye has angle closure glaucoma, the other eye *must* be treated with an iridectomy or iridotomy. If the affected eye has secondary glaucoma, the other eye probably requires no treatment, as it is likely to be a unilateral condition. If the affected eye has primary open angle glaucoma, the other eye is likely to have early glaucoma or may develop it in the future. It will require careful observation and possibly a trabeculectomy operation or life-long medical treatment.

Open angle glaucoma

This is an important cause of blindness all over the world, particularly in old people and black people. Early detection followed by effective treatment is the only way to prevent blindness from glaucoma. However, even in areas with good ophthalmic services, patients sometimes go blind. Planning an early detection scheme for glaucoma in a poor country is therefore a major challenge, and must involve non-doctors working in the community.

Sometimes patients do not seek early treatment because they mistake glaucoma for cataract. Traditionally, cataracts are not treated surgically until the vision is considerably reduced. Therefore old patients with glaucoma often wait until they are almost blind before they come for treatment.

The ways of screening for open angle glaucoma have already been described. A screening test for glaucoma should be part of the routine eye test for any patient over 40. Relatives of glaucoma patients and people over 60 are especially at risk.

Angle closure glaucoma

In areas such as South East Asia where narrow drainage angles and angle closure glaucoma are common, the population and eye care professionals are much more aware of the disease, and may be trained to look for eyes with shallow anterior chambers. These patients can then be given prophylactic surgical iridectomies or YAG laser iridotomies. However, in most poor countries, it is impossible to predict and prevent angle closure attacks, because patients with healthy, normal eyes never encounter an eye-care professional who would notice the shallow anterior chamber. Therefore until the attack occurs, the patient and their eye are entirely normal. However, an iridectomy operation is a relatively straight-forward procedure, and a YAG laser iridotomy is even simpler. If given quickly this may treat the affected eye, and perhaps more importantly guarantees complete protection from acute glaucoma to the second eye.

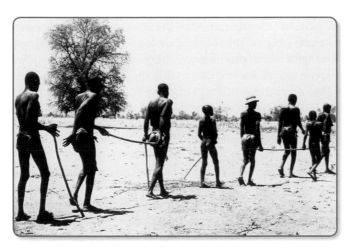

Blindness from onchocerciasis destroyed many communities in Africa 30 years ago. Thanks to mass treatment with ivermectin these scenes of destitute blind people in rural Africa are rarely seen today.

Infections by parasites are common in tropical climates. Although a few ocular parasitic infections are also seen in cooler climates (toxoplasmosis, acanthamoeba, toxocara), a huge number of parasites cause infection in hotter countries. Most of these are spread either by insect vectors or eating contaminated food. There are several reasons why parasitic diseases are found mainly in the tropics:

- Warm climates encourages:
  - the survival, growth and reproduction of many parasites and enables their larvae and eggs to survive outside the human body.
  - the survival of the insect vectors which transmit parasitic infections.
- Poor sanitation and poor water supplies increase the risk of:
  - food being contaminated by faeces.
  - food and particularly meat not being properly cooked. Good cooking eliminates almost all parasites.
- People who are subsistence farmers often live in close contact with the domestic animals that are involved in the life cycle of some parasites.

Some of these parasites have complex life cycles living in two or even three different hosts to complete their life cycle. Therefore, many parasitic diseases are confined to certain geographical areas where the climate and ecology will support these life cycles. One particularly interesting feature of parasitic diseases is how long some of the organisms can survive inside the body.

Therefore, these diseases sometimes appear in people who have left endemic areas many years previously.

As far as the eye is concerned onchocerciasis is by far the most important parasitic disease in the tropics. However it is never seen outside the tropics, where toxoplasmosis and toxocara are the most commonly seen parasitic diseases.

Onchocerciasis

Onchocerciasis is a parasitic disease caused by the filarial worm, *Onchocerca volvulus*. Large numbers of larval microfilaria are found in the skin and eye, and it is these microfilaria which produce the symptoms. **Figure 16.1** shows where onchocerciasis is found. The main focus is in the Savanna zone of west Africa, spreading across central Africa and into the Yemen. Onchocerciasis was also a problem in parts of Central America, and may have arrived with the slave trade.

Local names for onchocerciasis often describe the symptoms. For example, 'craw-craw' in west Africa describes the itching of the skin; 'sowda' (black) in the Yemen describes the increased pigmentation. The disease affects the whole body, but it can be particularly devastating to the eye.

About a quarter of a million people are blind and many more are visually impaired from onchocerciasis, with up to 20 million having significant symptoms. Altogether about 100 million people are at risk. Onchocerciasis is mainly a problem in isolated and rural communities in poor countries. For this reason attempts to eradicate the disease have made little progress, until recently. In the past, WHO has organised programmes to control the fly especially in the Volta river basin, one of the worst affected areas. The drug ivermectin (available since 1987) is very effective at controlling the disease and has made a dramatic difference in the fight against this devastating disease.

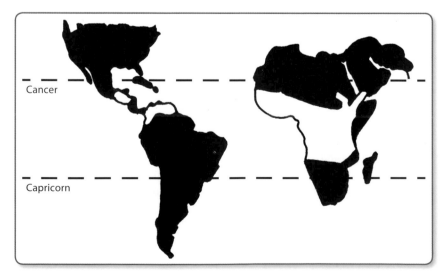

Figure 16.1 Areas of the world where onchocerciasis is found. These are shown in white.

The life cycle of *Onchocerca volvulus* in man and the *Simulium* fly (Figure 16.2)

The adult worms are mainly found in the subcutaneous tissues, but they may also occur in deep structures. Several worms usually coil together in a mass surrounded by fibrous tissue, and are called an 'onchocercoma' (**Figure 16.4a** and **16.4b**). The male is about 4 cm long and 0.2 mm in diameter. The female is larger, up to 40 cm long and 0.4 mm in diameter. The worms may live for up to 15 years, and during that time the female produces a vast number of living larvae (microfilaria), which are 300 microns long and 8 microns wide. These microfilariae can live for up to 2 years in the human host. The microfilariae move actively out of the nodules where the adult worms are found, and spread throughout the skin and into the eye by their own movements. They are often found in the urine and sputum of infected patients, and almost certainly spread into the bloodstream and lymphatics also. If the microfilariae remain in the human host, they die without further development. Microfilaria must pass through the insect vector to complete their life cycle.

The insect vector is a biting black fly of the genus *Simulium,* which is sometimes called the 'buffalo gnat'. Different species can carry the disease, but the most important species is *Simulium damnosum*. These flies lay their eggs in well-oxygenated water, such as fast flowing rivers and streams. Here larvae

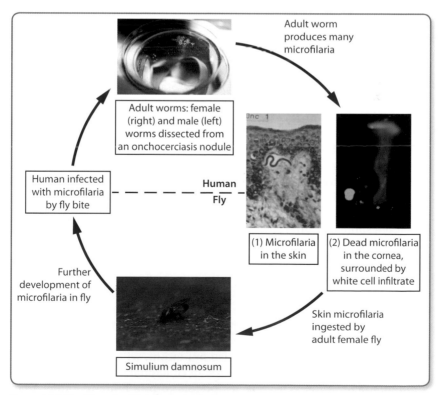

Figure 16.2 The life cycle of Onchocerca volvulus.

hatch and eventually develop into adult flies. This explains why the disease is commonly called '*river blindness*'.

Female flies feed on human blood. They feed during the day, and they cut the skin open in a messy way, which explains the description 'open-cast mining'. If a fly feeds on blood from an infected person, it may also ingest some microfilaria. The microfilaria can escape digestion by migrating to the thoracic muscle of the fly. Over a period of about a week, the microfilariae undergo further development, and migrate from the thoracic muscle to the haemocele in the head of the fly. They are now infective microfilaria, and are ready to enter another human host when the *Simulium* fly bites again.

It is not clear what happens to the infective microfilaria in the human host. They somehow develop into adult worms, which come together and undergo sexual reproduction. The fertilised female then starts to produce very large number of microfilaria.

People who live or work in areas where both the black biting fly and the disease are present are at risk of contracting onchocerciasis. The risk increases with the number of infected flies in the area.

Epidemiology of onchocerciasis

In hyperendemic areas, such as parts of the Savanna zone of west Africa, over 60% of the population suffer from onchocerciasis. However, in recent years the mass distribution of ivermectin has greatly reduced the burden of the disease in most areas, except in northern Uganda and South Sudan where the incidence is increasing. This probably reflects the difficulty of getting treatment to these dangerous or war-torn areas. Around 17 million people (mostly in Africa) remain infected.

The disease is acquired at an early age, although significant visual loss from the disease is rare below the age of 15 years. The prevalence rises gradually with age. Males are more likely to develop visual loss than females, but in a hyperendemic area <5% of the whole community and 30% of males over 40 will be blind (visual acuity worse than counting fingers at 3 metres).

The risk of blindness varies greatly from community to community, even if the `black-biting fly' is equally abundant. For example, the fly is common in the forest zone of west Africa and the prevalence of onchocerciasis is about the same as in the Savanna zone, but the risk of blindness is usually much lower (1.5%) and often not much more than in non-onchocercal areas. The prevalence of both infection and blindness varies widely even between neighbouring villages.

This great variation in prevalence is probably because even a slight alteration to one of the many factors important in the life cycle of the parasite, changes the local pattern of the disease, e.g. proximity to a fly breeding site or how much clothing an individual wears.

The species of *Simulium* fly is also important, with some species being more efficient vectors than others. In Guatemala, the main vector is *Simulium ochraceum*. This species prefers to bite humans rather than animals and prefers the upper parts of the body. In Venezuela, however, the fly *Simulium metallicum* bites both humans and animals, preferring the lower parts of the body. In some parts of Africa, the vector is *Simulium naevei*, a species that is easier to eradicate than *Simulium damnosum*. There is evidence of different strains of *Onchocerca*, some of which are more pathogenic than others. This may explain why the disease is more severe in the Savanna areas of Africa.

Climate may be a significant factor as well. In the Savanna the cornea is more exposed to sunlight, dust and drying, and sclerosing keratitis is more severe. It is unclear why men have a higher risk of blindness, but it may be because they spend more time outside exposed to sunlight, or simply that the inflammatory effects are more destructive. Racial and nutritional differences between communities may also be significant factors affecting prevalence, but there is no direct evidence for this..

Clinical signs and symptoms

The symptoms of onchocerciasis are mostly caused by the microscopic larval microfilaria rather than by the adult worms. These microfilariae may be found all over the body. However, they are concentrated in the skin and the eye, and it is here that they cause the most damage. It appears that it is the death of the microfilaria and the resultant inflammation that is the major cause of the symptoms and signs, as people who are heavily infected with living microfilaria do not seem to have any obvious reaction to them.

Skin changes

There is chronic dermatitis, sometimes with a papular rash, and often with itching (**Figure 16.3a**). This may be very severe and persistent in some cases. The symptoms are thought to be caused by the dying microfilaria. In advanced and burnt-out cases there may be atrophy and scaling of the skin, and the skin loses its elasticity. This is sometimes called 'lizard skin' (**Figure 16.3b**). There can be patches of skin depigmentation especially on the legs called 'leopard skin' (**Figure 16.3c**).

Nodules

Nodules, called onchocercomas are collections of adult worms, coiled together and surrounded by fibrous tissue (**Figure 16.4**). These onchocercomas are firm, well-defined, subcutaneous nodules. They vary from 0.5–10 cm in diameter, are painless and rarely produce any other symptoms. An average adult in a highly infected area might have about ten of these nodules. In Africa, the nodules are usually around the pelvis and on the body, and only occasionally on the limbs, head and neck. In Central America, however, about half of the nodules are on the head and neck. It is not yet known what percentage of the total adult worm load is in these nodules, and what percentage lies free in the subcutaneous tissues or in deeper structures, where they cannot be palpated.

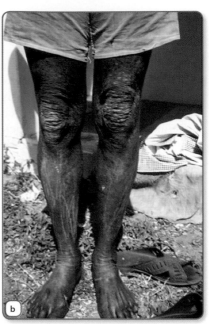

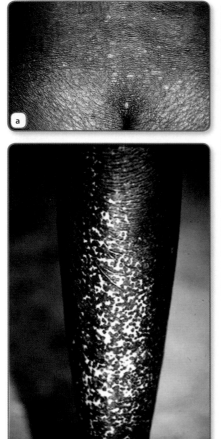

Figure 16.3 Skin changes. (a) Chronic skin rash. (b) Atrophy and scaling of the skin, sometimes called 'lizard skin'. There are scratch marks all over the skin from the intense itching. (c) Areas of skin depigmentation, sometimes called 'leopard skin'.

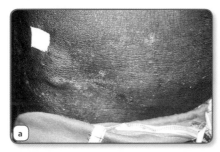

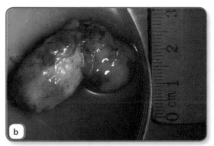

Figure 16.4 Nodule. (a) An abdominal nodule (onchocercoma). (b) The nodule has been excised.

Lymphadenopathy

The lymph nodes are often enlarged, and sometimes there may be chronic lymphoedema of the groin and scrotum (called 'hanging groin') from involvement of the inguinal nodes.

The brain

Onchocerciasis probably affects the brain and there is increasing evidence of an association with epilepsy, although a direct link has not yet been established. The 'nodding-disease' form of epilepsy, seen in areas with a high prevalence of onchocerciasis, is quite likely to be caused by the microfilaria.

Systemic

Heavily infected people have lower than average body weight.

Eye changes from onchocerciasis

The microfilariae are found in nearly every part of the eye, but it is not certain exactly how they enter. One route is likely to be from the skin and conjunctiva into the cornea. Microfilariae probably enter the back of the eye along the ciliary vessels and nerves, because the fundus changes usually start where the vessels pierce the sclera. Another possibility is that the microfilaria enter the eye via the bloodstream or the cerebrospinal fluid along the optic nerve sheath.

There is a great difference between the presence of living microfilaria, and the inflammatory reaction that they produce when they die. It is quite common to see an eye which contains many microfilariae, but which shows very little evidence of inflammation. The pathological changes develop slowly. Even in an area, which is heavily infested with *Onchocerca volvulus*, it usually takes many years of exposure to cause serious visual loss.

Most of the early changes in the anterior chamber need a slit lamp to see them properly, but the advanced changes are visible to the naked eye. An ophthalmoscope will show the changes in the fundus. The main eye changes are summarised in **Figure 16.5** and the details are listed below.

The cornea

The cornea may contain large numbers of living microfilaria. They are usually only visible with a slit lamp at high magnification and with retroillumination. Dead microfilariae are more obvious than living ones, because soon after death an inflammatory reaction around the larvae produces small, faint punctate opacities in the stroma of the cornea. These opacities are up to 0.5 mm in diameter, and usually require a slit lamp to be seen. However, with good illumination, they are just occasionally visible using a magnifying loupe, or even the naked eye. These are called 'snowflake', 'fluffy',

---

Box 16.1 Summary of non-ocular changes in onchocerciasis
Dermatitis
Itching
Atrophy and depigmentation of the skin nodules
Lymphadenopathy and lymphoedema weight loss
Epilepsy

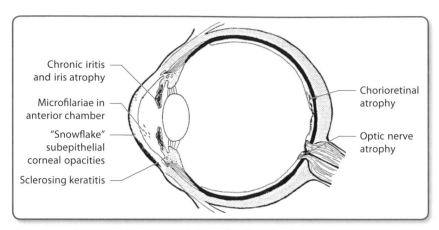

Figure 16.5 A summary of the common effects of onchocerciasis on the eye.

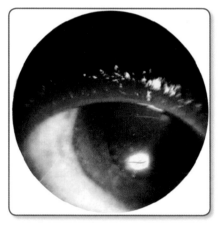

Figure 16.6 'Snowflake' corneal opacities. The opacities in this picture are much larger and more obvious than usual.

'cracked-ice' or 'cotton wool' opacities after their appearance (**Figure 16.6**), and will apparently disappear without scarring.

Patients who have been exposed to many microfilariae for a long time develop a pattern of corneal scarring called 'sclerosing keratitis' (**Figure 16.7**). This scarring is mainly peripheral, especially in the interpalpebral fissure and the lower cornea and can be seen with the naked eye. In advanced cases the scarring spreads to the centre and can cover the whole cornea.

There is often irregular pigmentation and occasionally calcification associated with the scarring. Patients with sclerosing keratitis usually have a very strongly positive skin snip (see below), but in older patients the microfilaria may have died. If the whole cornea is scarred, there is probably significant intraocular damage, and so corneal grafting is very unlikely to help.

The anterior chamber

The anterior chamber often contains living microfilariae, which move vigorously. They may sometimes adhere either to the endothelium of the cornea, or occasionally to the lens. They may also be visible in the anterior vitreous

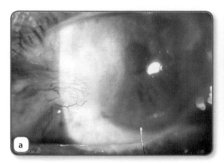 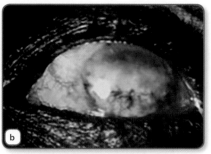

Figure 16.7 Sclerosing keratitis. (a) Early keratitis: the white opacity starts at the limbus in the interpalpebral fissure. (b) Advanced sclerosing keratitis causing blindness in this eye.

body behind the lens. One way of increasing the number of visible microfilaria in the anterior chamber is to ask the patient to bend their head down between their knees for 1 minute. Large volumes of microfilariae can even form a 'pseudohypopyon'.

A slit lamp is really required to see the microfilaria although they can sometimes just be seen as shadows with an ophthalmoscope if a slit lamp is not available. Hold the ophthalmoscope very close to the patient's eye using a +25 or +30 dioptre lens in order to focus on the anterior chamber. If the pupil is dilated, and there are no significant opacities in the cornea or lens, the microfilaria may be just visible as moving shadows against a clear red fundus reflex.

The iris and ciliary body and lens

The iris and ciliary body are often inflamed in heavily infected patients, causing a chronic non-granulomatous iridocyclitis. The usual features of onchocercal iridocyclitis are:

- Fine pigmented deposits on the back of the cornea, or at the front of the lens (these deposits can usually only be seen with a slit lamp).
- Atrophy of the iris.
- Irregularity of the pupil, which may be visible to the naked eye.
- Glaucoma. This is not a common complication, but it may cause blindness. It may result from the anterior and posterior synechiae, caused by the iridocyclitis, blocking aqueous circulation or by persistent inflammation in the trabecular meshwork.
- Cataract: the chronic inflammation is often responsible for secondary cataract. Very occasionally there can be microfilaria in the lens.

The back of the eye

Fundus changes such as choroidoretinal degeneration, optic neuritis and optic atrophy are common, and may cause profound visual loss. Both changes appear to be mainly inflammatory reactions to the microfilaria. Fundus changes are usually bilateral, but not always symmetrical in the two eyes.

The retina and choroid

Choroidoretinal atrophy usually starts as a mottling of the retinal pigment epithelium (**Figure 16.8a**). This mottling may then progress to atrophy of the

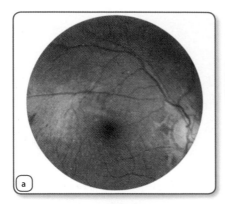
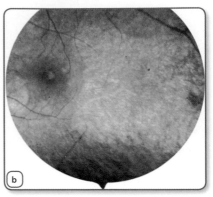
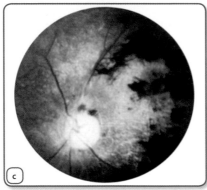

Figure 16.8 Choroidoretinal atrophy. (a) Early choroidoretinal atrophy from onchocerciasis. There is 'mottling' and early atrophy of the pigment epithelium on the temporal side of the macula. There are some early pigmentary changes around the optic disc. (b) More advanced atrophy of the pigment epithelium and choroidal capillaries on the temporal side of the macula. (c) Advanced onchocercal chorioretinal atrophy. There is excess pigmentation and extensive chorioretinal atrophy and also optic atrophy.

pigment epithelium, and atrophy of the choroidal capillaries (**Figure 16.8b**). Increased pigmentation, subretinal fibrosis and sheathing of the retinal vessels may also be seen (**Figure 16.8c**). Typically, the changes first appear temporal to the macula, then spread around the macula. Finally, the entire posterior retina, including the macula is affected. Onchocercal chorioretinal atrophy may be confused with other inflammatory or degenerative changes in the retina. However, choroiditis causes more localised, well-defined lesions (see Figure 11.13), and senile macular degeneration usually starts centrally in the macula (see Figure 13.25 and Figure 13.27).

The optic nerve

Optic nerve inflammation *(optic neuritis)* occurs, which can sometimes be seen clinically as optic nerve head swelling (**Figure 16.9**). Usually however, the patients are seen long after this stage by which time they have progressed to having a pale disc with few active nerve fibres: *optic atrophy*. At this stage patients may also have peri-papillary pigmentation and atrophy from previous inflammation, sheathing of the retinal vessels, and some glial tissue on the disc (**Figure 16.10**). Glial tissue in the central nervous system is the same as fibrous tissue elsewhere in the body, and represents scarring from inflammation. Optic atrophy may be compounded by the glaucoma. Primary optic atrophy with no signs of any previous inflammation is uncommon in onchocerciasis. Optic atrophy is the most devastating visual complication of the

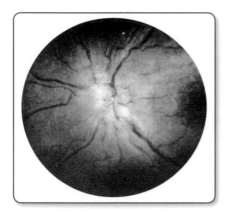 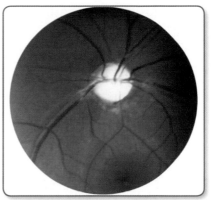

Figure 16.9 Optic neuritis from onchocerciasis. causing oedema and swelling of the optic disc.

Figure 16.10 Optic atrophy in onchocerciasis. Note the white scar tissue spreading from the disc along the retinal vessels.

disease, although is often missed because recognising it on fundus examination requires considerable experience and practice.

Visual loss

As onchocerciasis can cause damage to most parts of the eye, the pattern of visual loss is very variable. With early optic atrophy there may be constriction of the visual fields ('tunnel vision') and night blindness. If there is only choroidoretinal atrophy, and the optic nerve is healthy, the macula and the peripheral retina may be undamaged, and some useful central vision may remain. Visual loss from onchocerciasis is nearly always irreversible although if it is treated in the early stages it will prevent further visual loss.

Diagnosis

In advanced cases, the characteristic changes in the eye and skin are enough to make a clinical diagnosis. However, in less advanced cases it is best to demonstrate the microfilariae or the adult worms, especially in younger patients who may be quite severely infested but without any obvious clinical changes.

There are a number of different methods of demonstrating the microfilaria. Some of these methods can also indicate how severe the infection is. This is important both for the treatment and the prognosis.

Slit lamp examination

If possible a slit lamp should be used as direct viewing of microfilaria is the quickest and simplest way to make the diagnosis. However, this does not give a good indication of disease severity. There is often not a correlation between the number of microfilaria and pathological damage, particularly in young people.

A 'skin snip' examination

This is the best laboratory test for onchocerciasis (**Figure 16.11**). A small piece of skin is suspended in water or saline. After a few minutes, the microfilariae emerge, and they can be seen moving actively under the low power of a microscope. Although, very little skin is required (approximately 1 mg), it should include the outer part of the dermal papillae, where the microfilariae are most concentrated. There should therefore be faint blood staining of the wound after a few seconds. Ideally samples should be taken from several sites. A skin snip examination from just outside the lateral canthus will give the best indication of how many microfilariae there are in the eye. Another recommended site is the iliac crest, which in Africa, is the area with the highest concentration of microfilaria. The technique for taking a skin snip is to lift up the skin (ensuring there is no blood) with the point of a needle and cut a tiny fragment with a blade, fine scissors, or with a corneoscleral punch. The fragment is left on a slide in a drop of physiological saline. If no microfilariae have emerged after a few minutes, the skin sample should be 'teased' and re-examined after half an hour. In scientific surveys the method can be adapted for counting the numbers of microfilaria. The skin snip can be sent for histological assessment to confirm the diagnosis. The instruments must be properly sterilised between patients to prevent the spread of blood-borne viruses.

Unfortunately, other microfilaria may be present in the skin, especially *Dipetalonema* and *Streptocerca*. These other filarial worms do not seem to produce any specific pathological changes in the body. To identify the microfilaria, it may be necessary to stain them and examine them under the high power of a microscope.

Looking for skin nodules

This is a good way of making a rapid epidemiological assessment (REA) of a village or community, to decide how badly that community is affected by onchocerciasis. Thirty adults should be examined. If 9 or more have nodules, the village is hyperendemic, if 5–8 have nodules it is mesoendemic, and if 1–4 have nodules it is hypoendemic.

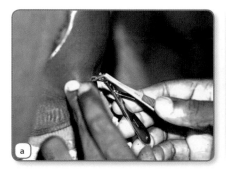
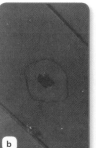
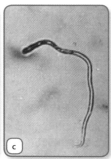

Figure 16.11 A skin snip examination. (a) Taking the skin with a needle and razor blade. (b) Mounting the skin on a microscope slide. (c) A microfilaria emerging from the skin seen through the microscope.

Other tests

The Mazzotti test

This test detects the presence of microfilaria by the patient's reaction to the drug diethylcarbamazine (DEC). DEC somehow removes the protection that the microfilariae have to the immune systems in the body. A small dose (50 mg) affects the microfilaria and produces a reaction in the patient with erythema, oedema and itching. However, the test is no longer recommended because on a few occasions, the reaction in heavily infected patients has caused visual loss.

Antibody and DNA tests

Antibody tests are relatively easy to perform, but they cannot distinguish between past and current infection and are therefore not very useful for people living in endemic areas. They can be used for visitors who return to a non-endemic area. DNA tests are more sensitive for current infection but are expensive and require good laboratory facilities.

Immunology

The immunological responses of the body to the parasite are not fully understood. It seems likely that there is a reaction to the adult worms, because they are usually surrounded by inflammatory and fibrous tissue. However, the microfilariae have a protective mechanism against the host antibodies and do not seem to provoke an inflammatory reaction while they are alive. When they die there is a severe reaction. The drug DEC, which is no longer used in treatment or diagnosis, probably kills the microfilaria in the body by interfering in some way with the protective mechanism of the microfilariae. DEC does not affect microfilaria *in vitro*.

It has also been found that commensal bacteria called *Walbachia* live inside the microfilaria. These are released when the microfilaria die and may cause many of the symptoms. If this theory is correct the symptoms of onchocerciasis may be lessened with broad-spectrum antibiotics such as doxycycline. This has recently been suggested as a supplementary or alternative treatment.

The immunological reaction of the body to the infective microfilaria transmitted from the fly is even less clear. It is not certain how many of these infective microfilariae survive the body defences to develop into adult worms. Microfilariae in pregnant women may invade the fetus across the placenta thus desensitising a subsequent immunological reaction to later infection by the parasite.

Treatment

Patients with a severe infection require treatment. Sterilising or killing as many of the adult worms and microfilariae as possible will prevent the irreversible progressive changes in the eye. A good macro filaricide (which kills adult worms) is the most effective method. The microfilariae then gradually disappear from the skin, interrupting transmission.

In the past, the treatment for onchocerciasis was a course of DEC and suramin. DEC killed the microfilaria but not the adult worms. Suramin was a rather toxic drug given by injection, which killed the adult worms. This treatment, however, was prolonged and unpleasant and could have serious and dangerous side effects. Therefore, it has been abandoned.

Ivermectin (Mectizan) has been the mainstay of treatment since 1987. It is available free of charge direct from its manufacturers Merck for those who will use it responsibly and carefully, and the company has undertaken to continue with this policy until onchocerciasis is eradicated. Ivermectin has a direct effect in killing microfilaria, but unlike DEC somehow kills them without causing a severe inflammatory reaction. Ivermectin also appears to make the adult female worms sterile so that they stop producing microfilaria. There is therefore a gradual but very profound and long-lasting fall in the number of living circulating microfilaria. It is relatively non-toxic and is taken by mouth once every 6–12 months. The dose is 150 µg/kg and it is available as 3 mg tablets (**Table 16.1**). Extreme care must be taken when treating patients in areas of loa-loa infection, where treatment can cause loa-loa encephalopathy (see below).

Unfortunately, and perhaps unsurprisingly, due to the enormous use of ivermectin, resistance is starting to appear. Other drugs are being tried, e.g. Moxidectin; a microfilaricidal that sterilises or kills the adult worms. Trials of Moxidectin are in progress.

In certain areas, it has been the practice to excise onchocercal nodules (nodulectomy). This is worthwhile in areas where the majority of the onchocercomata are on the head and neck. Otherwise, it is not beneficial.

Patients who have onchocerciasis and glaucoma are especially difficult to treat. There is a high risk that the death of the microfilaria will make the glaucoma worse. Topical steroid treatment is probably advisable to reduce inflammation, although some patients can have a pressure rise from steroid treatment itself. If the intraocular pressure does not respond to reducing inflammation, it may then be advisable to perform glaucoma surgery.

Onchocerciasis control programmes

Blindness due to onchocerciasis is only a problem in certain, fairly limited, areas of the world. The unnecessary and avoidable blindness and

Table 16.1 The dose and side effects of ivermectin	
Weight	**Dose**
15–25 kg	3 mg
26–44 kg	6 mg
45–64 kg	9 mg
65 kg +	12 mg

Contraindications
- Children under 5 years or weighing less than 15 kg or less than 90 cm tall
- Pregnant women.
- Breastfeeding mothers with children less than 1 month old.
- People with serious, acute or chronic illness, especially if meningitis is suspected.
- Use with great caution in areas where loiasis also exists.

burden on communities from this disease, is enormous. Therefore disease control programmes are critical. Before ivermectin was available, most onchocerciasis control programmes tried to control the Simulium fly, which carries the disease. Various pesticide sprays have been used, including dichlorodiphenyltrichloroethane (DDT), which was effective at eliminating the fly in parts of Kenya, but it is very toxic. Insecticide spray needs to be implemented weekly to break the life cycle of the disease. It has now been decided that future control programmes should be directed at mass ivermectin treatment in affected communities rather than fly eradication.

At present, the main strategy for delivering ivermectin to the people who need it is the Community Directed Treatment with Ivermectin (CDTI) plan. This plan tries to involve the community in planning and distribution of treatment. In hyper- or mesoendemic areas, there is mass treatment of the entire community; in hypoendemic areas where the risk is less, only affected individuals are treated.

It was hoped that onchocerciasis would be eliminated by 2020 as part of the Vision 2020 programme. Despite the success of the mass treatment programme, onchocerciasis remains a significant public health problem. Computer modelling suggests that mass treatment will be required for at least 20–25 years, and possibly 35 years if therapeutic coverage is less than 65%. Although the ivermectin is free, running community or even countrywide treatment programmes requires a vast amount of resources and is currently impossible in some poor and war-torn areas.

In areas like the Volta river basin, where the disease has been controlled, village communities are coming back to life. However, in other areas like parts of Uganda, surveys have shown that onchocerciasis is more prevalent than previously thought. Great strides have been made in controlling and treating onchocerciasis, but there is still a long way to go.

Loiasis

Loiasis is only found in the equatorial rain forests of central and west Africa, and it is caused by the filarial worm, *Loa loa*. It is the only other filarial infection that causes ocular complications. These occur quite frequently, but are not usually a threat to the sight.

The life cycle of *Loa loa* and *Onchocerca volvulus* are in many ways similar. A biting fly of the genus *Chrysops* ingests microfilaria (which are found in the blood) when it bites, and transmits them when it bites another person. The microfilariae develop into adult worms and move around fairly freely in the connective and subcutaneous tissues. Unlike onchocerciasis, however, it is the adult worms that cause the symptoms, and not the microfilaria.

The *Loa loa* worms often appear under the conjunctiva (**Figure 16.12**). They can move quite vigorously, and can cause severe pain, irritation or itching. Sometimes the body reacts to the worms with an acute attack of localised inflammatory oedema. This usually means that the worm is dying. The body produces a much more severe reaction to a dying worm than a live one. The swelling is often called 'Calabar swelling' because of the high

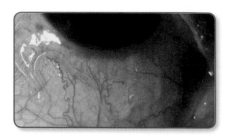

Figure 16.12 A *Loa loa* worm under the conjunctiva.

incidence in the Calabar region of Nigeria and is classically seen on the back of the wrist. Another common site for a Calabar swelling is the orbit and eyelids. The characteristic feature is a sudden and severe episode of oedema (**Figure 16.13**), but the patients feel well in themselves. After a few days, the oedema subsides, and the tissues return to normal just leaving some small, firm lumps, which are the dead fragments of the worm (**Figure 16.14**). A Calabar swelling looks alarming, but it does not seem to damage the vision or leave any permanent scarring although the patients will need reassurance that the swelling will subside.

The diagnosis of loiasis is usually obvious from the history and the physical signs. Blood samples may show variable number of microfilaria, and the eosinophil count usually increases, especially during an attack of oedema.

Ivermectin and DEC both kill the *Loa loa* microfilariae. However, patients with a load of over 10,000 microfilariae/mL of blood have a risk of developing encephalopathy with treatment, which can be fatal. The encephalopathy may be due to dead microfilarial micro-emboli entering the cerebral circulation. The risk of *Loa-loa* encephalopathy can hinder onchocerciasis treatment programmes in areas of co-endemicity. If there is a pronounced reaction to the treatment, antihistamines should be given urgently. Steroids have been given in the past, they may in fact be detrimental, as they can increase the risk of infection and/or cause gastrointestinal bleeding.

Sometimes it is possible to catch and remove a worm moving across the conjunctiva. In order to do this, after instilling topical anaesthetic drops, one should grasp the worm through the conjunctiva with artery forceps and then

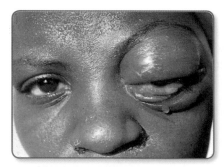

Figure 16.13 Calabar swelling. In spite of the oedema and proptosis the eye and orbit were not painful and the patient was not seriously ill.

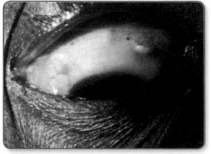

Figure 16.14 After a few days the Calabar swelling subsided and fragments of a dead worm were visible under the conjunctiva.

make a small incision in the conjunctiva through which the worm can be removed with forceps.

Toxoplasmosis

Toxoplasmosis is systemic infection by the protozoan parasite, *Toxoplasmosis gondii*. It can cause a wide range of systemic and ocular symptoms and signs. Its most damaging effects occur in congenital infection and when it infects the retina and chorioid (see Chapter 13).

Toxocara

Toxocara canis is a nematode worm, which lives in the intestine of the dog. A similar species lives in the cat and is known as *Toxocara cati*. Most puppies and kittens are heavily infested with Toxocara and their faeces will contain toxocara eggs. If humans ingest these eggs they can hatch to produce larvae that can migrate through the human tissues. These larvae however will not develop into adult worms. The larvae may migrate throughout the body particularly in the liver and lungs causing general malaise, hepatomegaly, pulmonary symptoms, lymphadenopathy and eosinophilia. This collection of symptoms and signs is called *visceral larva migrans* and occurs more frequently in young children who probably have quite large numbers of larvae and the disease. Occasionally, a single larva may penetrate the eye. Although this may occur in association with *visceral larva migrans*, usually there are no associated systemic symptoms. Therefore, it is likely that there are just a few larvae in the body one of which happens to enter the eye. Once inside the eye the larva may cause very varying degrees of damage. The most common change is an inflammatory mass in the retina or choroid with associated anterior or posterior uveitis (**Figure 16.15**) which then settles down to leave a scar (**Figure 16.16**). A clinical diagnosis can

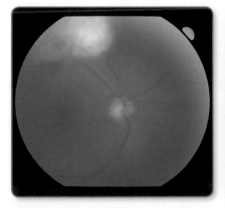

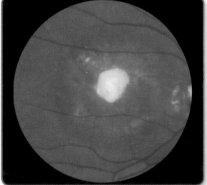

Figure 16.15 Toxocara of the retina. The view is very hazy because of vitreous inflammation.

Figure 16.16 Toxocara scar. A raised white scar at the macula with some surrounding disturbance of the retinal pigment epithelium. Toxocara lesions are often larger than this.

be made, although this can only be confirmed by histological examination. Sometimes eyes have been enucleated with a suspected diagnosis of an intraocular tumour, but then histological examination has demonstrated the toxocara worm. Most of the reported cases of toxocara have come from rich countries, but it is likely that it is a more common but under-diagnsosed disease in poor countries.

Treatment

The larvae are thought to be sensitive to the anti-helminthic drugs albendazole, mebendazole, thiabendazole and possibly diethylcarbamazine. These are used for the treatment of *visceral larva migrans*, but are unlikely to have much benefit for ocular toxocara of the eye when a solitary larva has entered the eye. Topical or systemic steroid treatment may be helpful in limiting the inflammatory changes inside the eye.

Other parasitic infections

Thelazia

These are small nematode worms, which can live in the conjunctival sac and are probably spread directly from person to person by flies. In the conjunctiva they provoke quite severe irritation and can occasionally cause corneal scarring. The only treatment is mechanical removal.

Gnathostomiasis and angiostrongyliasis

Gnathostoma is a parasite, which lives in the intestinal wall of various animals, particularly cats and dogs. It has a very complicated life cycle. The larvae hatch from eggs and invade a small water living crustacean called *cyclops*. It then enters a further intermediate host such as a fish or frog, which eat *cyclops*. Man can become infected by eating uncooked or poorly cooked meat of various animals such as fish, frogs, snakes, etc. The larvae migrate through the tissues causing an acute inflammatory reaction in the tissues. They may pass through the eyelid or orbit causing inflammatory swelling and oedema or they may enter the eye to cause endophthalmitis.

Angiostrongylus is a rather similar parasite to *Gnathostoma* of which the main host is the rat and the secondary hosts are snails. Humans can become infected by eating contaminated or raw snails and the migrating larvae cause similar but less severe symptoms to *Gnathosthoma*. Both *Gnathostoma* and *Angiostrongylus* are most common in south East Asia.

The treatment of both parasites is uncertain but antihelminthic drugs, in particular mebendazole, have been recommended.

Trichinosis

Trichinosis is caused by the larvae of *Trichinella spiralis*. The disease is caught by eating infected meat, particularly pork, and the larvae mature in the stomach and intestine to form the adult worms. The adult worms lay eggs, which hatch and migrate through the intestinal wall and become disseminated throughout the body, particularly in the muscles. During the phase of migration through the muscles patients feel unwell with myalgia, fever and marked eosinophilia and may specifically develop eyelid oedema and conjunctivitis. Retinal haemorrhages and optical neuritis have also been described. Mebendazole is probably effective in killing the migrating larvae, and topical and systemic steroids may relieve the local symptoms.

Cysticercosis

Cysticercosis is caused by eating infected, poorly cooked pork, which contains the larvae of the tapeworm, *Taenia solium*. The adult tapeworm then lives and breeds in the human intestine. The pig is the secondary host and the immature larvae develop into small cysts in the body tissues of the pig. However, it is possible for man to become a secondary host rather than a primary host, either by eating food contaminated with human faeces, or by the patients contaminating themselves with their own faeces or possibly through intestinal regurgitation. The larvae develop in the human body into small cysts that contain a protoscolex, which is the earlier stage in development of the head of the tapeworm. These cysts may remain dormant for some years before they die. The symptoms of cysticercosis depend upon where the cysts are found. For example in the brain, a variety of neurological symptoms can occur, while in the eye and surrounding tissues, the intra-ocular cysts may be seen or if they rupture a vigorous inflammatory reaction may occur.

The cysticercosis worms are treated with albendazole or praziquantel and topical or oral steroids may be required if there is significant inflammation. Surgical removal of the cyst may be indicated sometimes if it is seen before a severe inflammatory reaction has developed.

Hydatid disease

Hydatid disease is caused by cysts of the dog tapeworm, *Echinococcus*. The tapeworm lives in the intestine of the dog, and sheep or other animals are the usual secondary hosts. However, man may become the secondary host by eating food contaminated with infected dog faeces. Usually, only one egg develops inside the body to form quite a large cyst, which becomes surrounded by a fibrous capsule. Hydatid cysts may occur anywhere in the body. The most common site is the liver and occasionally they occur in the orbit. They present as a space-occupying orbital mass and the treatment is surgical removal. It is important not to rupture the cyst but to remove it whole as it contains numerous living daughter cysts, which will cause a severe tissue reaction if exposed. Again albendazole or praziquantel are the treatments of choice and need to be given both pre and post-operatively in case a cyst is ruptured. Hydatid disease is found in many parts of the world, especially northern Kenya, the Middle East and central Asia.

Sparganosis

This is an intestinal worm that lives mainly in dogs and cats and is most common in China and Southeast Asia. The life cycle of the worm is complex. The eggs from contaminated faeces are ingested by the same water-borne crustacean as in gnathostoma, *cyclops*, where they develop further. This crustacean is then eaten by fish, frogs or ducks where the larva develops further in the tissues. This form is known as a second stage larva. If a cat or a dog eats this it develops into an intestinal worm but if it is eaten by humans the larva again enters the tissues to form another cyst or an immature worm. These may cause swellings to form in the conjunctiva, eyelids or orbit. It is thought that this may occur particularly in some areas of Southeast Asia, where frog flesh is applied to the eye as a form of traditional treatment.

Myiasis

Myiasis is the infection of humans by the larval maggots of flies. Various different species of fly can cause myiasis. In some cases, they lay their eggs only on diseased, necrotic tissue, but in other cases they lay their eggs in normal healthy tissues. Myiasis is predominantly seen in sick or debilitated patients, especially the very old or very young, and particularly in people who live close to farm animals. It can present as conjunctival, orbital or intraocular myiasis.

Conjunctival myiasis

The maggots live in the conjunctival sac. They may also be found in the lymph nodes or the nasal sinuses or nasal passages and they may invade the eyelid. The treatment is to manually remove the maggots under local anaesthesia.

Orbital myiasis

The maggots are buried more deeply into the orbital tissue causing extensive tissue destruction and secondary infection. For example, the *Tumbu* fly lays a solitary egg that becomes a maggot, which lives in the subcutaneous tissues. It requires oxygen from the air. Therefore, they can be treated by covering the site with petroleum jelly, forcing the maggot to 'come out for air' when it can be grasped and removed.

Intraocular myiasis

The eye is usually only invaded by one solitary larva. In some cases this may be asymptomatic, and the larva may die without causing serious intraocular damage. However, in other cases, there may be a severe inflammatory reaction inside the eye causing extensive damage. If this occurs, the larva should be removed if at all possible. It is also possible to attempt to destroy the larva with laser photocoagulation.

Other ocular parasitic infections

Apart from the parasites described above, there are numerous other rare causes of ocular parasitic disease. The majority of these infections are transmitted either by insect bites or by eating contaminated or poorly cooked food. If the parasite is inside the eye, the symptoms are usually of transient disturbance in the vision or intraocular inflammation. If the parasite is outside the eye, it usually presents with inflammation of the lid, orbit or conjunctiva. The inflammation is often quite transient and the patient may sometimes be aware of the movement of the parasite through the tissues. In many cases there will be an increase in the eosinophil count and often there is evidence of parasitic infection elsewhere in the body. One surprising feature of many parasitic infections is the length of time for which the parasites may survive. It is not uncommon for people to develop symptoms many years after leaving the area where the infection was acquired. Local treatment may involve attempts to remove the parasite or suppressing the inflammatory reaction with steroids, and in many cases a suitable antiparasitic drug can be given. In communities where parasitic infections are common it may be possible by health education to find ways of preventing the spread of the infection by cooking food, disposal of faeces or preventing insect bites.

Diffuse unilateral subacute neuroretitinis (DUSN)

DUSN is the ophthalmic manifestation of infection by a nematode (**Figure 16.17**). The specific nematode that causes is not clear, or it may be caused by several different worms. It is usually a unilateral disease characterised by visual loss, vitreous inflammation and retinitis, which is seen as peri-papillary inflammation and exudate and transient and recurrent patches of grey-white outer retinal lesions. Occasionally, the nematode can be seen on fundus examination.

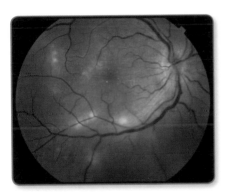

Figure 16.17 Diffuse unilateral subacute neuroretinitis. Note the clusters of white outer retinal lesions. Each of these lesions will fade and new ones will erupt as the nematode moves around under the retina.

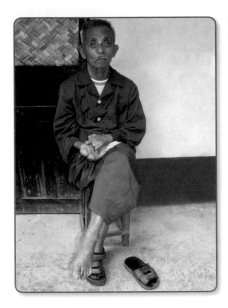

Leprosy is much less common than 20 years ago, but still causes terrible suffering.

Leprosy is a chronic infectious disease caused by the bacteria *Mycobacterium leprae*. It can cause terrible cosmetic and physical disability and frequently causes eye disease. To this day the word 'leper' is sadly used to describe people who are excluded from society. The disease was known and feared in ancient times, but the cause remained unknown until 1873, when Hansen, a Norwegian doctor, identified the bacterium that causes the disease. For this reason, leprosy is sometimes called 'Hansen's disease'.

Leprosy is a communicable disease, which is passed from person to person by inhaled droplets. In most cases there is close contact, usually in childhood, with an active 'open' case. These open cases probably excrete large number of organisms, especially in their nasal discharges. Sneezing is probably a very effective way of spreading the organisms from an active carrier. However, it is not clearly understood why some people become infected and others do not. Leprosy disappeared spontaneously in richer countries, before any antibacterial treatments became available. This was probably because improved living standards and hygiene restricted its spread and better health and nutrition improved the immune response that can clear the disease. In those countries where it still exists, it seems to be more prevalent among the poor. The peak age of onset of symptoms is in young adults (20–30 years old), although these patients actually became infected many years previously. Clinically apparent leprosy is very rare in children.

Mycobacterium leprae survives best at temperatures below the normal body temperature. Therefore, the bacteria are found mostly in the cooler surface tissues. After they have entered the body, the organisms multiply and spread in the superficial nerves (especially the Schwann cells), the skin and superficial organs such as the testes, nose, mouth and eye. In the eye, the organism is only found in the anterior parts: the iris, cornea, sclera and eyelids.

The different clinical types of leprosy

Leprosy bacilli multiply very slowly. It takes about 2 weeks for leprosy bacilli to double their number when growing in an ideal situation (by contrast most bacteria will double their number every 20 minutes). Accordingly, the incubation period before symptoms appear is about 2–7 years. When symptoms do eventually occur, the clinical appearance varies greatly, according to the cell-mediated immunity (CMI) of the patient towards the organism (**Figure 17.1**). There are two main subtypes of leprosy:

Multibacillary (MB) leprosy

In patients whose CMI is low, the organisms spread and multiply throughout the tissues. They are taken up by the macrophages but not killed by them. Histological examination of infected tissue shows many infiltrating macrophages, which are filled with living, active leprosy bacilli. This is the more severe form of the disease and clinically is characterised by having multiple (more than five) skin lesions, nodules, plaques or areas of thickened skin. Also there may be involvement of the nasal mucosa, which causes nasal congestion and bleeding. It used to be called lepromatous leprosy.

Paucibacillary (PB) leprosy

At the other extreme, where the CMI is high, there is a localised inflammatory reaction in the infected tissues, with thickening of the superficial nerves and depigmentation of the skin. A histological examination will reveal very few or

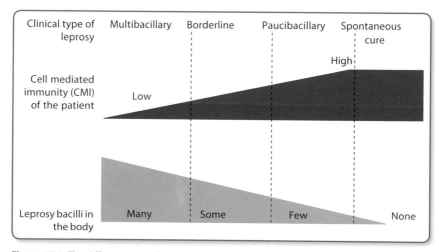

Figure 17.1 The different types of leprosy and the immune reactions of a patient.

even no organisms. This is a milder form of the disease and clinically it is defined by having few (up to five) hypopigmented, anaesthetic skin lesions. It used to be called tuberculoid leprosy.

Other clinical scenarios

In people whose resistance is very high, the disease may even heal itself spontaneously without producing any symptoms or signs at all. This may explain why so many people in endemic areas are exposed to the disease but do not develop leprosy and why the disease has disappeared in richer areas of the world.

Many patients are somewhere between these two extremes of MB and PB leprosy, and may show varying degrees of resistance to the organism. These are called 'borderline cases'. Leprosy specialists divide these borderline cases into several different subgroups. There is 'borderline lepromatous' leprosy (BL), which is closer to the MB end of the spectrum, and 'borderline tuberculoid' (BT) which is closer to the PB end of the spectrum. There is also 'borderline borderline' (BB), which is in the middle.

Leprosy reactions: reversal, downgrading and erythema nodosum leprosum

The reactional state is a common and important stage of leprosy when the symptoms become worse, often quite suddenly. There are several different subtypes but they are usually caused by changes in the CMI, and they may occur spontaneously or during treatment. If the CMI improves, the disease is pushed towards the PB end of the spectrum, i.e. the immune system is reacting more effectively to the leprosy bacteria. This is called a *reversal reaction*. It can provoke a facial palsy. If the CMI is reduced the disease is pushed towards the MB end of the spectrum. This is called downgrading. The final type of reaction is called *erythema nodosum leprosum (ENL)*. This only occurs in MB cases. There is thought to be an immune reaction to circulating protein from the leprosy bacilli, causing painful skin nodules, fever, joint pains and acute anterior uveitis. It is very important to recognise these reactions and treat the clinical complications of them because it is during these periods that most of the permanent damage occurs. In the eye, most of the blinding complications occur during a reversal or an ENL reaction.

Treatment for leprosy

The first effective chemotherapy for leprosy was Dapsone, which became available in 1940. Dapsone is still used in leprosy treatment, but it is now part of multiple drug therapy (MDT) usually with the antituberculous drug rifampicin and in MB cases with clofazimine as well (**Table 17.1**). MDT minimises the risk of drug resistance and shortens the time for which treatment is required. If the full course is taken it will cure 98% of patients. However, the treatments can have side effects. Clofazimine causes a reddish discolouration of the skin, conjunctiva and urine, although this returns to normal at the end of treatment. For patients who cannot tolerate any of these drugs or

Table 17.1 Leprosy multiple drug therapy (MDT) regimen		
	Adult	Child (10–14 years)
PB infection		
Once monthly (day 1)	Rifampicin 600 mg Dapsone 100 mg	Rifampicin 600 mg Dapsone 50 mg
Once daily (days 2–28)	Dapsone 100 mg/day	Dapsone 50 mg/day
Total treatment	24 weeks (6 cycles)	24 weeks (6 cycles)
MB infection		
Once monthly (day 1)	Rifampicin 600 mg Dapsone 100 mg Clofazimine 300 mg	Rifampicin 600 mg Dapsone 100 mg Clofazimine 150 mg
Once daily (days 2–28)	Dapsone 100 mg Clofazimine 50 mg	Dapsone 50 mg/day Clofazimine 50 mg alternate days
Total treatment	48 weeks (12 cycles)	48 weeks (12 cycles)

have side effects, ofloxacin 400 mg daily for 6 months, minocycline 100 mg daily for 6 months, or clarithromycin 500 mg daily for 6 months are second line drugs which may be used.

Ideally the patient should come every 4 weeks for treatment. On the first day, they take their medication under direct supervision and are then given their drugs for the next 4 weeks. This treatment method is known as Directly Observed Treatment Schedule (DOTS). Regular supervision, ideally by someone with experience in the management of leprosy, is important to ensure that the drugs are being taken correctly, to check the progress of the disease and to look for side effects, complications and reactions.

The patient's relatives and contacts should also be examined carefully as they may be infected and this also helps to prevent spread of the disease. Modern treatment aims to keep the patients in the community and not treat them in institutions or hospitals unless necessary. Remember that even after 'successful' treatment, patients can have peripheral neuropathy and immune-mediated complications for many years after. Ocular leprosy requires other medical and surgical treatments (see below).

Leprosy reactions

Leprosy reactions need urgent additional treatment to prevent permanent complications. A course of systemic steroids such as prednisolone (40 mg initially decreasing by 10 mg every 2 weeks, until 10 mg when it is decreased to 5 mg for 2 weeks before stopping) is used to reduce the inflammatory response, and analgesia (e.g. aspirin and paracetamol) should be given to reduce pain and fever.

Leprosy control

The basis of modern leprosy control in the community is early diagnosis and treatment as an outpatient. WHO initiatives have allowed MDT for leprosy to be available free of charge at health centres throughout endemic countries. This, and the huge leprosy initiatives led by health ministries, charities and NGOs as well as improvements in living conditions in some endemic countries has had two profound effects:

1. Many less patients are developing severe deformities and mutilation from long-standing leprosy.
2. The early treatment of open active cases has greatly reduced the spread of the disease in the community.

The control of leprosy in the past few years has been one of the great success stories of community health and modern medical treatment. The prevalence of leprosy has fallen by about 90% in recent decades. Between 1985 and 2005, over 14 million people were treated for leprosy. Very few relapses were reported. Never the less new cases continue to occur and incidence has increased in some countries, particularly those with recent or active civil wars such as Sudan, Somalia and Liberia. Also, some countries are probably not reporting as many as half of their active cases. Currently there are probably about half a million people with leprosy (around 200,000 registered with leprosy + 230,000 new cases per year, + unknown number of non-registered cases). They mainly live in Africa, Asia and South America, with the highest prevalence being in central and west Africa. However, these figures do not include the huge number of patients who have been 'cured' but still have severe disability from the disease; a many patients with chronic leprosy who have received treatment late are blind and have other serious disabilities.

Periodically there is excitement about the possibility of a leprosy vaccine. Although this has become a step closer since the organism has been successfully grown in an animal model (the armadillo), there is as yet no available leprosy vaccine. However, the BCG vaccine that is given for tuberculosis, does give some protection for leprosy.

Interestingly, unlike most other infectious diseases of poverty, the HIV epidemic does not seem to be having an effect on either the number or the severity of cases. This is possibly because the leprosy bacterium multiplies too slowly to be greatly affected by the immunocompromise caused by HIV.

Eye disease in leprosy

Leprosy can produce many changes in the eye. As it favours the surface parts of the body these changes are usually confined to the face and the eyelids, cornea, conjunctiva, anterior chamber and iris of the eye. *The two most important changes in the eye from leprosy reactions are **facial palsy** and **acute anterior uveitis.***

Leprosy does not always involve the eye. Reports of eye involvement range from 6–90% of leprosy patients. There are several reasons for this wide variation:

*   The risk of eye complications has decreased greatly in recent years, because of earlier diagnosis and more effective treatment of leprosy. Eye disease is much more likely in patients who have had leprosy for a long time. The complication rate in chronic patients in a leprosy

settlement is therefore much higher than in a group of less advanced cases who are receiving treatment as outpatients.

- The clinical pattern of leprosy may differ from area to area. PB leprosy seems to be more common in Africa and MB leprosy more common in east Asia and south America.
- Many of the early eye changes are not obvious to the naked eye. Some cases of ocular leprosy can only be diagnosed by a careful examination with a slit lamp. Therefore, some studies probably underestimate the prevalence of eye disease.

Awareness of the signs of leprosy in the eye is particularly important in two situations:

1. An eye problem may be the first sign in a patient with undiagnosed leprosy.
2. Patients with known leprosy, especially those who have had it for a long time often develop eye complications requiring assessment and treatment.

Early diagnosis is essential for leprosy. The health practitioner working in endemic areas must consider the diagnosis of leprosy in patients with particular signs and symptoms.

Unfortunately, the early changes are as difficult to detect in the eye as in the rest of the body. The advanced changes are much more obvious, but by this time the damage is irreversible. One study in the US found that patients who first went to the doctor with eye symptoms waited for an average of 6 years before leprosy was correctly diagnosed. It is particularly important to consider the diagnosis of leprosy in patients with facial palsy or with acute anterior uveitis. Always remember that any unusual eyelid or corneal lesion may be caused by leprosy. The diagnosis of leprosy can be particularly difficult if other diseases affecting the skin are also present such as onchocerciasis, chronic fungal infection or eczema.

Giving a patient a diagnosis of leprosy is likely to cause great anxiety and fear, because of the social stigma attached to the disease, the potential complications of the disease and because they will have to take quite toxic treatment for many months. Therefore, the diagnosis must be conveyed very sensitively and if there is any uncertainty, it is wise to seek a second opinion and further investigations before suggesting a diagnosis of leprosy.

The eyelid and skin around the eye

Loss of eyebrows (madarosis) and eyelashes

Madarosis is one of the most common eye changes in MB leprosy. It is usually symmetrical and it is more common in the lateral part of the eyebrows (**Figure 17.5**). Loss of the eyelashes is slightly less common (**Figure 17.8**).

Skin changes

In MB leprosy, the facial skin may be diffusely thickened and inflamed or have nodules (**Figure 17.2**). These changes are often found on the eyelids and/or the eyebrows. After treatment, baggy folds of skin may persist on the

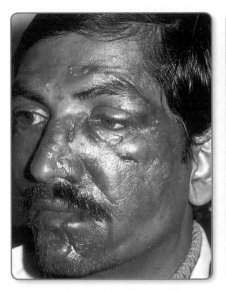

Figure 17.2 Thickened and inflamed facial skin in MB leprosy.

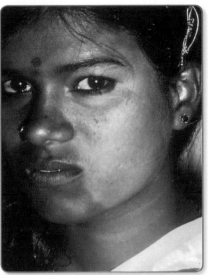

Figure 17.3 Depigmented patch on the face of a patient with leprosy.

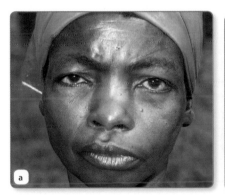

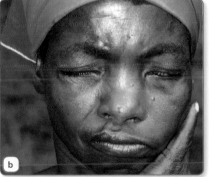

Figure 17.4 A patient with partial facial palsy from leprosy. (a) In resting position the face appears fairly normal, although the left side is slightly lower than the right causing slight asymmetry. (b) In attempted eye closure, the left-sided weakness of the face becomes obvious and the face is drawn towards the right side. The right eyelid just closes but the left eyelids do not close properly. There is some loss of the outer eyebrow hair (madarosis).

lids, and there may be loss of skin elasticity and some atrophy of the subcutaneous tissues. An anaesthetic or depigmented patch of skin on the face is extremely suspicious sign of leprosy (**Figure 17.3**).

Facial nerve palsy

This is by far the most important change in the eyelid (Figures 17.4, 17.5 and 17.7). The facial nerve is a motor nerve supplying most of the facial muscles including the orbicularis oculi, which closes the eyelids. The branches of the facial nerve run quite superficially under the skin, where they are very susceptible to lepromatous damage. It is common for the facial nerve and other superficial nerves to thicken making it possible to feel them just under the surface of the skin. Patients with PB or borderline leprosy are at particular risk as inflammatory changes during a reversal reaction may cause a facial palsy. We will now discuss the important signs of a facial nerve palsy:

Clinical appearance

If a facial palsy is unilateral, the face drops on one side and the face is pulled over to the undamaged side. This is usually obvious. However, facial palsy in leprosy is often bilateral and incomplete. The clinical changes are much less obvious because the muscles are weakened but not completely paralysed and the face remains symmetrical because both sides are affected. However, the face does lose much of its expression and character because of the general weakness of the facial muscles. This is known as a 'leprous stare' (**Figure 17.6**). Very often this is not recognised and the health worker just thinks the patient is a bit slow or non-responsive.

Lagophthalmos and corneal exposure

The most important defect in a facial palsy is the inability to close the eyelids (lagophthalmos). This may be obvious in a complete palsy, but in an incomplete palsy, two simple tests will demonstrate the weakness:

- Ask the patient to close the eye gently as in sleep. The eyelids may not come together properly.
- Ask the patient to close the eyes tightly. The health practitioner can then try to force open the eyelids. In a patient with partial facial nerve palsy they can usually be opened relatively easily, but in an unaffected patient, it is very difficult to prise them apart. Alternatively, one can hold the patient's eyes open and ask them to close the eyes against this resistance. One can usually feel the weakness of the lids.

When a patient with a facial palsy attempts to close his eyes, the eyeball usually turns upwards spontaneously (**Figure 17.7**). In this way, the cornea is protected under the upper eyelid. This is probably a protective reflex to prevent corneal damage during sleep. It is called the 'Bell's phenomenon'. However, in some people the lower cornea often still remains exposed and

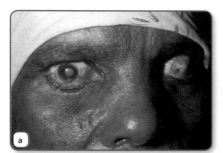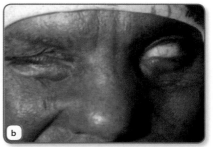

Figure 17.5 Advanced facial palsy and corneal scarring from leprosy. (a) In resting position, corneal exposure has caused severe corneal scarring. Note the mature cataract in the right eye. Cataracts are more common in leprosy. (b) On attempting to close the eyes, the left eye does not close at all. The right eye almost closes, although the cornea is still likely to scar from exposure. There is also a lower lid ectropion as a complication of the facial palsy.

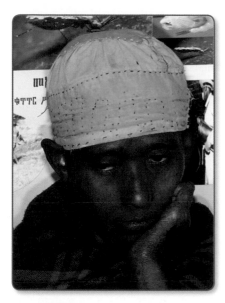

Figure 17.6 Leprous stare. The patient has severely damaged fingers and hands.

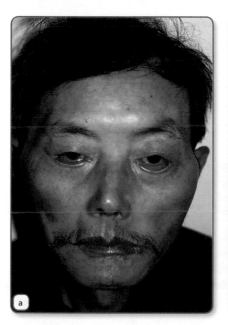
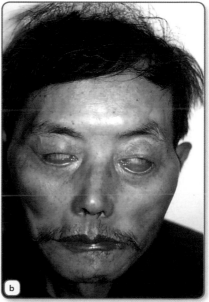

Figure 17.7 Bell's phenomen and lagophthalmos. (a) This patient's severe bilateral facial nerve palsy is not particularly obvious in the resting position because it is symmetrical. However, note that he does have marked lower lid ectropion from the facial weakness and the characteristic lack of facial expression of patients with leprosy. (b) When the patient attempts to close his eyes, the severe facial palsy and lagophthalmos are obvious, but note that the eyes have rolled upwards which does give some protection to the corneas. This is called a positive Bell's phenomenon.

other people do not have a good Bell's phenomenon and more of the cornea stays exposed. Exposed cornea is at risk of drying and ulceration. Therefore, patients with facial palsy often develop corneal ulceration and scarring, which is typically in the lower part of the cornea.

Ectropion

In a complete facial palsy, the lower eyelid will sag, and may eventually become floppy and everted (ectropion) (**Figure 17.7**). The red conjunctiva of the inner surface of the lid can sometimes seen facing outwards.

Watering eye (epiphora)

The lower eyelid loses its tone and the lower punctum draining the tears does not rest against the eyeball because of ectropion (see above). The pumping action of the orbicularis oculi muscle that helps to squeeze the tears to the punctum and down the drainage channels into the nose is lost. Furthermore, leprosy can cause damage inside the nose, which may obstruct the drainage outflow from the nasolacrimal duct.

Reduced blinking and dry eye

A facial palsy will prevent blinking and this prevents the precorneal tear film from forming. The exposed part of the cornea does not get coated with tears and becomes dry. This worsens the effect of lagophthalmos making the cornea even more susceptible to damage. The eye may also be dry because occasionally leprosy involves the lacrimal glands.

Upper lid entropion

Sometimes patients with facial palsy may develop entropion of the upper eyelid. This may be from loss of tone of the orbicularis muscle causing the upper lid skin to become lax and the lashes to hang down against the cornea. If the eyelashes are rubbing against the cornea, serious damage can occur because the eye has a poor protective tear film and the protective corneal sensation is often absent in leprosy.

The cornea

Leprosy can affect the cornea in two different ways. Firstly, there can be primary involvement from infection with leprosy bacilli and a resultant inflammatory reaction. Secondly, corneal damage occurs from exposure and loss of sensation caused by the nerve palsies (see above).

Primary changes

The *primary changes* of leprosy bacilli invading the cornea are often hard to see and may be only temporary. These changes are:

- Beading and thickening of the corneal nerves is an early and specific sign of leprosy, which is only visible with the magnification of a slit lamp.
- Punctate keratitis is a localised inflammatory reaction to bacillae in the superficial layers of the cornea.
- Interstitial keratitis (or stromal keratitis) is a more extensive inflammatory reaction to leprosy organisms in the corneal stroma (**Figure 17.8**). It may subside to leave a diffuse corneal scar or pannus (**Figure 17.9**).

Secondary changes

The *secondary changes* come from corneal ulceration and scarring (**Figures 17.2** and **17.4**). These secondary changes are a very important cause of visual loss in leprosy. They occur because the protective corneal reflexes are damaged or destroyed by disease of the following nerves:

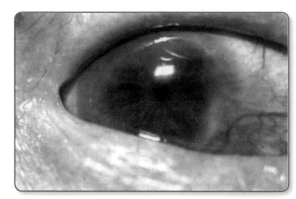

Figure 17.8 Interstitial keratitis: white appearance of the margin of the margin of the cornea. Note also the inflamed episcleral blood vessels, constriction of the pupil from chronic anterior uveitis and the loss of the eyelashes.

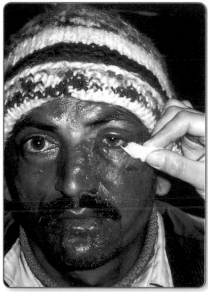

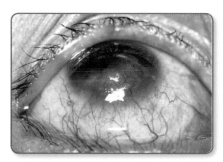

Figure 17.9 Corneal scarring caused by exposure from facial nerve palsy in leprosy.

Figure 17.10 The corneal sensation being tested with cotton wool.

- The fifth cranial nerve (trigeminal nerve) supplies the sensation of the cornea. Therefore, damage causes corneal anaesthesia. Every leprosy patient should have the corneal sensation tested by touching the cornea with a fine wisp of cotton wool (**Figure 17.10**). This is uncomfortable and causes immediate blinking in the normal eye, but is not felt or reacted to in a desensitised eye. The loss of corneal sensation destroys the sensory part of the protective blink reflex that is essential for protecting the eye and clearing debris.
- Damage to the seventh cranial nerve (facial nerve) causes facial palsy (see above). Damage destroys the motor part of the blink reflex, which prevents blinking and eyelid closure.

If there is either corneal anaesthesia or a facial palsy, secondary corneal damage is common. If both are present, then secondary corneal damage is inevitable. The damage may be increased by eye rubbing. Often patients have anaesthetic rough hands as well as anaesthetic corneas and rubbing the eyes may cause corneal ulcers. These provoke irritation in the eye and further rubbing. Keratitis and corneal ulceration will progress to corneal scars or total destruction of the eye.

Iris and anterior chamber

Anterior uveitis is a common and damaging ocular complication, especially of MB leprosy. It tends to present in two different ways: either as a chronic gradual and insidious inflammation, or as an acute sudden and severe inflammation.

Chronic anterior uveitis

The first sign of chronic anterior uveitis is usually that the iris dilator muscle atrophies and becomes too weak to oppose the action of the sphincter muscle. The pupil therefore becomes progressively more constricted (**Figure 17.11**). Whitish lepromatous nodules ('iris pearls') may appear on the iris, which are probably diagnostic of leprosy, but they are a rare sign. There may also be a chronic granulomatous anterior uveitis with 'mutton fat' keratic precipitates on the inner surface of the cornea. All these changes occur slowly and gradually in a quiet, white eye.

Acute anterior uveitis

Acute anterior uveitis may develop in erythema nodosum leprosum (**Figure 17.12**). It results from a reaction between systemic antibodies and antigen, which is released when the microorganisms break up. This reaction often occurs during treatment, but it may occur in untreated cases. There is acute anterior uveitis with a red painful eye, ciliary vasodilatation, and protein exudate and inflammatory cells in the anterior chamber. Any of the complications of acute anterior uveitis may develop, e.g. secondary glaucoma, pupil block and iris bombé, diminished secretions of aqueous fluid, and phthisis bulbi (see Chapter 11). Permanent visual loss is common if it is not treated urgently.

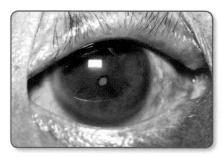

Figure 17.11 A pinpoint pupil caused by iris dilator atrophy. Note also the dense cataract.

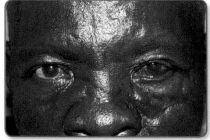

Figure 17.12 Acute anterior uveitis in leprosy. This patient's left eye is acutely inflamed. Note the thickened facial skin caused by the leprosy.

Conjunctiva, sclera and episclera

The leprosy bacilli may invade any part of the anterior segment of the eye and can cause inflammatory or degenerative changes. Therefore conjunctivitis, scleritis and episcleritis are often found. Nodules in the sclera may occur in MB leprosy especially at the limbus (**Figure 17.13**).

The lens

Cataract is quite common in leprosy patients (**Figure. 17.5**), probably as a complication of anterior uveitis. The cataract may have a much greater effect in leprosy patients than other patients because of the pupillary constriction caused by iris atrophy also greatly restricts light entry into the eye. An eye which is blind from cataract, but which has no other serious damage, is of course treatable.

Blindness from leprosy

There is unfortunately a high prevalence of blindness in long-standing leprosy. Surveys of settlements have found 10% or more of the patients to be blind. The most common causes of blindness are cataract with iris atrophy, intraocular inflammation and its complications, and corneal scarring from facial palsy and corneal anaesthesia.

The diagnosis of leprosy is basically clinical. However, if the facilities are available, skin smears and nasal discharges can be examined for the presence of leprosy bacilli. These are more likely to be found in MB cases where large numbers of bacilli are present. It is not usual to find any bacilli in PB cases, but the thickened paralysed nerves and the skin changes make the clinical diagnosis easier.

Treatment of the complications of ocular leprosy

The treatment of leprosy in general has already been discussed above. This section discusses how to treat the complications in the eye.

Uveitis

The treatment of acute anterior uveitis consists of topical steroids and mydriatics. It is described in detail in Chapter 11. Treatment of secondary glaucoma may also be required.

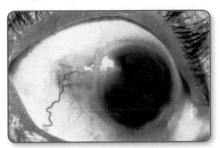

Figure 17.13 A lepromatous nodule at the corneal limbus. The pupil is also distorted from anterior uveitis.

Chronic iritis in a quiet eye, which is often found in MB leprosy, is very difficult to treat. Steroid drops may be advisable but long-term treatment is needed. Because the inflammation is slight and prolonged steroid drops cause many complications, in some cases steroids should be given only intermittently or not at all. The long-term use of mydriatics (e.g. atropine 1% daily) may help to keep the pupil dilated, and some people advise the intermittent use of 2.5% phenylephrine drops to try to stimulate the dilator muscle of the iris.

Cataracts

Cataracts should be treated by lens extraction. However, surgery will only be beneficial if there is clear evidence of light projection (see Chapter 3). Cataract extraction should only be performed in MB leprosy when all the organisms have been killed by drug treatment. This may take some time, and can be confirmed by a skin smear examination. If cataract extraction is performed while MB leprosy is still active, prolonged postoperative uveitis may occur. However, the patient cannot wait forever if they are blind with cataract. Therefore, choosing the best time to operate is difficult. The careful use of pre- and post-operative systemic and topical steroid will reduce the risk of post-operative uveitis. It is almost always safe to use an intra-ocular lens (IOL) in cataract surgery, particularly if the IOL is placed in the capsule. In eyes with lagophthalmos but no corneal ulcers, some people advise performing a tarsorrhaphy soon after (a few days or weeks) the cataract surgery to protect the exposed and possibly anaesthetic cornea during the recovery period. In eyes that do have corneal ulcers it is not advisable to perform cataract surgery until these have been treated.

Damage to the corneal protective reflex

Patients with a facial palsy and/or corneal anaesthesia have a high risk of corneal ulceration or scarring. The eye should be examined regularly, and the patient must be asked to attend a clinic at the first sign of a red or watering eye. The following measures are helpful for preventing corneal damage:

- Frequent applications of a water-based lubricant eyedrop (e.g. methylcellulose) help to preserve the precorneal tear film, which protects the cornea. If the eyelids do not close completely in sleep, any thick ocular lubricant or antibiotic ointment will help to protect the eye at night.
- Close-fitting dark glasses may be helpful. They protect the eye from foreign bodies and stop the patients rubbing their eyes. They may also help preserve the tear film from evaporation.
- Protective goggles at night may be helpful if the cornea is exposed when the patient is asleep.
- Blink exercises. If the patient has an anaesthetic cornea, the desire to blink goes away. Blinking is vital as it spreads the tear film over the cornea and keeps it moist. The patients must be encouraged to blink consciously and regularly, (e.g. advising the patient to deliberately close their eyes very frequently).

- It is best to avoid padding the eye. The eyelid may open under the pad causing the cornea to rub against the pad. Also, padding increases the number of bacteria in the conjunctiva.

If the cornea has ulcerated, immediate treatment is required with intensive antibiotic drops and ointment. Also the eyelids must be held together in order to protect and cover the cornea. They can be closed either with surgical tape or they can be sutured together until the ulcer heals (a temporary tarsorrhaphy).

Facial palsy

If the facial palsy has come on recently, it is probably due to inflammatory changes in the facial nerve from a reactional state. It should be treated urgently with systemic steroids and will probably recover. A permanent and complete facial palsy must be treated surgically and frequently even a temporary or partial palsy requires surgical treatment to protect or treat the cornea.

If corneal anaesthesia is also present, the risk of corneal ulceration increases, and the need for surgical correction of the facial palsy becomes more urgent. Many surgical techniques can be used to reduce the corneal exposure caused by a facial palsy (**Table 17.2**). The simplest and often most effective operation is called a lateral tarsorrhaphy. This sews together and often overlaps the lateral part of the upper and lower lid. It will shorten the palpebral fissure both lengthwise and from top to bottom. If a greater effect is needed in more severe cases, the medial side of the lids can also be sutured (medial tarsorrhaphy or canthoplasty). However, great care must be taken not to damage the lacrimal puncta and canaliculi. Other more complicated procedures that are carried out by more specialised surgeons include:

1. Tightening the lower lid which has become lax and out-turned, by either hitching it tightly up to the lateral orbital rim (lateral tarsal strip) or removing a section of the lower lid (wedge excision).
2. Increasing the weight of the upper lid to assist with closure. Gold and platinum weights have been designed for inserting in the upper lid.
3. Cheek lift. This can be done with sutures or specially designed meshes or even donor tendon tissue and helps to support the lower lid and make the face look more normal.
4. In a few very specialised centres nerve, tendon and muscle transplants (usually temporalis tendon and muscle transplants) are used with some success in recovering partial function.

Table 17.2 Summary of possible treatments for eye protection following facial palsy and corneal anaesthesia	
Medical treatments	**Surgical treatments**
Systemic steroids for acute facial palsy Topical antibiotic ointment Lubricant drops or creams Taping shut the eyelids, particularly when sleeping Dark glasses Regular deliberate blinking	Lateral tarsorrhaphy Medial tarsorrhaphy (also known as medial canthoplasty) Lower lid tightening, e.g. wedge excision (can be combined with tarsorrhaphy.

Madarosis

Madarosis can be treated by performing an eyebrow graft. A free graft of hair skin is used from the nape of the neck. However, this is a skilled technique which requires considerable experience to perform well.

Squint and other disorders of eye movement

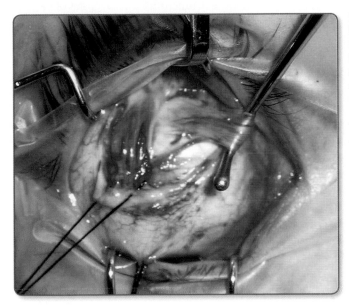

Squint is common. Early detection can help preserve sight in the eye and surgical correction can make a child much happier and more confident in their community and school.

A squint means that the two eyes are looking in different directions, i.e. they are not directed at the same object, either for near vision, far vision or both. It is also known as strabismus, from the Greek word for squinting. Squint is in fact a very complex subject because the control of eye movements and keeping the two eyes pointing in the same direction requires precise communication between the eyes and multiple areas of the brain. Fortunately the management and treatment of most cases of squint can be carried out by following a few basic rules, and without a detailed knowledge of all the factors controlling eye movement. Squints are quite common all over the world, and do not have any special association with poverty or a tropical environment, except of course that poor patients are much less likely to be able to access treatment for their condition and poor patients are much more likely to lose the vision in one or both eyes, which can result in a squint.

The extraocular muscles

The anatomy of the muscles that control the movements of the eye are described in Chapter 2. We will now look at the functions of the muscles (**Figure 18.1**). There are 6 muscles that move the eyeball: 4 recti and 2 obliques.

The recti are superior, inferior, medial and lateral and their main movements are straightforward, i.e. superior moves the eye upwards, inferior downwards, etc. The obliques are slightly more difficult to imagine. The superior oblique is at the top of the eye, but as its origin is anterior and it travels posteriorly to attach behind the equator of the eye it pulls the eye ball downwards. The inferior oblique works in the opposite way; it attaches behind the equator at the bottom of the eye and therefore rotates the eye upwards. Most of the muscles have secondary and even tertiary functions. The strength of each of these actions depends greatly on the position of the eyeball. Their range of movements are shown in **Table 18.1** and **Figure 18.1**.

How does a squint develop?

There are many possible causes of a squint. In every case a cause should be looked for although often an obvious one cannot be found. The two eyes are normally kept looking in the same direction by a complex set of reflexes called the 'binocular reflexes'. Using these reflexes the brain takes the two images from each eye and joins them into one image. The binocular reflexes also ensure that the two eyes are constantly looking in the same direction. If for any reason these reflexes fail then a squint will develop. These reflexes involve both the sensory and the motor parts of the nervous system:

- *The sensory part of the reflex:* this takes the two images produced by the two eyes and joins them together in the brain. The eyes are in slightly

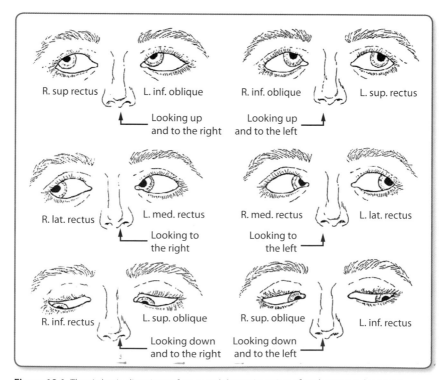

Figure 18.1 The six basic directions of gaze and the main action of each extraocular muscle.

Table 18.1 Actions of the extraocular muscles			
Muscle	Primary function	Secondary function	Tertiary function
Medial rectus	Adduction (inwards)		
Lateral rectus	Abduction (outwards)		
Superior rectus	Elevation	Incyclotorsion	Adduction
Inferior rectus	Depression	Excyclotorsion	Adduction
Superior oblique	Incyclotorsion	Depression	Abduction
Inferior oblique	Excyclotorsion	Elevation	Abduction

In Figure 18.1 the inferior and superior oblique muscles move the eye respectively upwards and downwards when it is adducted (i.e. looking towards the nose), but they have this tertiary action of abduction (i.e. turning the eye away from the nose). This is because of the way they are inserted into the eye. When the eye is adducted towards the nose the oblique muscles have a much stronger action in moving the eye up and down, which is their secondary function. When the eye is abducted away from the nose then the oblique muscles lose their power to turn the eye up and down, and this power is taken over by the superior and inferior rectus muscles.

different positions on either side of the head; therefore if they are looking at the same object, they will have a slightly different image to each other. These two images are superimposed (fused) to build a single three-dimensional or stereoscopic image. However, for this to occur, the eyes need to be directed at the same object and have an approximately similar degree of image clarity and size.

- *The motor part of the reflex:* this makes sure that the two eyes always move together, so that they are always pointing in the same direction.

The binocular reflexes are much weaker in children, and therefore squints usually start in early childhood, or occur after disease or injury cause significant visual loss in one eye and interferes with the binocular reflex. Disorders of the vision will affect the sensory part of the reflex, and disorders of the eye movements will affect the motor part of the reflex. Refractive errors in children are also an important cause of squint, because they can affect both the vision and the binocular reflexes.

The effects of a squint

The effects of a squint are very different in adults and children. If the squint starts in adult life, the two most common effects are *double vision (diplopia)* and *abnormal head posture*. If the squint starts in childhood the most common effect is *amblyopia* in the squinting eye, commonly called a 'lazy eye'. **Amblyopia is a very important subject and we will discuss it in detail below.**

Adult onset squints

When the squint first begins, the patient sees everything double. This is very confusing, and in order to prevent it, the patient may shut or cover one eye. Double vision may be present only when the patient looks in certain directions, especially with a squint caused by the failure of one or more of the extraocular muscles (paralytic squint), which is the most common cause of adult onset squints. The patient then turns their head in order to avoid looking in the direction that produces double vision and the patient gradually develops a persistent abnormal head posture.

Child onset squints

If a squint begins in early childhood, the child's brain appears to be able to quickly learn to ignore the image from one of the eyes in order to prevent double vision. The lack of use of one eye in the first few years of life causes reduced visual development of this eye: 'amblyopia' or a lazy eye (see below). Amblyopia can result in varied loss of vision ranging from just a slight difference between the eyes to count fingers vision in bad cases. It should be noted that amblyopia only affects the visual acuity and not the overall visual field or the pupil reflexes.

Amblyopia

Amblyopia is the failure for the vision in one eye to fully develop during childhood because the eye is not receiving a clear image. The vision in each eye and the binocular vision continue to develop until the age of about 7 years. For both eyes to fully develop their vision, the brain depends on receiving unimpaired and symmetrical images from both eyes. If there is any obstruction or restriction to the image coming from either eye, the vision does not develop normally and the other eye is favoured. Amblyopia can be treated (see below) until the age of 6 or 7 years, but after that it is not reversible.

The three groups of conditions that prevent an eye receiving a clear image and therefore cause amblyopia in children are described in **Box 18.1**.

Box 18.1 The causes of amblyopia

1. *Stimulus deprivation amblyopia:* an obstruction to light rays reaching the retina, e.g. from cataract or corneal opacity will prevent a clear image forming on the retina. Even prolonged application of an eye pad or a ptosis can cause stimulus deprivation amblyopia in an infant. This is why the eyes of young children should only be padded when it is absolutely necessary.

2. *Anisometropic (refractive error) amblyopia:* uncorrected refractive error in one eye (anisometropia) will reduce the clarity of the image in this eye. If there is symmetrical refractive error in both eyes, amblyopia does not develop in either eye. Similarly, astigmatism in one eye causes amblyopia. Unfortunately, even if the refractive error is corrected at a later stage, the visual acuity of the amblyopic eye is still likely to be poor.

3. *Strabismic (squint) amblyopia:* a manifest squint (i.e. a squint that is present all or most of the time) causes the two images to be different in the two eyes. The child's brain will favour one of the images, allowing the other image to be blurred and the eye to become amblyopic.

Diagnosing amblyopia

It can be difficult to test the vision in very young children, making it difficult to diagnose amblyopia. However, there are several methods for estimating the visual acuity in young children which are described in Chapter 3. If a child has a constant squint in one eye and no apparent eye disease (in particular no cataract or refractive error), it can be assumed that the squinting eye is probably amblyopic and treatment for amblyopia should be started.

Problems of having amblyopia

Amblyopia in one eye doesn't seem to cause any serious difficulty for the patient. However, there are problems associated with amblyopia:

- The patient will not have normal stereoscopic vision. This may affect depth perception and prevents people doing some jobs in later life.
- Any injury to the good eye in later life is a disaster. Therefore, amblyopic adults must be particularly careful if they have occupations or hobbies that put the good eye at risk. Interestingly although amblyopia is not treatable after childhood, it has been observed that when an amblyopic adult has a sight impairing injury to their better eye, there is sometimes a small improvement in vision in the amblyopic eye.

Treatment of amblyopia

Before starting any treatment the eye must be fully examined to look for refractive error or eye disease such as cataract that must be corrected. There is no point in patching the good eye, if there is a cataract or other disease in the bad eye! The aim of treatment is to force the brain to accept the image from the poorer eye by occluding the good eye. This is normally done with an eye patch. Alternatively, atropine drops can be used to fog the good eye, if a patch is not tolerated. Occlusion of the good eye allows the poorer eye to develop and not be 'ignored' by the brain. The younger the treatment is started, and the better the compliance of the child, the more effective it will be. If patching is being used, it should be worn for a few hours every day. If atropine is used, drops should be put in twice a week in the better eye. The vision in both eyes must be monitored every few weeks during the patching period, as it is possible for the amblyopia to switch to the better eye, in which case the amount of occlusion should be reduced. Also, if there is no improvement in vision, the eye should be re-examined, in case other pathology has been missed. Although it is difficult to measure the visual acuity of the child, one clue that the vision has improved is that a constant squint will become an alternating squint. If this occurs the patching can be stopped, as the brain is now favouring both eyes equally. Amblyopia treatment is not usually very effective in children over 5 years, and is useless in children over 8 years. Children often resent this treatment because they cannot see well when the good eye is covered, but it is very important for parents and health professionals to be persistent, but gentle with the child. It can be helpful to allow them do activities they enjoy, e.g. playing with games or toys if they wear their patch, as this can help them to forget about the patch.

Classification of squint

Several different systems of classification are used and there is no one system that will include all causes or types of squint. The classification systems are based on either the cause of the squint, the type of squint or whether the squint is permanently or intermittently present. Full classification systems are beyond the scope of this book, and we will therefore give a simple overview of the ways of classifying squints and look in more detail at understanding the fundamental cause of a squint.

The following classifications may be helpful when you see a patient with squint. You may find, e.g. that classifying by cause is helpful in making a diagnosis, while classifying by eye position may be more helpful when planning treatment.

Comitance

Concomitant (or non-paralytic) squints have the same angle of deviation in all positions of gaze. These are more common in children and carry a high-risk of amblyopia. They can also be the presenting symptom of refractive error, and therefore. Incomitant (paralytic) squints result from a paresis or restriction of one or more muscles and therefore cause different degrees of squint in different positions of gazes. In fact the eye position may be completely normal in many positions of gaze, but if a patient tells you that they only have diplopia in certain positions of gaze, you should try to determine if there is a paretic muscle. For example, if the patient has a problem with lateral rectus of the right eye, when they look to the right, they will report double vision and you will see the squint, but when they look to the left they will be fine. Incomitant squints are discussed in more detail below.

Eye position

The two eyes can be exotropic (divergent, **Figure 18.2**), esotropic (convergent, **Figures 18.3** and **18.4**), hypertropic or hypotropic (**Figure 18.5**) to each other. They can also be excyclotorted or incyclotorted. Horizontal squints are much more common than vertical squints. Some squints may have both horizontal and vertical components. We will discuss the major causes of each of these below.

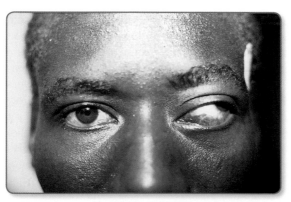

Figure 18.2 A very large left divergent squint. The corneal light reflex is the reflection of a light which is shone into the eyes from the surface of the cornea. In this case it is the reflection of the flash bulb of the camera. The left eye is so divergent that no corneal light reflex can be seen from the left eye. The light is reflected from the white opaque sclera and so does not show.

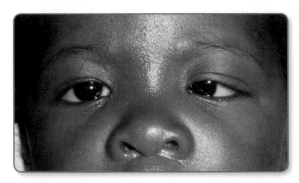

Figure 18.3 Large convergent squint.

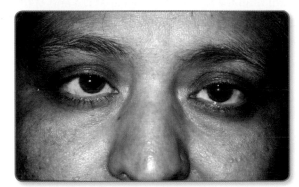

Figure 18.4 A small right convergent squint. In this patient, the corneal light reflex in the left eye is in the centre of the cornea. In the right eye it is displaced laterally demonstrating a right convergent squint.

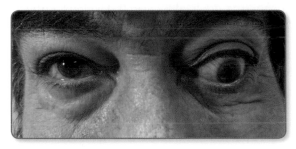

Figure 18.5 Left hypotropia. In this patient, we know that the left eye is the abnormal eye because we have asked the patient to look straight at the camera. If we had asked the patient to look down, it would have been the right eye that was abnormal because it could not look down.

Alternating or non-alternating

In an alternating squint either eye can take up fixation with the other eye becoming the squinting eye. In alternating squints the vision is usually equal in the two eyes. If the squint does not alternate then it is likely that the squinting eye will have worse vision.

Manifest or latent

A manifest squint is present all the time. It is called a 'tropia, e.g. esotropia. A latent squint (phoria, e.g. exophoria) can usually be controlled by the patient and appears when fusion is broken down. This is tested with an alternate cover test, which alternately covers one and then the other eye in order to interrupt fusion. Fusion may also break down in daily life with tiredness, alcohol or simply not concentrating on looking at something. A small latent squint is normal and is almost always asymptomatic, as with both eyes open the brain can still fuse the two images. You can check whether you have a phoria simply by looking at an object and alternately closing each eye and seeing if the object jumps slightly to the left and right.

Constant or intermittent

Some squints are present all the time while others are intermittently present. For example a squint may only appear when the patient looks at a near object. This will usually be a convergent squint. By contrast the squint may only appear when the patient looks in the distance and this will usually be a divergent squint. In some children the squint may appear at the end of the day when they are tired.

Classification by underlying pathology

This is perhaps the most important thing to think about when seeing a squint as it will help you to avoid missing a potentially serious or treatable cause of a squint. We will therefore focus on this classification system and will discuss the major pathological causes of a squint.

The causes of squint

Disorders of vision

If one eye has poor vision, the brain may not be able to join this blurred image with the normal image from the healthy eye. It develops a preference for using the image from the 'good' eye and ignores the poorer image. There is no stimulus for the diseased eye to remain pointing in the same direction as the healthy eye, and in time the diseased eye may drift away from fixation, i.e. it develops a squint. Any disease that affects the vision of one eye (e.g. a corneal scar, cataract, disease of the retina or optic nerve) may ultimately end up causing a squint in that eye (**Figure 18.6**). By contrast, squint is much less likely to develop in patients with bilateral symmetrical disease. For example, patients with bilateral congenital cataract are much less likely to have a squint than those with unilateral cataract.

In early childhood, convergence is very active. Therefore, a young child with defective vision in one eye will usually develop a convergent squint in that eye. However, if in adult life an eye becomes blind, that eye is more likely to develop a divergent squint.

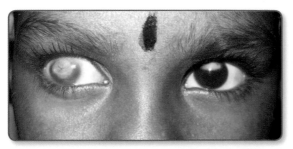

Figure 18.6 Right exotropia secondary to visual loss. This patient has corneal scars in both eyes. The left corneal scar does not interfere with the central vision. However, the right scarring has blinded this eye which has now drifted away from fixation (it has become exotropic).

Central disorders of the eye movements

Many neurological problems cause defective eye movements which often result in a squint. The most common diseases are strokes in older patients and multiple sclerosis in young and middle aged adults. Many of these central disorders and the eye movement abnormalities that they cause are very complex.

Disorders of the extraocular muscles

There are many possible disorders of the extraocular muscles, but the four most common are as follows:

- *Congenital abnormalities.* These will cause squints from early childhood.
- *Fractures of the orbital walls.* The extraocular muscles may become trapped in the fracture or adhere to the bone, causing limitation and restriction of the eye movements.
- *Thyroid eye disease.* This causes inflammation and fibrosis in the muscles, and therefore restricts eye movements.
- *Neurological disorders* affecting the muscle function, such as myasthenia gravis, Guillain Barré syndrome, muscular dystrophy and chronic external ophthalmoplegia. Some of these diseases will affect the whole body causing widespread muscle weakness, while others may only affect the eye muscles.

The cranial nerves

The third (oculomotor), fourth (trochlear) and sixth (abducent) cranial nerve supply specific extraocular muscles, and so damage to these nerves will cause an incomitant squint. The fourth and sixth nerves are more commonly damaged, probably because they have a long intracranial course and are very thin. They also supply only one muscle each. Therefore, damage to either of these nerves will cause a very specific squint. The oculomotor nerve supplies four of the extraocular muscles as well as the iris sphincter muscle and the levator palpebrae superioris muscle of the upper lid. Therefore, any damage usually has a much greater effect on eye movements. The effects and symptoms of the different cranial nerve palsies are shown in **Table 18.2**.

Cranial nerve palsies are the most common cause of acute onset squints in adults, but can also occur in children when they are likely to be a sign of significant or dangerous pathology. There are numerous causes of cranial nerve palsies. When you see a patient with a cranial nerve palsy remember both the most common causes and those that may be a sign of serious or even fatal disease. The most common causes of cranial nerve palsies are:

- Vascular occlusion. This is more common in patients with the following risk factors:
  - Older age
  - Hypertension
  - Diabetes
  - Known atherosclerotic disease elsewhere, e.g. angina, previous stroke
  - Smoking

Table 18.2 Squints caused by cranial nerve palsies				
Nerve	Eye muscle affected	Defect in movement	Main symptom	Emergency causes
Oculomotor (3rd)	• Superior, medial and inferior recti • Inferior oblique • Levator palpebrae superioris of the upper lid • Sphincter pupillae	• All movements paralysed except abduction and depression. The eye is therefore 'down and out' • Ptosis • Mydriasis (dilated pupil)	• Diplopia, in all positions of gaze • Ptosis • Dilated pupil	• Expanding cerebral aneurysm. This can be rapidly fatal and is a surgical emergency
Trochlear (4th)	Superior oblique	Limitation of depression when the eye is adducted. The eye is seen to be hypertropic in adduction	Vertical diplopia on downgaze (e.g. reading)	
Abducent (6th)	Lateral rectus	Limitation of abduction	Horizontal diplopia on looking to affected side	Increased intracranial pressure, meningitis and skull fracture which all can compress this long nerve as it passes over the sphenoid bone

- Head injuries
- Space-occupying lesions (mainly tumours) inside the skull
- Meningitis

Refractive errors

There are two reasons for refractive errors to cause squints. Firstly, a refractive error in one eye only will obviously blur the vision in that eye, and therefore may result in a sensory deprivation squint (see above).

Secondly, long sight (hypermetropia) in both eyes is also a common cause of childhood squints. The best way of understanding this is to think about what happens when a normal sighted person looks at a near object. Two things happen at the same time:

1. Each eye must focus on the near object. The lens within the eye changes shape to enable this. This is called accommodation.
2. The two eyes must turn inwards so that they are both looking at the object. This is called convergence.

These two actions, accommodation and convergence, are linked together in the brain, to form the 'near reflex'.

Now, if we consider a long-sighted or hypermetropic child. They have a smaller than average sized eye, causing images to focus behind the retina. They can compensate for this by accommodating, i.e. changing the shape of their lens in order to make images come into focus on the retina. However, accommodation is linked to convergence in the near reflex and therefore the eyes will also converge, i.e. squint.

Other causes of squint

Squints sometimes develop in children when there is no obvious defect or refractive error in the eye. Sometimes they first appear when the child is ill. There is often a family history of a similar squint. Many squints are only seen, or are worse when the patient is tired, when their ability to maintain binocular vision is reduced.

Clinical examination and assessment of squints

The corneal light reflex test

This is the quickest and simplest test for a squint. It is easy to do and easy to interpret and only requires a torch. The cornea is transparent, but its front surface reflects enough light to act as a convex mirror. If the patient looks at a bright light, such as a torch or an ophthalmoscope, a reflection of that light can be seen from the corneal surface. If the two eyes are straight, then the two corneal light reflexes are central and symmetrical (**Figure 18.7a**). If one eye is not straight, then the reflex deviates from the centre of that cornea (**Figure 18.7b**). The deviation can be approximately measured with this test; the cornea has a radius of approximately 5.5 mm and each millimetre of displacement of the reflection is equivalent to approximately 7° or 15 prism dioptres of deviation. For example if the light reflection is at the corneal limbus, the deviation is 5.5 mm, i.e. 38.5° (5.5 × 7). The Krimsky test is an extension of the corneal light reflex test in which prisms are used to bring the displaced image to the centre of the eye. The strength of prism required determines the amount of deviation.

The cover-uncover-alternate cover test

The cover test is a quick way of determining if there is a squint and whether this is manifest or latent. You just require your hands and a small object for the patient to look at for this test! Very small squints can be detected and if you also use prisms you can accurately measure them. For the cover test

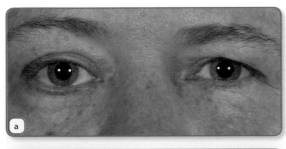
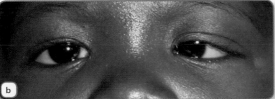

Figure 18.7 Corneal reflex test. (a) The corneal reflexes (note that this camera flash has created two reflexes in each eye) are in exactly the same place on both corneas, therefore, this patient does not have squint. It is easier to accurately assess the reflex position in people with lighter coloured irises. (b) The corneal reflexes are not symmetrical. The reflex in the left eye is lateral and higher than the one in the right eye, therefore, the eye must be deviated inwards and downwards.

to work the patient must have fairly good vision in each eye, and be old enough to cooperate. The patient must look at a small object. If you use your pen for this, ask them to look at the very tip of the pen-nib rather than the whole pen. Although these seem like simple tests, they are in fact surprisingly difficult to do well and require practice. All three parts of the test should be done first with the patient fixing on a distant object, and then also on a near object.

The cover test (Figure 18.8)

The examiner covers each of the patient's eyes in turn. If there is a squint, the eye that is not covered will move to take up fixation of the object. This movement of the uncovered eye demonstrates a positive cover test. If the eye moves inwards, it must have been resting in an outwardly deviated position, i.e. exotropic and vice versa. If there is no movement, then binocular fixation is present.

The uncover test (Figure 18.9)

As the cover is being taken away from an eye, this eye is examined for any movement. If it moves, then a latent squint is present. Again, the direction of the latent squint can be determined by the direction that the eye moves on removing the cover.

The alternate cover test (Figure 18.10)

In this test the cover is alternately moved from one eye to the other eye. This breaks down fusion and allows assessment of the total deviation, i.e. both the latent and manifest parts combined.

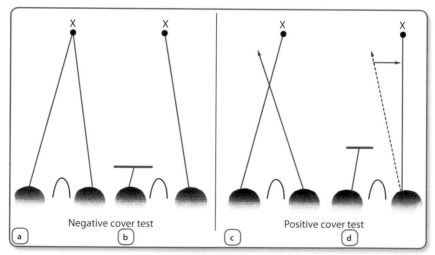

Figure 18.8 The cover test. (a) Both eyes are straight looking at the object X. (b) The left eye is covered but the right eye does not move. There is no squint and the cover test is negative. (c) The left eye is fixating on object X, but the right eye has a small convergent squint. (d) The left eye is covered so the right eye now moves to fixate the object X. The cover test is now positive and demonstrates the squint.

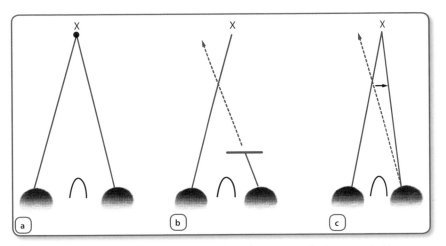

Figure 18.9 The uncover test. (a) The patient does not have a squint. Both eyes are looking at the object X. (b) On covering one eye, in this case the right eye, there is no stimulus for the right eye to remain looking straight ahead and so it turns a little. (c) On removing the cover or uncovering the eye, it moves back to fixate the object X. There is a latent convergent squint (an esophoria); a squint that only appears when the two eyes are forced to look at different things.

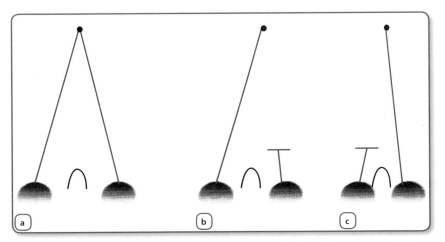

Figure 18.10 The alternate cover test. (a) The eyes are straight. (b) The right eye is covered. (c) The cover is quickly transferred from the right eye to the left. This can be repeated back and forth, so the two eyes don't have the chance to work together. In this way small latent squints will be demonstrated.

Testing the ocular movements

Versions

Versions are movements of both eyes in the same direction (*ductions* are movements of a single eye, i.e. adduction – towards the nose, abduction away from the nose). There are six extraocular muscles, and each one produces most of the movement in a particular direction. There are therefore six main directions of gaze (**Figure 18.1**). The patient should be asked to fix on a small target or a light and their gaze should be slowly taken into each of these six directions. They should be asked to inform you if they have any double vision or pain in any particular directions of gaze. If diplopia is found in a particular position of gaze, it is very helpful to conduct the cover test (see above) to confirm the presence of the squint and help determine which muscle(s) are affected.

Convergence

Convergence is tested by asking the patient to keep looking at a small object and slowly bringing it closer to their eyes.

Assessing squints in children

As well as the above tests, the eyes must be examined very carefully for any disease that might explain the squint. Three tests are especially important:

1. The visual acuity should be tested in both eyes to see if there is any amblyopia (see Chapter 3, visual acuity measurement). This requires both skill and patience, especially in young children, but it is very important.
2. The refraction of the eyes should be measured. Cycloplegic drops (atropine or cyclopentolate), are needed to dilate the pupil and paralyse the ciliary muscle, which is very active in young children. However, always remember to check the pupil light reflexes before dilating the pupil. A retinoscope and a set of trial lenses can then be used to measure the refraction.
3. A dilated ocular examination to assess for any intraocular pathology, which might explain the squint or reduced vision.

Prominent epicanthal folds

Prominent epicanthal folds of skin on the nasal side of the eye are often mistaken for a squint in young children (**Figure 18.11**). These occur because the ethmoid sinuses develop before the other sinuses, so that many young children have a broad nasal bridge relative the rest of their face. The fold of skin covers much of the white sclera on the inside or nasal side of the eye and can give the appearance of the eyes being in-turned. However, the corneal light reflex and cover tests will both show that this is not a true squint. As the rest of the skull grows, these folds become less marked and the apparent 'squint' disappears.

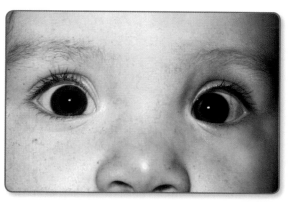

Figure 18.11 Epicanthal folds. This child appears to have a left convergent squint because less white sclera is visible on the medial side of the left eye than on the right eye. However, the corneal light reflexes show that both eyes are in fact looking in the same direction.

The management and treatment of squints

The management and treatment of squints is very different in children and in adults.

Squints in children

The following steps must be taken when assessing and treating squint in children:

Assess and treat the cause of the visual impairment or squint

Remember that serious and potentially fatal diseases such as retinoblastoma and meningitis can present as squint in childhood.

Correct refractive errors with spectacles (see Chapter 5)

Most common childhood squints improve with the correction of refraction. Young children usually happily wear their glasses if they improve their vision. A few types of squint will become more prominent with refractive correction and may require complicated spectacle lens planning such as bifocal lenses. Such patients will require management by a specialist ophthalmologist and optometrist.

Treat amblyopia (see above)

Covering the 'good' eye for a few hours a day is enormously effective at improving the vision in the amblyopic eye as long as there is no other pathology that requires treatment. Both patching or atropine can be used to occlude the 'good eye' and trials have shown them to be similarly effective.

Straighten the eyes with surgery

Squint surgery should not be undertaken until all the previous steps have been completed. If the squint is of recent onset or is intermittent, then surgery might restore full binocular vision and bring about a complete cure. However in most cases the surgery is primarily cosmetic, i.e. it will improve the appearance but not the function of the eyes. In some cultures, a squint is a serious defect, while in others it is ignored. It is therefore very important that the clinician determines the impact of the squint on the child and their family and whether surgical correction is indicated or desired. Surgeons differ as to what is considered the best age to correct squints and also each case is different. In general many surgeons and the parents of children with squints will consider surgery at around 5 years old, just before school starts. Remember that convergent squints may improve gradually as children grow older, especially if the squinting eye is amblyopic or the patient hypermetropic. The surgeon can straighten the eye by either weakening, strengthening or re-aligning the extraocular muscles.

Treatment of squints in adults

If the squint has been present since childhood there is unlikely to be a treatable diagnosis. Surgery to improve the appearance may be considered. If however the squint has come on recently an underlying diagnosis must be looked for. There may be a serious neurological or general medical disease. Double vision can be temporarily relieved by covering one eye or in some cases by fitting a prism on or in the glasses lens of one eye. Some squints such as those caused by vascular cranial nerve palsies frequently recover some months after their onset. Therefore, surgery must not be undertaken until persistence and stability of the squint is confirmed. One may need to measure the squint on a few occasions over a year. In some cases, squint surgery can re-align the eyes and cure diplopia but in other cases the surgery is primarily cosmetic.

Nystagmus

Nystagmus is involuntary, repeated bilateral oscillation of the eyes, i.e. both eyes flick back and forth or up and down, or even in a torsional motion. Nystagmus is a complex condition, which is beyond the scope of this book. However, we will try and briefly outline the main forms of nystagmus as accurate documentation of the nystagmus will help identify the pathology if you have the opportunity to discuss the patient with a specialist. We will also identify some key types of nystagmus and nystagmus 'red-flags' to look out for to help avoid missing potentially dangerous pathology.

Classification

1. *Classify type of movement:*
   a. Jerk: the eyes move slowly in one direction, followed by a quick movement in the other direction. The direction of nystagmus is recorded as the direction of the fast phase.
   b. Pendular: the eyes move in one direction and then back in the other direction at a similar speed.
   c. Mixed: a mixture of jerk and pendular nystagmus depending on eye position.
2. *Classify the direction of movement:*
   a. Horizontal
   b. Vertical
   c. Torsional
3. *Classify other features of the movement:*
   a. Fast/slow
   b. Manifest (present when the eyes are open), latent (present when one or other eye is occluded) or manifest latent (present with both eyes open, but more pronounced with one eye occluded).

Types of nystagmus

Sensory deprivation nystagmus (SDN)

This is caused by a defect in the sensory visual pathway in children, e.g. cataracts. SDN accounts for the majority of early onset nystagmus. It is not a cause of nystagmus in adult-onset reduced vision as they have already developed a fixation point. It may be the consequence of a disease that the child is already known to have, but it also may alert you to previously undiagnosed disease; look for corneal opacities, aniridia, cataracts and retinal and optic nerve pathology. For example, consider a child of 10 years old with cataracts, if they also have nystagmus, it indicates that the cataracts have been there since an early age and the fixation point did not develop normally. It is therefore very unlikely that the visual acuity will recover to normal with cataract surgery. However, if there is no nystagmus, the cataracts probably developed later, and the visual prognosis from cataract is excellent.

Congenital Idiopathic nystagmus (CIN)

CIN is horizontal in all positions of gaze, becomes less obvious ('dampens') with convergence, disappears during sleep and is usually associated with only mild visual impairment. Patients may have a head turn which brings their eyes to a position with the nystagmus is least pronounced and therefore the vision better. It is a reassuring diagnosis and does not require further investigation.

Up and downbeat nystagmus ▶

Vertical nystagmus is often a sign of significant neurological pathology, such as tumours or other space occupying lesions, the Arnold-Chiari malformation and drug intoxication.

Spasmus mutans ▶

Spasmus mutans is asymmetrical rapid binocular nystagmus (or sometimes even monocular) and usually presents within the first year of life. It is associated with head nodding and sometimes an abnormal head position. It is usually benign and resolves by the 4th year of life, but can be the presenting sign of a tumour in the suprasellar or hypothalamic region.

▶ The conditions marked with a red flag are potentially fatal or rapidly blinding and should be investigated urgently.

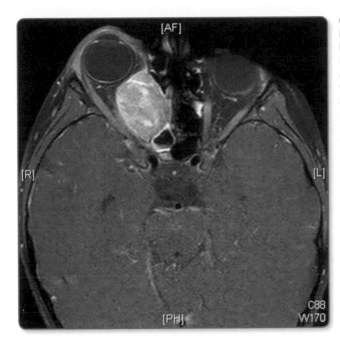

Orbital disease is rare, but it can be very serious. It is diagnostically and surgically very challenging and sometimes needs high-tech investigations to guide the management.

Orbital diseases are not very common. However, they are often serious, and may cause blindness or even death. A patient with orbital disease is always a difficult clinical problem for at least four reasons:

- The symptoms and signs are often variable, non-specific and in the early stages of the disease, quite mild. Therefore, orbital disease is often missed.
- MRI and CT scanning are the major methods for investigating orbital disease. However, they are expensive and required skilled technicians and radiologists and are therefore only available in the major cities of poor countries. Remember that if a CT scan or MRI is not available, even a plain X-ray can be useful, especially in detecting any underlying nasal sinus disease, and sometimes subtle changes in the orbital wall can be seen on a plain X-ray.
- Even when the diagnosis is known it may be difficult or even impossible to treat the patient.
- The treatment of orbital disease is often surgical. Orbital surgery is technically difficult and very few people are experienced in it.

There are three main types of orbital disease:
1. Space-occupying lesions in the orbit.
2. Acute orbital cellulitis (infection in the orbit).
3. Thyroid eye disease.

Space-occupying lesions in the orbit

Symptoms and signs

There are many different orbital space-occupying lesions. The major symptoms and signs are eye ache, displacement of the eyeball which is usually forward (proptosis) but can be in other directions as well, visual loss, double vision, corneal ulceration, conjunctival swelling (chemosis) and dilated blood vessels. Therefore, every patient with proptosis must have a careful examination of the optic nerve function, the ocular movements, the pupil reflexes, the conjunctiva and the cornea.

Proptosis (exophthalmos)

Proptosis is forward displacement of the eye. Patients often describe it as their eye becoming 'larger', although it is of course exactly the same size but looks larger because the eyelids become wider apart as the eyeball moves forward. The proptosis is often accompanied by an ache behind the eye or pressure sensation. The ache is usually made worse by pressure on the eyeball. Proptosis can be measured with an instrument called an 'exophthalmometer' (**Figure 19.1**). This measures how far forward the cornea is in relation to the bony orbital rim. Although exophthalmometers are not particularly expensive, they are often not available in eye clinics in poor countries. However, the presence of proptosis can be easily detected simply by looking from above the patient (**Figure 19.2**) or with a ruler as described in **Box 19.1**. Lesions inside the extraocular muscle cone usually displace the eye forwards only ('axial proptosis', **Figure 19.4**). Lesions outside the muscle cone or in the wall of the orbit usually displace the eye in the opposite direction to the lesion (non-axial proptosis). For example, a lesion

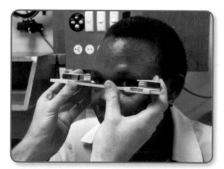

Figure 19.1 Examining a patient with an exophthalmometer.

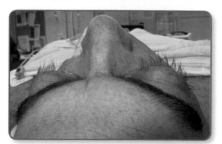

Figure 19.2 To show how a proptosed eye can be recognised by sitting a patient down and looking down from above the head. This patient has bilateral proptosis but it is more prominent on the right.

Box 19.1 Detecting proptosis and measuring displacement of the eyeball

Detecting and measuring axial (forward) proptosis (**Figure 19.2**)

1. Sit the patient down.

2. Stand over him, and look down at his forehead from above.

3. A simple and quick way to check for proptosis is to hold a straight edge (e.g. a ruler) vertically from the bone of the eyebrow to the bone of the upper cheek. Then look from the side and you can see how close the eyeball is to the ruler (in some cases the eyeball can be touching the ruler). A more proptosed eye will be closer.

4. If available, an exophthalmometer is used to measure the proptosis (**Figure 19.1**).

Measuring vertical displacement in non-axial (i.e. not just forward) proptosis of the eye (**Figure 19.3**)

1. Place a ruler horizontally over the bridge of the nose at the level of the outer corners of the eyes.

2. Horizontal displacement: measure the distance of the corneal light reflexes from the centre of the nasal bridge.

3. Vertical displacement: place a second ruler vertically and use it to measure the distance of the corneal light reflex from the horizontal reflex.

Remember that if the patient has a squint the vertical or horizontal measurements will be unequal but this is because the eyeball is rotated, unlike in orbital disease in which the eyeball is displaced.

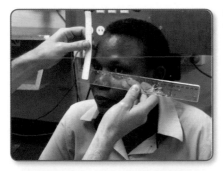

Figure 19.3 Measuring vertical displacement with two rulers.

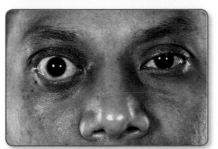

Figure 19.4 Axial proptosis of the right eye. This patient had a haemangioma inside the extraocular muscle cone, pushing the eye forwards. There is no vertical or horizontal displacement.

of the frontal sinus in the roof of the orbit usually displaces the eye downwards (**Figure 19.5**).

Reduced vision

The vision can be reduced from pressure on the optic nerve (and its blood supply) and pressure on the eyeball. Pressure on the nerve usually causes reduced colour vision and an enlarged blind spot initially and then reduced visual acuity. Continued pressure that starts to damage the optic nerve will also cause an afferent papillary defect (see Chapter 3). Pressure on the eyeball may cause the eye to become more hypermetropic or astigmatic (see Chapter 5) and to develop choroidal folds (**Figure 19.6**), both of which reduce the visual acuity.

Corneal and conjunctival ulceration

There may be so much proptosis that the cornea becomes exposed and ulcerated (**Figure 19.7**). The exposed conjunctiva can also become very swollen (chemosis) and even ulcerated (**Figure 19.8**).

Double vision (diplopia)

The function of the extraocular muscles may be affected by the orbital mass and the eyeball may not be able to move normally in some or all directions. This causes double vision.

Differential diagnosis of space-occupying orbital lesions

The most common orbital lesions are: tumours, cysts, inflammatory orbital masses and vascular lesions.

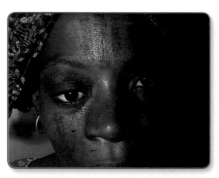

Figure 19.5 Non-axial proptosis of the right eye. This patient had a mucocele of the right frontal sinus, pushing the eye downwards.

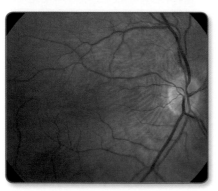

Figure 19.6 Choroidal folds caused by an orbital mass.

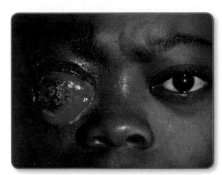

Figure 19.7 Leukaemic deposits in the orbit of a young boy. The right cornea has ulcerated away completely and there is chemosis of the conjunctiva.

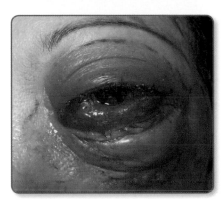

Figure 19.8 Conjunctival swelling (chemosis). In this patient the proptosis, which has caused the chemosis, has been caused by orbital cellulitis. The pen marks around the inflamed area were drawn to monitor whether infection improved or worsened after antibiotics had been started.

Tumours

There are many types of orbital tumour, both benign and malignant, but they are all rare. The orbit contains muscles, connective tissue, blood vessels, fat, bone and periosteum, the dural and arachnoid sheath surrounding the optic nerve, and the lacrimal gland, as well as the eye itself. A tumour can arise from any of these. The tumours can be broadly divided into benign and malignant ones.

Benign orbital tumours

Benign orbital tumours all present with a very slow and gradually increasing proptosis. The most frequent benign tumours are haemangiomas, benign lacrimal gland tumours (pleomorphic adenomas, see Figure 6.26b) and neurofibromas.

Malignant orbital tumours

Malignant orbital tumours grow more rapidly. They may infiltrate and destroy the surrounding tissues, or spread to other parts of the body. They may originate from the orbit itself or from adjoining tissues (e.g. brain, skin or sinus), or be a metastasis from a cancer elsewhere in the body. The most frequent malignant tumours are:

In children:
- Retinoblastoma which has spread outside the eye (see Figure 13.39).
- Lymphoma or leukaemic deposits (**Figure 19.9**). Burkitt's lymphoma, which usually starts around the maxilla in children is an important

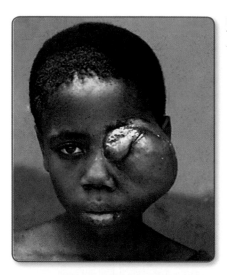

Figure 19.9 A child with Burkitt's lymphoma. The tumour started in the maxilla and spread to the orbit.

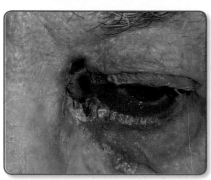

Figure 19.10 A basal cell carcinoma of the medial canthus and lower eyelid that is invading the orbit. This tumour was found to have eroded into the lacrimal sac and ethomoid sinuses.

cause of orbital tumours in Central Africa. Orbital lymphomas also occur more commonly in patients with HIV/AIDS.

- Rhabdomyosarcoma arising from the extraocular muscles.

In adults:

- Lacrimal gland tumours, e.g. adenocarcinoma. When lacrimal gland tumours become larger they push the eyeball downwards and outwards, but the patient is often not aware of this until it is very advanced because it happens gradually.
- Lymphomas.
- Malignant tumours of the skin (e.g. squamous cell carcinoma, basal cell carcinoma (**Figure 19.10**) and malignant melanoma) and the nasal sinuses (e.g. squamous cell carcinoma, adenocarcinoma and malignant melanoma), which may spread into the orbit.

Cysts

Cysts present clinically in the same way as benign orbital tumours. They are also quite rare. The most common types are dermoid or epidermoid cysts (**Figure 19.11**), or parasitic cysts such as a hydatid cyst. Sometimes the cyst may rupture or leak, particularly after trauma, and this will cause inflammation in the orbit.

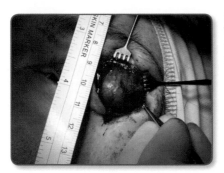

Figure 19.11 A dermoid cyst being excised. This dermoid cyst is situated in the most common location: the lateral side of the eyebrow.

Inflammatory orbital masses

Inflammatory orbital masses are typically more spread out than tumours and are sometimes associated with systemic disease elsewhere. The causes of orbital inflammation include:

- A parasitic granuloma, usually from a nematode worm
- A chronic infection, e.g. fungal or tuberculosis.
- Sarcoidosis.
- Granulomatosis with polyangiitis (previously known as Wegener disease). This is usually associated with severe nasal sinus inflammation, lung disease and other systemic symptoms.
- Inflammation around a leaking dermoid cyst or hydatid cyst.

Idiopathic orbital inflammation

Often, in spite of many investigations, the cause of the orbital inflammation remains unknown. This is called idiopathic orbital inflammation (IOI). Many of these idiopathic inflammatory lesions seem very like tumours and are therefore sometimes called pseudo-tumours. They are quite common in tropical climates and especially in young Africans.

Recent studies have found that some of these 'idiopathic' cases may be a relatively recently described condition called IgG4-related disease. This diagnosis is made on histopathological examination where a large number of IgG4 inflammatory cells are seen with a characteristic microscopic appearance. However, the clinical significance of this subtype is not yet clear.

Tolosa Hunt syndrome is inflammation due to an unknown cause at the very apex of the orbit or in the superior orbital fissure. There is little or no proptosis but there is marked pain and one or more of the cranial nerves coming through the superior orbital fissure (third, fourth, fifth or sixth) will usually be affected. Therefore the eye movements are likely to be restricted. Tolosa Hunt syndrome responds extremely well to steroids.

The typical clinical findings of all these inflammatory lesions in the orbit are:

- A history of pain or some discomfort in the orbit.
- Proptosis, often with limitation of eye movements.
- Evidence of inflammation, with some oedema or vasodilation of the conjunctiva or the eyelids.

- Systemic symptoms: many of the diseases that cause orbital inflammatory masses are systemic diseases. Therefore, ask the patients about systemic symptoms such as breathlessness, urinary or bowel problems, skin rashes, joint and back pain and fever and night sweats.

Vascular lesions

The orbit has a very good blood supply. Vascular lesions may cause proptosis, but they are very rare. One very serious vascular disorder is an arteriovenous fistula between the carotid artery and the cavernous sinus. Very rarely, abnormal blood vessels may rupture and cause a sudden orbital haemorrhage which is seen as proptosis and a 'red' eye with dilated scleral and episcleral blood vessels.

The treatment of space-occupying lesions in the orbit

It is often very difficult to decide what treatment to give and also how to give it. The treatment plan is much easier if histology services are available. However, even trained pathologists may have difficulty in identifying exactly what a lesion is. For example, it may be difficult to decide whether a biopsy specimen is a lymphoma (needing chemotherapy) or idiopathic orbital inflammation (needing steroids). The following plan is a simple guide to a complex subject (**Box 19.2**):

Does the disease originate in the nasal sinuses?

A plain X-ray and a simple clinical examination should be able to determine this. If it does, the nasal sinuses should be explored surgically. Sinus infections and mucoceles need to be drained (**Figure 19.12**), and nasal tumours need a biopsy.

Does the disease originate in the orbit itself?

In this case the following options should be considered:

    a. *Leave untreated:* orbital surgery is very difficult and has a high-risk of serious complications such as complete visual loss or even meningitis and death. Lesions that do not appear either to be growing or harming the eye can often be left untreated.

    b. *Remove the entire lesion:* Benign tumours and cysts that are causing significant symptoms should be removed completely. This is usually done either by lateral orbitotomy, in which the orbit is entered by removing the bony lateral wall, or through the eyelid skin crease.

Box 19.2 Possible treatment plan for orbital tumours

1. Leave untreated
2. Remove the entire lesion
3. Biopsy
4. Exenteration
5. Chemotherapy/radiotherapy
6. Medical treatment

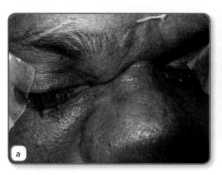

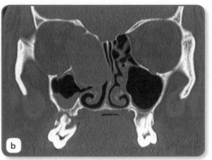

Figure 19.12 A sinus mucocele. (a) A lump can be seen supero-nasal to the right eye. This lump is causing proptosis on this side. (b) A CT scan of the area shows that this lump is in fact a large mucocele coming from the sinuses. It would have been possible to see this on a plain X-ray.

The tumour can then be removed without disturbing the eye. However, there is a risk of damaging important orbital structures during the operation, including the extra-ocular muscles and optic nerve and its blood supply, and the operation is technically difficult.

c. *Biopsy:* Suspected malignant tumours or inflammatory masses need a biopsy. For a biopsy the orbit should be entered through the eyelid skin or conjunctiva. Further treatment depends on the result of the biopsy.

d. *Exenteration (removal of all the orbital contents including the eyeball):* This is a mutilating operation, but it is the best treatment for some malignant tumours (e.g. most carcinomas) and may save the patient's life, or make their final months of life more comfortable (**Figure 19.13**).

e. *Non-surgical treatments:* some tumours, such as lymphomas are sensitive to chemotherapy and/or radiotherapy. This requires very specialised facilities.

f. *Medical treatment:* Chronic infection requires antibiotic treatment with appropriate antibiotics. Idiopathic orbital inflammation and some other inflammatory lesions should be treated with systemic steroids. In ideal circumstances systemic steroid treatment for a pseudotumour or chemotherapy for a lymphoma should never be started until the diagnosis has been confirmed with a biopsy. In

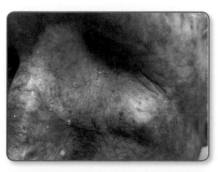

Figure 19.13 Exenteration. This patient has a skin squamous cell carcinoma that had spread into the orbit. The orbit and maxillary sinus below the orbit were excised and a large flap of muscle and skin placed to fill in the defect. The skin graft comes from the arm and has a different colour to the sundamaged surrounding skin of the face.

practice such a 'text book' approach is not always possible, and it is reasonable in a case of suspected orbital inflammation to give a short course of systemic steroids as a treatment trial. Many cases of orbital inflammatory disease respond very well to systemic steroids. However, remember that lymphomas also initially shrink with steroids. This can cause false reassurance and the wrong diagnosis to be made.

Is the orbital lesion part of a systemic disease?

In this case, other treatment is likely to be required, e.g. for lung or kidney disease.

Acute orbital cellulitis and pre-septal cellulitis

Acute orbital cellulitis is one of the few emergency conditions in ophthalmology. There are pyogenic bacteria, or fungi and pus in the orbit that can rapidly cause visual loss and even death if the pus spreads to the cavernous sinus and brain to cause meningitis and encephalitis.

Symptoms and signs

Orbital cellulitis (**Figure 19.14**) must be distinguished from pre-septal cellulitis (Figure 6.3) (**Table 19.1**). Pre-septal cellulitis means there is infection in the eyelid but it has not spread behind the septum which is a layer in the eyelid (see Chapter 2), which is preventing the infection entering the orbit. Pre-septal cellulitis often comes from a meibomian cyst that has become infected or a small wound or scratch to the eyelid, although frequently, no cause can be found.

Orbital cellulitis often comes from sinus or dental infection. The infection usually reaches the orbit through the very thin bone between the nasal sinuses and the medial wall of the orbit. Young children are especially at risk. This is because upper respiratory tract infections are very common in young children, and the walls of the sinuses are less well developed. They are also at risk of pre-septal cellulitis turning into orbital cellulitis, because they do not have a well-developed septum.

The difference between the two conditions is shown in **Table 19.1**. The most significant difference is that in pre-septal cellulitis the symptoms and signs are of the eyelid and skin around the eye, but in orbital cellulitis there are symptoms and signs of infection in the orbit. However, if the eyelids are very swollen, the orbital signs can easily be missed. Also, in early orbital cel-

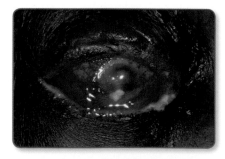

Figure 19.14 Acute orbital cellulitis. This is a severe case, but in the early stages of the infection it can be very difficult to distinguish it from preseptal cellulitis.

Table 19.1 The differences between orbital cellulitis and pre-septal cellulitis		
	Pre-septal cellulitis	Orbital cellulitis Not all the signs below need to be present
Systemic	Well, no fever	Fever and malaise
Pain	In eyelid	Behind eye and worse with eye movements
Eyelids	Swollen, but often one lid only or mainly. It may be possible to identify a chalazion in the lid	Both lids usually very swollen and tense
Eyeball	No proptosis	Proptosis
Eye-movements	Full	Restricted (but may not have double vision particular if swollen lids occlude the eye)
Pupils	Normal reactions	Relative afferent pupillary defect (RAPD)
Conjunctiva	Not inflamed (white)	Inflamed (red)
Vision	Normal	Reduced
Colour vision	Normal	Reduced
Blood tests	Normal or mildly raised white cell count and inflammatory markers	High white cell count (usually neutrophilia), very raised inflammatory markers
Nasal examination	Normal	Pus in the middle nasal meatus
X-rays	Normal	Nasal sinus infection

lulitis, some of the signs may not be present, making it much more difficult to diagnose.

Disease course

Sometimes, the infection resolves without treatment, or an abscess forms and discharges itself through the skin at the orbital margin. However, there is a significant risk especially in orbital cellulitis that the infection will spread backwards along the orbital veins into the cavernous sinus at the base of the brain. There is then a risk of septicaemia, cavernous sinus thrombosis or intracranial infection. **These are all very serious, life-threatening complications**. Inflammation and oedema in both orbits indicates that the infection has reached the cavernous sinus.

The treatment for orbital cellulitis is systemic antibiotics in large doses usually intravenously. The choice of antibiotic depends on what is available and what is recommended locally but ceftriaxone (50 mg/kg/dose up to 2 g twice daily) is recommended in many places. Metronidazole (500 mg 8 hourly) is also recommended because anaerobic organisms from the nasal sinuses may be the cause. Fungal infections require treatment with high dose antifungals, such as amphoteracin B. If an obvious abscess can be seen it should be drained, and most of these patients have a severe infection in the ethmoid sinuses which need draining also.

A similar picture to orbital cellulitis can also be caused by an acute allergic reaction to parasites in the orbit or eyelids, especially the *Loa loa* worm (**Figure 16.13**). However, the patient usually feels well and there is very little localised pain or tenderness. A white cell count will show increased eosinophils in parasitic infections.

Thyroid eye disease

Thyroid eye disease (TED) is associated with primary thyrotoxicosis (Graves's disease). It is more common in women and in smokers. Circulating antibodies cause an auto-immune inflammatory reaction in the orbit. It is not known why these antibodies particularly affect the orbital tissues. In the early (inflammatory) phases of the disease the orbital and peri-ocular tissues (in particular the extraocular muscles and orbital fat) become inflamed and swell. This phase can last many months or even a few years. Gradually the inflammation reduces and the disease becomes 'quiescent' but the patient can be left with severe eye problems or even visual loss.

Symptoms and signs

Patients with TED have a variety of symptoms and the severity can be very varied, ranging form very mild dry eye to severe orbital swelling causing optic nerve compression and visual loss. The severity of the TED often does not relate to the severity of the thyroid dysfunction and TED can even occur in patients whose thyroid function tests are normal, because they may still have the circulating antibodies. The symptoms that should be looked for are:

- *Inflammatory eyelid and conjunctival signs:* in the early and active stages of TED, the eyelids and conjunctiva can become very red and swollen (**Figure 19.15**).
- *Dry eyes:* this is often the only sign of mild or early TED. It probably occurs because mild proptosis and lid retraction cause increased exposure and inflammatory changes in the lacrimal gland reduce tear secretion.
- *Proptosis* (**Figure 19.16**): the enlargement of the extraocular muscles and the swelling of the orbital fat pushes the eyeball forwards. The proptosis is often asymmetrical and sometimes unilateral (**Figure 19.17**). In these patients it is easy to confuse TED with an orbital tumour.
- In some patients with TED, proptosis does not occur. These patients may have a firmly attached orbital septum which is preventing the eyeball moving forwards even though the orbital pressure is high.

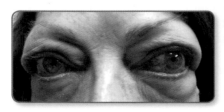

Figure 19.15 The inflammatory stage of thyroid eye disease.

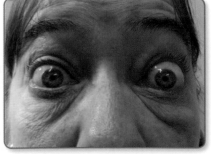

Figure 19.16 Bilateral proptosis and retraction of both the upper and lower eyelids.

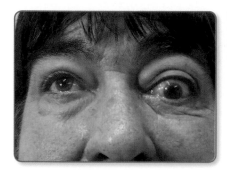

Figure 19.17 Many patients with dysthyroid eye disease do not have symmetrical proptosis and one eye may be more proptosed than the other.

These patients without proptosis are at particular risk of optic nerve compression.

- *Restricted eye movements with diplopia:* this is caused by inflammation, swelling and fibrosis of the extraocular muscles. The inferior and medial recti are most commonly involved. Therefore, there is usually limitation of upward gaze or abduction of the eye. The eyeball can be very markedly displaced by the enlarged muscles (**Figure 19.17**).
- *Eyelid retraction:* this causes the palpebral fissure to widen and the sclera above and/or below the cornea to be visible; the patient looks like they are staring or startled (**Figure 19.16**). This is caused by contracture of the sympathetic muscle fibres in the eyelids and contracture of the levator palpebrae superioris muscle, which opens the upper eyelid.
- *Visual loss:* in severe cases, there may be visual loss either from pressure or lack of blood supply to the optic nerve, or from ulcers in the exposed cornea.

Treatment of thyroid eye disease

The usual sequence for the treatment of TED is:

1. **Treat the inflammatory symptoms and protect the vision.**
   This is sometimes an emergency. High dose steroids (e.g. IV methylprednisolone 500 mg weekly, or 1 g/day for three days, or oral prednisolone up to 100 mg/day) are usually very effective at reducing the inflammation. Occasionally emergency orbital decompression surgery is required to relieve the pressure in the orbit. This requires removal of parts of the walls of the orbit and is complex and specialised surgery. Radiotherapy, if available can also be effective treatment for reducing active inflammation. If the active phase is not treated, the disease eventually burns itself out, but the patient may be left with serious damage to the sight from optic nerve compression or corneal exposure.
2. **Treat proptosis if very prominent.** Once the active inflamed phase of the disease has been controlled, the patient may still have very marked proptosis. Orbital decompression may then be considered as a carefully planned, elective procedure.
3. **Treat the double vision.** This can be managed with patching of one eye or prism spectacles. A more permanent solution can sometimes be

achieved with squint surgery to improve the alignment of the eyes, but this should not be done until the squint has stabilised.

4. **Treat the eyelid position.** The lower eyelids can be raised with lid tightening surgery and the upper eyelids lowered with surgery to weaken the levator muscle.

Most patients with TED have dry eyes probably from the proptosis and reduced tear production. Any artificial teardrops can be used to treat this and prevent any exposure changes in the cornea.

Human immunodeficiency virus and the eye

20

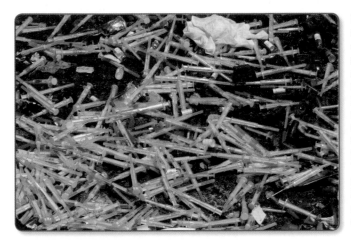

HIV has become a worldwide epidemic. It remains a deadly disease despite modern treatment. A healthy lifestyle and good medical practice are both essential to stop the spread in the community. These syringes and needles have not been properly or safely discarded and are a HIV hazard.

In 1981, some very unusual infections were noted in the USA and became known as 'acquired immune deficiency syndrome (AIDS)'. Shortly afterwards the 'human immunodeficiency virus (HIV)' was recognised as the underlying cause of the disease. Despite the short history of this disease it is now a major worldwide cause of morbidity and mortality and it can have severe effects in the eye. Although it is seen worldwide, HIV is much more prevalent in poor countries and particularly in Africa, where it has spread rapidly and until recently treatment has been much less widely available.

Epidemiology

Prevalence and incidence

Since the disease was first described in 1981, the world has seen an exploding epidemic of HIV infection and deaths from AIDS. At the end of 2012 there were approximately 35 million people living with HIV/AIDS and about 1.6 million people died from AIDS related disease in the year. However, these figures hide the enormous variation in prevalence in the world. The epidemic is most severe in sub Saharan Africa where about 25 million people are thought to be infected (prevalence: 4.7%) (2012 data). In some African countries over 10% of the adult population are estimated to have HIV infection. This compares to 3.9 million in South and South East Asia (prevalence: 0.3%) and 860, 000 in Western Europe (prevalence: 0.2%) In Africa, the infection is most commonly transmitted either by heterosexual intercourse or by vertical transmission from mother to child and it is therefore prevalent in many communities. Also Africa is the only continent in which the infection is more common in women than men, highlighting the huge challenge of reaching women (and their male partners) with effective healthcare and education. However, in most countries outside of Africa, the infection is more common in people who partake in high-risk behaviour, such as intravenous drug users and promiscuous homosexual men who do not use condoms. India may be an exception to this, where there seems to be an increasingly large burden of HIV, which is not restricted to particular groups. There is some good news; it does appear the incidence of new infections is gradually decreasing, with about 3.5 million new infections in 2001 and around 2.3 million new infections in 2012. This is probably due mainly to education, awareness and anti-retroviral treatment programmes. The rates are decreasing fastest in sub-Saharan Africa and the Caribbean. However, about 1.8 million people are still becoming infected each year in sub-Saharan Africa (down from 2.4 million in 2001), and worryingly the rate is continuing to rise in young women and adolescent girls.

HIV transmission

The HIV virus can be spread in two ways:
1. Sexual intercourse, either heterosexual or homosexual. HIV infection can be spread by vaginal, oral and anal intercourse.
2. Direct inoculation into the bloodstream. This may happen in various ways:
- Intravenous injection using unsterile needles. This mainly occurs in people who use illegal intravenous drugs, because they sometimes share needles and syringes. However, needle-stick injuries occasionally cause HIV infection in health professionals. Sharps disposal is very poor in many health clinics, particularly in poorer areas or the world (**Figure 20.1**). This puts health workers at great risk.
- Blood transfusions with contaminated blood. This was a major cause of infection before the routes of transmission were well-understood. In the past many patients with haemophilia (who require regular blood transfusions and received it from pooled donors containing contaminated blood before careful checks for HIV were made) became infected with HIV. Nowadays, all blood and blood donors should be checked for HIV infection, although sadly, HIV is still occasionally spread by blood transfusion, when testing is not carefully performed.
- Mother-to-child (vertical transmission). This can occur in-utero, during birth or from breastfeeding.

HIV is not spread by normal social contact, such as shaking hands, hugging, kissing or normal clinical examination of patients. There is however a small risk of transmission via items that are exposed to infected blood, such as shaving razors and toothbrushes. Medical staff do not need to wear gloves or protective clothing when examining or treating patients with HIV unless there is a risk of a needlestick injury, e.g. during cannulation or surgery.

Some people prefer to wear two pairs of gloves ('double-gloving') when performing surgery in patients with HIV. Others prefer not to as they find this that this reduces dexterity and furthermore in some places, as many as half the patients may have HIV. Patients with HIV certainly do not need to be isolated or segregated as occurred in previous years.

If someone does receive a needlestick injury whilst treating a patient who is HIV positive, the overall risk of then becoming HIV positive themselves is probably about 0.3%. However, the risk varies greatly depending on the volume of blood inoculated and the viral load of the patient. The viral load depends on whether a patient is receiving anti-retroviral drugs and the stage of the disease. For example, the blood of an untreated patient in the latter stages of the disease will have a much higher load of virus particles.

When the patient first becomes infected with HIV, there may be a flu-like illness but often there are no symptoms at all. However, the virus is multiplying and very gradually destroying the patient's immune system. If the infection is not treated with anti-retrovirals, ophthalmic symptoms will start to appear, although sometimes these do not occur for as long as 10 years, even without treatment.

HIV pathophysiology

HIV is a ribonucleic acid (RNA) retrovirus. This means that it has RNA as its genetic material. The other main type of virus contains deoxyribonucleic acid (DNA). DNA viruses include adenovirus that causes conjunctivitis and herpes virus. Retroviruses use their own enzymes (reverse transcriptase) to make a DNA copy of its RNA, which becomes integrated into the host (human) DNA. HIV can infect various human cells, but the failure of the immune system that results in AIDS is caused by HIV infection of CD4 positive (CD4+) T lymphocytes. These are white blood cells that are an essential part of the immune system. The CD4 part is simply a protein on their surface which is important for their disease preventing function, but is also probably how HIV enters the cells. Once inside these lymphocytes, the precise way in which HIV affects them is complex and incompletely understood, but the ultimate effect is to dramatically reduce the number of circulating CD4+ T lymphocytes. Therefore, the body's ability to fight many infections is greatly decreased, and the patient will eventually start to develop infections. Some of these infections are by organisms that are not normally pathogenic and called opportunistic infections. If the HIV is untreated this may occur about 2–10 years after infection, but this can be delayed by decades with careful antiretroviral treatment. HIV infection also increases the risk of developing cancers, including rare cancers. This is probably through its immunosuppressive activity and the increased risk of patients becoming infected with viruses that promote cancer formation such as some of the human papilloma viruses. In fact, it was the clusters of cases of Kaposi's sarcoma and non-Hodgkin's lymphomas in young men in America that led to the discovery of HIV, as these groups are normally rarely affected by these very unusual cancers.

Laboratory tests and the definition of AIDS

Many HIV tests are available. They generally detect the body's antibodies to HIV, HIV antigens or HIV nucleic acid. Different tests can be used for whole blood, serum, plasma, saliva and urine. There are also rapid tests which can give a result within 30 minutes. These can be particularly useful after a needle-stick injury or if it is likely a patient will not return for follow up. Some HIV tests will only give a positive result several weeks after someone contracts the infection. Diagnostic tests are not 100% reliable, therefore repeat testing may be required. After the diagnosis has been made specialised tests can be conducted in laboratories to measure the number of CD4+ lymphocytes in the blood and the HIV load. These tests give a good indication of how advanced the disease is and the risk of getting HIV associated infections and AIDS.

A patient is defined as having AIDS if he/she is infected with HIV and also has one of the following:

- A CD4+ count of less than 200 cells/mL (or a CD4+ T-cell percentage of total lymphocytes of less than 15%)
- An AIDS defining illness: there are 26 conditions in adults, and a further two in children less than 13 years old. **Box 20.1** contains a list of the AIDS defining conditions that may be first diagnosed in the eye. The reference for the full list is given in the further reading section in the front of the book.

Treatment and prevention of HIV

Anti-retroviral therapy (ART)

The treatment of HIV has changed dramatically and rapidly in recent years. HIV treatment has become increasingly safe, effective and easily

---

> ### Box 20.1 AIDS defining conditions that affect the eye, periocular area or vision
> 1. Coccidioidomycosis,
> 2. Cryptococcosis, extrapulmonary
> 3. **Cytomegalovirus retinitis (with loss of vision)**
> 4. Encephalopathy (HIV-related)
> 5. Herpes simplex: chronic ulcer(s) (for more than 1 month); or bronchitis, pneumonitis, or esophagitis
> 6. Histoplasmosis, disseminated or extrapulmonary
> 7. Kaposi's sarcoma
> 8. **Lymphoma, Burkitt's**
> 9. Lymphoma, immunoblastic (or equivalent term)
> 10. Lymphoma, primary, of brain
> 11. Infection with non-tuberculous species of Mycobacterium
> 12. Progressive multifocal leukoencephalopathy
> 13. **Toxoplasmosis of the brain**
> 14. **Tuberculosis, disseminated**
>
> The conditions that are more common in the eye are listed in bold.

administered and taken. Perhaps most importantly, treatment is now widely available for poor people. The recommended drugs and combinations of drugs is constantly changing and being updated, and treatment needs to be administered by an appropriate specialist. It is beyond the scope of this book to discuss treatment in detail, but it is important for eye care practitioners to have a basic understanding of the types of drugs that are used and how these may affect eye health. Currently there are six different classes of ART drugs. The three most widely used classes are: nucleoside reverse transcriptase inhibitors (NRTIs), the non-nucleoside reverse transcriptase inhibitors (NNRTIs) and the protease inhibitors (PIs). Each of these classes of drugs attacks a different step in the viral life cycle as the virus infects CD4+ T lymphocytes or other cells. Although, a complete cure has not yet been achieved, patients taking combination anti-retroviral treatment can now live relatively normal and healthy lives for many years. The specific infections and diseases that a patient with HIV/AIDS suffers from have their own treatments, which must be used as well as the ARTs.

Health education

By far the best way of fighting the epidemic of HIV and AIDS is with a vigorous campaign of public health and public education, especially amongst school children and young sexually active adults. The first African country to report a fall in the incidence of HIV infection was Uganda. This is very likely to be due to its comprehensive programme of public education and awareness about HIV, which started relatively early in the epidemic.

Needlestick injuries

Needlestick injuries happen relatively frequently in health clinics. Occasionally, these infect people working in the clinic with HIV or hepatitis. All individuals from cleaners to professors must take responsibility for safe sharp disposal in the clinic or hospital in which they work. Many clinics in poor countries do not have conveniently located sharps disposal bins, despite these now being widely available. **It is simply not acceptable anywhere in the world to use needles or sharps without a safe disposal system (Figure 20.1).** It is also not acceptable to assume that someone else will dispose of your sharps.

If a needlestick injury does occur, a short course of ART prophylaxis greatly reduces the likelihood of acquiring HIV infection. Clinics must have within date ART prophylaxis readily available. The current guidelines are that

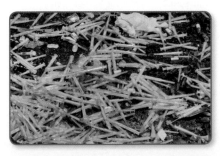

Figure 20.1 A collection of used needles discarded in the soil behind a clinic. This should never be seen.

treatment should be given for a duration of 28 days and within 72 hours of the exposure (although they should be started as soon as possible after the injury). However, the guidelines may change and the current local, national and WHO guidelines should always be consulted.

HIV counselling

In many cases, the eye signs may be the first to occur and so the eye doctor or nurse may be the first person to realise that the patient could be HIV positive and be suffering from AIDS. For example, if a young patient presents with herpes zoster ophthalmicus (shingles around the eye) (**Figures 20.2** and **20.3**), there is a high likelihood of the patient having HIV infection. This situation requires great tact and sympathy. If an HIV test is recommended, the patient must first be counselled to discuss the implications of the test, to discover if they really want to be tested, and if they are prepared for the possibility of the test being positive. A positive test will have life long effects both on the patient, and also their relatives who may be positive as well.

HIV disease epidemiology

The HIV epidemic causes particular infections and tumours to develop in patients who are HIV positive (**Figure 20.2**). It has also affected the whole pattern of disease in the wider community. For example, until recently tuberculosis was declining quite rapidly in the world and some years ago there was the hope that it might disappear altogether. The HIV epidemic has brought about another epidemic of tuberculosis, because patients with HIV are much more vulnerable to TB and it is often much harder to treat. They

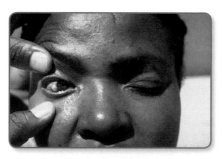

Figure 20.2 A patient with two of the likely signs of being HIV positive. There is a conjunctival carcinoma in one eye and a small scar from a previous herpes zoster infection on the other forehead.

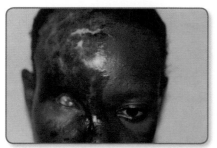

Figure 20.3 Ophthalmic herpes zoster scarring. This patient is young and had very severe disease that left the skin terribly scarred. It caused viral retinitis which ultimately resulted in loss of the eyeball. Such severe disease in a young person, makes HIV very likely. They are likely to have immune compromise. Note that the scarring extends down the side of the nose. This means that the nasociliary branch of the ophthalmic nerve was affected and the eye more likely to be affected also.

then actively spread the infection in the community and therefore, tuberculosis is becoming much more common in both HIV positive and HIV negative patients. Another example is conjunctival carcinoma which was previously an extremely rare cancer (**Figures 20.2, 20.6** and **20.7**). However, with the HIV epidemic it is being seen much more often both in HIV positive and negative patients (see below).

There is a significant difference between the type of diseases seen in AIDS patients in rich countries and in AIDS patients in poor countries, especially in Africa. In rich countries, it is common to see patients with opportunistic infections like CMV and Pneumocystis, which only occur when the patient's CD4+ count has fallen to very low levels. In poor countries, infections with normal pathogenic organisms like herpes zoster, tuberculosis and toxoplasmosis are more common, probably because these diseases are more common in the community and will first develop with higher levels of immunity and CD4+ count. Generally, the opportunistic infections are less widely seen in poor countries because the patients have often died from the pathogenic infections before their immune system is weak enough to be vulnerable to them. However, the picture is changing as more poor patients are able to receive effective ART treatment. Interestingly, the cancers that are associated with the HIV epidemic are also more common in Africa. This is probably because the triggering viruses are more common, although the exact reason is uncertain.

Ophthalmic complications of HIV/AIDS

About 70–80% of people with HIV will develop eye conditions. For many people these will be the first signs of HIV infection, therefore anyone examining eye patients must know how to recognise these signs so that ART treatment can be started. Tact is equally essential. If the patient learns that they are HIV-positive it will have life changing implications for them and their family. The most common complications are summarised in **Table 20.1**. In brief these are:

- Pathogenic infections. These are infections that healthy people can suffer from, but are more common in patients with reduced cellular immunity.
- Opportunistic infection. These are infections that only attack people whose immune system is very depressed.
- Tumours. There are certain tumours that develop as a response to a viral infection.
- The HIV virus itself can also affect the eye but the changes are not severe.
- Side effects of treatment. These can be severe in the body, but not in the eye.

The eyelids and conjunctiva

Herpes zoster ophthalmicus (HZO, ophthalmic shingles)

Shingles is a localised reactivation of the varicella-zoster virus (VZV) that causes chicken pox. After chicken pox, the virus remains dormant in nerve endings. During an episode of shingles it travels down the nerve to the skin

Table 20.1 A summary of the more common eye complications in HIV infection and AIDS

Disease process	Effect on eye
Pathogenic infections	
Human immunodeficiency virus	Microvascular occlusion • Retinal cotton wool spots • Conjunctival vessel abnormalities
Herpes zoster virus	Ophthalmic shingles Keratitis Uveitis Retinal necrosis
Herpes simplex virus	Dendritic corneal ulcers Retinal necrosis
Toxoplasmosis	Chorioretinitis and vitreous inflammation Intracerebral complications
Tuberculosis	Uveitis: anterior and posterior Phlyctens Tuberculomas Optic atrophy
Syphilis	Uveitis and choroiditis Optic neuritis and atrophy
Opportunistic infections	
Cytomegalovirus	Retinitis Cranial nerve palsies Encephalitis
Cryptococcus neoformans	Papilloedema (from meningitis) Uveitis
Pneumocystis jiroveci	Choroiditis
Atypical (non-tubercular) mycobacteria	Uveitis
Yeasts and fungi	Uveitis Suppurative keratitis (possibly associated with HIV)
Tumours	
Ocular surface neoplasia	Conjunctival tumours
Kaposi sarcoma	Eyelid and subconjunctival tumours
Lymphoma	Orbital tumour
Treatment complications	
Immune recovery uveitis	Uveitis causing cataract, epiretinal membrane, cystoid macular oedema, retinal neovascularisation

to cause a vesicular rash and pain. It usually occurs in the area of skin associated with one particular sensory nerve (a dermatome). When this nerve is the ophthalmic branch of the trigeminal nerve (the fifth cranial nerve), it is called HZO (**Figure 20.3**). The virus tends to 'awaken' in elderly patients and patients whose immune system is weak, and particularly in patients with HIV. If HZO is seen in a young patient, HIV infection must be suspected. HZO often occurs quite early in the disease before there are any other signs of HIV and while the patient is still feeling well and healthy with a reasonable CD4+ count. The incidence of shingles does not seem to have changed greatly with the advent of ART.

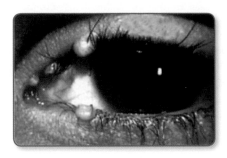

Figure 20.4 Molluscum contagiosum of the eyelids.

HZO is nearly always more severe in HIV positive patients and complications such as keratitis, uveitis (see Chapter 11) and retinitis (see below) are much more likely. In some studies over 30% of eyes have gone blind from severe complications, especially corneal scarring. Eyelid scarring and postherpetic neuralgia (chronic pain in the forehead long after the active episode has recovered) are also very common. Treatment is possible with oral or intravenous acyclovir, valacyclovir or famciclovir, but to be effective this must be given as soon as possible after the symptoms develop. Acyclovir is widely available and relatively cheap. The other antivirals are currently too expensive for most patients.

Molluscum contagiosum (Figure 20.4)

Although molluscum is a common condition in healthy children, there is a definite association between molluscum contagiosum and being HIV positive, particularly in adults. The treatment is discussed on page 150.

Kaposi sarcoma

Kaposi sarcoma is a vascularised tumour that mainly affects the skin and mucous membranes. It forms a painless purple-coloured lump or patch on the skin or red area under the surface of the conjunctiva (**Figure 20.5**). There are often other similar tumours in different parts of the body (it is 'multifocal'). At first, Kaposi sarcoma may not require treatment if there are no symptoms. If it enlarges or becomes symptomatic, surgical excision is the only treatment possible in most places, although radiotherapy and chemotherapy are also used. There is uncertainty as to the best treatment for Kaposi sarcoma.

Ocular surface squamous neoplasia (OSSN)

The OSSN refers to a particular group of cancerous conditions of the conjunctiva and cornea (cornea-conjunctival intraepithelial neoplasia and

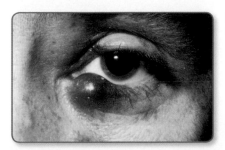

Figure 20.5 A Kaposi sarcoma of typical colour on the eyelid.

carcinoma) (**Figures 20.6** and **20.7** and Figures 7.26 and 7.27). Conjunctival squamous cell carcinomas are now widely seen in Africa. There has been a huge increase in the incidence of OSSN in the last 30 years. HIV positive patients have about 10 times the risk of developing OSSN, although interestingly about a third of patients with OSSN in Africa are HIV negative. However, since the HIV epidemic everyone is probably much more vulnerable to the Human Papilloma Virus that is thought to be responsible for triggering the cancerous change. There may also be an association with sunlight as these tumours have always been more common near in Africa and particularly near the equator. OSSN often occurs fairly early in the course of HIV infection. Conjunctival carcinoma should be excised with at least a 3-mm margin of clear tissue. The base and edges of the wound should probably be treated with cautery, cryotherapy or cytotoxic drugs like mitomycin to destroy any residual carcinoma cells.

Dilated conjunctival blood vessels (conjunctival microvasculopathy)

Conjunctival microvascular changes are frequently seen in HIV infection. These include segments of vessel narrowing and widening, microaneurysms and comma-shaped vascular fragments. The cause of these changes is not known, but it may relate to increased blood thickness and deposition of immune complexes, or even because of direct effects of the HIV virus on the vessel endothelium.

Trichomegaly (eyelash growth and thickening)

Trichomegaly usually occurs in the later stages of HIV infection. The cause is unknown.

The orbit

The most common orbital lesion associated with HIV/AIDS is orbital lymphoma, especially the B cell type and Burkitt's lymphoma (Figure 19.9). Kaposi sarcoma may also occur in the orbit. The management of these tumours is first a biopsy to confirm the diagnosis and then chemotherapy. Lymphomas usually respond very well to chemotherapy.

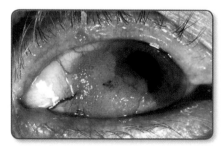

Figure 20.6 Conjunctival squamous cell carcinoma.

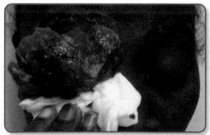

Figure 20.7 Advanced conjunctival squamous cell carcinoma.

The cornea

Infectious keratitis

Viral keratitis (herpes zoster and herpes simplex infections) is more common and recurs more frequently in HIV-positive people. They may also be more difficult to treat. Herpes simplex corneal ulcers in HIV positive patients are often at the edge of the cornea unlike in HIV-negative people.

Bacterial and fungal keratitis are both common in the tropics. They may be more common and possibly more severe in HIV positive people. If a patient has severe and persistent suppurative keratitis that is not responding well to treatment, the possibility of HIV should be considered.

Microsporidia is a protozoon which only very rarely causes cornea infection in healthy individuals. However, it is sometimes an opportunistic corneal pathogen in HIV-positive individuals.

Dry eyes

Dry eyes occur in about 10–20% of HIV positive patients, usually in the later stages of the disease. It can cause punctate keratitis. It is probably caused by HIV induced inflammation and scarring of the lacrimal gland and ducts.

Intraocular inflammation

Uveitis

Uveitis is a very common presenting symptom in HIV positive patients. The uveitis may be acute or chronic and either generalised or localised, and in most cases is caused by or is associated with ocular infection. There are two types of infection causing uveitis.

1. *Infection with a pathogenic organism.*
   Ocular toxoplasmosis (**Figure 20.8** and Figures. 13.42, 13.43), tuberculosis, syphilis and occasionally histoplasmosis, can all occur in HIV negative people. However, they occur more commonly and with greater severity in HIV positive people. These infections often cause very vigorous inflammation in the anterior chamber and in the vitreous. They are usually unilateral. The fundal view is often very hazy.

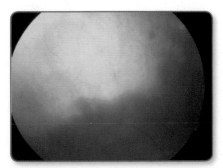

Figure 20.8 Toxoplasmosis chorioretinitis in a patient with immunocompromise caused by HIV. There are extensive changes a which can be compared to more the localised changes in Figures 13.42 and 13.43 from a patient with a healthy immune system.

2. *Infection with an opportunistic organism.*
These only affect patients with severe immune suppression, and a very low CD4+ count. Their life expectancy is very short if left untreated. There are many such organisms, some of which are listed in **Table 20.1**. If a good laboratory is available these different infections can be diagnosed, and in most cases treatment is available, but it is usually very expensive. For example, pneumocystis can be treated with atovaquone and cryptococcus with amphotericin B.

In known or suspected HIV positive patients, an infective cause of the uveitis is highly likely and steroids should not be used. A search for an infection must be done, as intraocular infection can be rapidly destructive if it is not treated and will worsen with steroids. Good laboratory services are often required to assist the diagnosis as aqueous or vitreous need to be examined microscopically. Unfortunately, these are not available in many places where HIV is prevalent.

Immune recovery uveitis (IRU)

Some patients with regressed CMV retinitis (see below) that start ART develop a vigorous uveitis as their immunity recovers. This is caused by an immune response to CMV antigens which only becomes possible with the improved immune system. When this response is severe, it can cause cataract, epiretinal membrane, retinal/optic disc neovascularisation and cystoid macular oedema. It is particularly likely to occur in patients who have large areas of CMV retinitis and a history of cidofovir treatment for their HIV. In some patients it is important to start ART and CMV treatment at the same time. Systemic or local (peri/retrrobulbar or intravitreal) steroids are the main treatment for IRU.

Retina

HIV retinopathy

Patients with HIV infection can develop occlusions in small retinal blood vessels (microangiopathy). This results in infarcts in the retinal nerve fibre layer that are seen as cotton wool spots (**Figure 20.9**). These microvascular changes were seen in 50–70% of HIV patients, but are now less commonly seen probably because of the widespread use of ARTs. They are usually

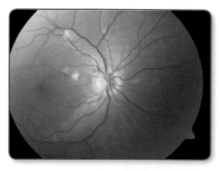

Figure 20.9 HIV retinopathy. The cotton-wool spots are caused by infarcts in the retinal nerve fibre layer.

asymptomatic unless the macula is involved, when the visual acuity may be slightly reduced.

Viral retinal infection

Acute retinal necrosis and progressive outer retinal necrosis

Acute retinal necrosis (ARN) is the rapid vaso-occlusive necrotising retinitis that sometimes occurs in patients with viral retinal infection (**Figure 20.10**). The viruses that typically cause ARN are varicella zoster virus (VZV), herpes simplex virus (HSV) and cytomegalovirus (CMV). In patients with a functioning immune system, there is vigorous inflammation in the vitreous as well which can greatly or even completely obscure the view of the retina.

The clinical picture is very different in immunocompromised individuals. In people with HIV/AIDS, viral retinitis is often bilateral. It can cause rapid retinal destruction with subsequent retinal detachment. Therefore, it can cause bilateral visual loss. Patients with these conditions who are not receiving ART usually have a short life-expectancy.

The retina may also be affected by a condition called progressive outer retinal necrosis (PORN). PORN is a rapidly progressive, necrotising retinitis in patients with advanced AIDS. Unlike in ARN there is minimal intraocular inflammation, probably because these patients are unable to mount a vigorous inflammatory response. PORN appears to be only caused by reactivation of VZV.

Cytomegalovirus retinitis (CMV)

Cytomegalovirus is the most common cause of retinitis in HIV positive patients. In healthy individuals CMV almost never causes retinitis. The reactivation of this opportunistic virus that remains dormant in most people can cause rapid necrotising destruction of the retina. On fundal examination one sees extensive exudates and haemorrhages in the nerve fibre layer of the retina. It usually starts along the main vessels and gradually spreads to involve the whole retina. The retinal appearance has been rather crudely although accurately described as looking like 'tomato ketchup and cream cheese' (**Figure. 20.11**). It causes progressive loss of vision and can even cause death. The damaged thin retina is likely to subsequently detach. CMV tends to occur at a very late stage in the progression of AIDS, when the CD4+

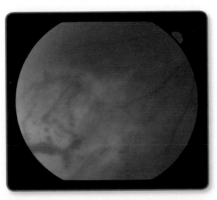

Figure 20.10 Acute retinal necrosis. the patient has extensive arteritis and viral retinal infection mainly affecting the arteries.

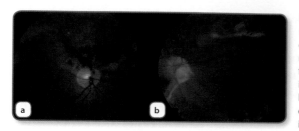

Figure 20.11 Cytomegalovirus retinitis. (a) There is typical distribution along the main retinal blood vessels going from the optic disc and there is a mixture of scattered haemorrhages and thick white exudates. This patient has the infection in both eyes, which further suggests they are very immunocompromised. (b) A very severe case of CMV retinitis in which the 'tomtao ketchup and cream cheese' appearance can be clearly seen.

count is below 50. CMV is less common in poor countries. The reason is uncertain, although it may be because before the widespread availability of ARTs, people with HIV in these countries died, before their CD4+ count was low enough to be vulnerable to CMV. Also, since the advent of these ART programmes, CMV retinitis is being seen less commonly as patients CD4+ counts are not dropping as low.

Treatment of viral retinal infection

Viral retinitis requires prompt and aggressive treatment with anti-viral agents. It is unknown if steroids are of any benefit; in some cases they reduce the inflammation, but in others they seem to trigger the attack. The retinal changes need to be watched closely as there is a high risk of retinal detachment, which would require surgery.

Other retinal infections

Bacteria

Ocular syphilis and TB are much more common in HIV positive people. They are discussed in Chapter 11. Remember that the clinical appearance can look atypical in immunosuppressed patients and syphilis can also rapidly progress to having neurological involvement.

Others infections

Pneumocystis jiroveci is a yeast-like fungus that is responsible for Pneumocystis pneumonia which is relatively common in patients with AIDS. It was originally thought to be the same organism as *Pneumocystis carinii* that was found in rats, but DNA analysis found host specific differences and it was renamed. It can cause choroiditis in patients with widespread systemic infection. Numerous other infections, such as toxoplasmosis (protozoa) (page 351), histoplasma (fungus) (**Figure 20.2**) and *Cryptococcus* (fungus) are more common causes of chorioretinitis in patients with HIV/AIDS.

Neuro-ophthalmic complications

There are many neuro-ophthalmological complications of HIV infection. It is beyond the scope of this book to discuss them in detail, but eye care professionals should be aware of neuro-ophthalmic presentations of ocular disease, such as cranial nerve palsies and papilloedema.

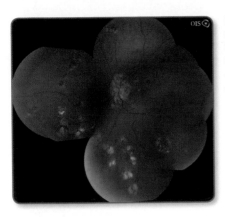

Figure 20.12 Presumed ocular histoplasmosis syndrome. The many causes of chorioretinal inflammation and scarring look very similar. However, the features suggestive of POHS are widespread peripheral spots and atrophy around the optic nerve.

Cranial nerve palsies

Cranial nerve palsies are common, especially in the later stages of AIDS. Double vision will develop if the third, fourth or sixth nerves are affected (Chapter 18). Visual loss will occur if the optic nerve is affected. The most likely cause of cranial nerve palsies is CMV infection, but other infective, malignant or inflammatory processes can also cause them. Syphilis, which can cause optic neuritis, optic atrophy or neurological disease is so often forgotten but is a frequent cause of neurological complications and can be relatively easily treated.

Meningitis and encephalitis

Meningitis and encephalitis can be caused by numerous opportunistic and pathogenic infections. *Cryptococcus neoformans* is a fungus, which is a frequent cause of cerebral infection. Eye care professionals can assist greatly with the diagnosis as patients often present to the eye clinic with headaches and visual symptoms, which is caused by papilloedema.

Ophthalmic side effects of ARTs

ARTs have numerous side effects and patients taking them need careful monitoring and supervision. Rifabutin and Cidofovir cause intraocular inflammation in about a quarter to third patients taking them. This can usually be treated with topical steroids, although if it is very severe, the ARTs must be changed before blinding disease and hypotony occur.

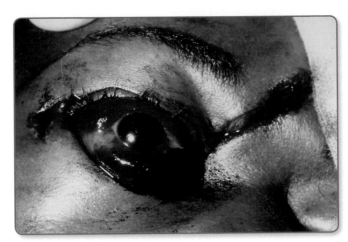

Severe face and eye injury following a road accident. Do you wear your seat belt regularly?

The eye is an external organ, and so is therefore easily injured. Eye injuries are common amongst people all over the world. All medical workers should be able to treat minor eye injuries, and should know something about serious eye injuries. Serious injuries usually require specialist surgical treatment, but often a non-specialist must make the initial diagnosis and may be obliged to treat these if no one else is available. The eye is so complex, that occasionally what seems like a minor injury may have serious complications.

It is helpful to try to answer three questions to assess an eye injury properly:

1. *What caused the injury?* Most patients will explain what happened. Occasionally, however, the patient is unaware of any injury, especially if a small, sharp fragment has penetrated the eye at high speed. Young children are unable to describe what happened and we depend on their parents or older children who may be too scared to tell the truth. However, always remember that occasionally parents or other guardians and relatives commit the injuries (*non-accidental injury*). Therefore, when examining eye injuries in children you should always consider if the injury you are seeing is consistent with the parent's report of the injury.

2. *When did the injury occur?* In some areas, patients may arrive days, or even weeks after the injury. This further complicates the treatment.

3. *Are there injuries to other parts of the body?* You have to decide which injuries are most serious and which require priority in treatment.

The exact history of the injury should be taken and very careful clinical notes of the injury made. After some injuries, such as road accidents, work injuries, non-accidental injury of children and assaults, there may be a medicolegal dispute or a claim for compensation. Detailed notes of exactly what the patient (or their parent) reported and your precise clinical findings are then very important.

Examination and assessment

The examination of an eye after an injury is essential, but may be difficult because of swelling, pain and bleeding. However, the upper and lower eyelids can usually be separated gently to allow measurement of the visual acuity and assessment of the pupils, eye movements and the eye itself. The examination may be difficult for several reasons: the patient may be shocked or frightened, and in pain. Topical anaesthetic drops and thorough drying of the area with clean gauze to stop your fingers slipping will make the examination much easier. Occasionally, it can be helpful to use a Desmarres retractor (after applying topical local anaesthetic drops) to open the lids. If there is a suspicion of a penetrating injury, it is important not to put too much pressure on the eyeball. Therefore, an examination under general anaesthetic may be advisable to allow a thorough search for any penetrations. Also, a general anaesthetic may be needed to examine children's eyes.

Eye injuries can be divided into seven common types:
1. Corneal and conjunctival foreign bodies, and corneal abrasions
2. Burns and chemical injuries
3. Non-penetrating, or blunt injuries to the eyeball
4. Penetrating injuries to the eye
5. Injuries to the eyelids
6. Orbital injuries
7. Cranial nerve injuries

Corneal and conjunctival foreign bodies and corneal abrasions

These are the most common eye injuries. They are especially common where there is dust, sand or other particles in the air and in people with exposure to lots of foreign bodies, such as farmers and tradesmen. Because the cornea is so sensitive, most patients are aware of any foreign body or abrasion. Some conjunctival and corneal foreign bodies are very small and need good magnification and a very careful examination to find them. In particular tiny hairs from certain caterpillars or insects or plants may become embedded in the conjunctiva or cornea. These are extremely hard to see except with the slit lamp, and they often cause great discomfort until they are found and removed.

Corneal foreign body

This may be on the surface of the cornea, or embedded in the cornea (**Figure 21.1**). Normally, it is easy to detect, but if it is dark-coloured, it may be more difficult to see against the pupil or a dark iris. Most corneal foreign bodies are very easy to remove. The method is described in **Box 21.1**:

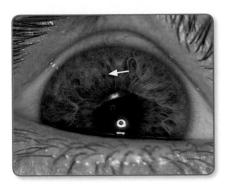

Figure 21.1 A small corneal foreign body just above the pupil (arrow). This is a fragment of metal that has rusted and therefore is brown in colour.

Box 21.1 Methods for removing and treating a corneal foreign body

1. Instill local anaesthetic drops in the eye.
2. Remove the foreign body with a sterile hypodermic needle
   - If the foreign body is on the cornea gently remove it with the edge of a sterile hypodermic needle.
   - If the foreign body is superficially embedded in the cornea, use the tip of the needle to pick it out
   - If the foreign body is deeply embedded in the corneal stroma, it may be necessary to use a sharp needle to lever it out, or it may be better to refer to a specialist.
   - If a fragment of iron is embedded in the cornea, it quickly forms an area of rust stained corneal stroma around it (a 'rust ring'). The rust ring will eventually disappear, but this can take months or even years and the rust may impair the healing of the cornea. It is therefore better to remove it either with the sterile needle or with a small dental burr.
3. Instill an antibiotic ointment, e.g. chloramphenicol and give the rest of the tube to the patient to use 3–4 times/day for 5–7 days.

Conjunctival foreign body

If the foreign body is on the conjunctiva covering the eyeball (the bulbar conjunctiva) it is usually easy to see. However it may be stuck to the inside of the upper eyelid when it is called a subtarsal foreign body. It will scratch the cornea each time the patient blinks and fine scratches may be seen on the surface of the cornea if it is examined with fluorescein stain and some magnification. Therefore, if a patient reports a foreign body sensation, but one is not immediately seen, it is always advisable to evert the upper lid (**Figure 21.2**). A cotton-wool bud is usually sufficient to wipe off bulbar or subtarsal conjunctival foreign bodies.

A corneal abrasion

This occurs when something rubs or scratches the eye, and removes some of the epithelium. Corneal abrasions are especially common among people

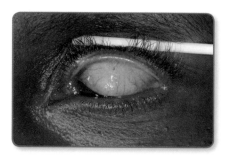

Figure 21.2 A subtarsal foreign body is easily seen by everting the upper lid.

who work in forests, and always produces severe pain and photophobia. There may be some redness of the eye, but otherwise it looks normal to the naked eye. However, fluorescein drops will immediately stain the corneal abrasion (**Figure 21.3a–c**).

Treatment of corneal abrasions

Most corneal abrasions heal without intervention. The patient can be given an antibiotic cream to minimise the risk of infection and slightly reduce the pain by protecting the raw corneal surface from being rubbed by the upper lid when blinking, although abrasions rarely get infected. If there is any risk of injury with vegetable matter, particularly in a hot humid climate, it is wise to apply a fungicide as well, if available (see page 206). Topical dilating drops can reduce the pain a little by preventing iris spasm, but are usually painful to instill. It is very important that the patient does not treat the pain with topical anaesthetic as this will impair the healing. The eye can be padded if the patient finds it more comfortable. The epithelium usually takes one or

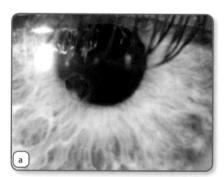

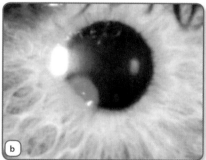

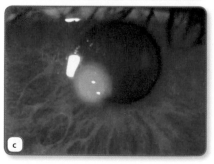

Figure 21.3 Corneal abrasion. (a) It is almost invisible with plain light. (b) The same corneal abrasion becomes obvious on applying fluorescein dye to the eye. (c) The fluorescein stain is even more obvious in blue light.

two days to recover. Specialist eye units sometimes stock very thin, soft contact lenses, with no refractive power, called 'bandage contact lenses' which may help a corneal abrasion to heal. They can be used if the abrasion is not healing after several days. They usually are left in for about 4–14 days. They must be used with topical antibiotics (ideally preservative free) as there is a risk of an infection developing under the lens.

Recurrent erosion (abrasion) syndrome

Occasionally, the epithelium of a corneal abrasion that has healed will lift up again without any trauma. This typically happens when the patient wakes up and opens their eyes in the morning, or if they rub their eyes. It can happen weeks or even months after the initial abrasion has healed. This is called recurrent abrasion syndrome. These patients should be given an antibiotic ointment or ocular lubricant cream or gel to use several times a day for several months to allow the epithelium to heal fully.

Burns and chemical injuries

Burns to the eyelids and eyes may be caused by open fires or chemicals. Most fire burns or scalds from boiling water occur in the home, either when small children have an accident or epileptics falling into the fire during a seizure. The eyelids will be damaged by heat or boiling water, but the blink reflex is so quick that the eyes themselves are often protected.

Treatment of eyelid burns

Topical antibiotics should be applied and also systemic antibiotics in severe cases. It is best not to pad the eye, but to let a firm scab develop. Severe burns will cause secondary skin contractures, and will need skin grafting later. If the eyelids do not cover the cornea at rest, then skin grafting is required as an emergency, and sometimes needs to be done several times during the recovery period. The blood supply to the eyelids is so good that partial thickness skin grafting is usually effective even if there is some infection in the burnt tissues.

Corneal and conjunctival chemical injuries

The eyes and conjunctiva can be seriously damaged by toxic fluids especially acids and alkalis. Chemical burns are common in industries that use irritant fluids such as acids, alkalis, cement or lime. Cement or wet plaster from buildings and acid from car batteries are the commonest chemical injuries at work. Chemicals are sadly sometimes used in assaults on people (**Figure 21.4**).

Alkali burns are particularly serious. Alkalis pass deeply into the tissues causing extensive melting, disruption and inflammation. In the acute stage, the cornea appears oedematous and the conjunctiva inflamed. If the burn is serious the limbal blood vessels become occluded causing the limbus to appear white, rather than red and inflamed as would be expected (**Figure 21.5a–c**). This is a bad sign and indicates severe tissue disruption which will progress to dense scarring and vascularisation of the cornea. Apart from corneal scarring there may be symblepharon formation and scarring and

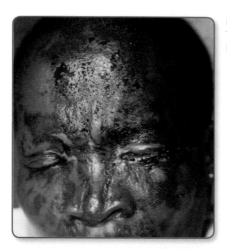

Figure 21.4 A lady assaulted with battery acid. The left eye was severely injured and the skin badly scarred.

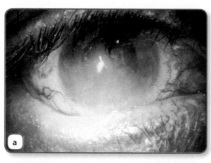

a

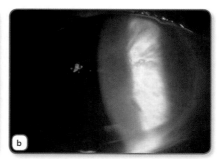

b

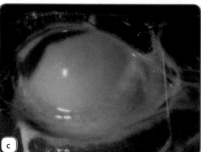

c

Figure 21.5 Alkali burns. (a) Initially this eye may not appear to be severely damaged. However, most of the limbus appears white from loss of the limbal blood vessels. The lower lid also shows some damage with destruction of the eyelashes. These signs are suggestive of a very severe injury. (b) This is another alkali injury. When the slit lamp is used to examine the eye, the cornea is seen to be oedematous. (c) This picture shows the same eye as (b) but with fluorescein dye instilled. This shows that the whole of the surface of the cornea has been damaged except for a very small part at the top.

contracture of the conjunctiva. If the whole epithelium has been dissolved by the chemical, it can be harder to detect with fluorescein dye than a localised area of loss. Therefore, if a generalised fluorescein haze is seen all over the cornea, it is likely that the whole epithelium has been dissolved and that it is a serious eye injury.

Emergency treatment of chemical burns to the conjunctiva and cornea

1. *First aid treatment.* First aid treatment is vital. The sooner the eye is irrigated with normal saline or even water, the better is the chance

of irrigating out the toxic chemical. The irrigation should be applied copiously for at least 10 minutes.

2. *Antibiotics.* Topical antibiotics as drops or ointment should be given to prevent secondary infection.
3. *Mydriatics* should be given to prevent iritis.
4. *Topical steroids.* These help to prevent some of the vascularisation and scarring and reduce the inflammation that occurs after a chemical injury. However, they also encourage the action of collagenase enzymes which are released from the damaged cornea and can cause further corneal destruction. A steroid drop should be used 2 hourly for about a week after the injury.
5. *Vitamin C tablets orally and ascorbic acid or citrate drops if available*: vitamin C is thought to reduce tissue destruction.

Long term treatment of eyes that have had severe chemical injuries

- *Delayed surgery:* Corneal scarring from burns does not respond very well to corneal grafting because the vascularisation causes graft rejection, and the damage to the corneal limbus prevents the graft developing a healthy epithelium.
- *Limbal autograft (**Figure 21.6**):* if only one eye has been damaged it may improve with a transplant of some of the limbus from the healthy eye to the damaged eye. The theory of this is that the limbal stem cells, which are responsible for producing healthy corneal epithelium, are destroyed in the injured eye. They are replaced with healthy stem cells from the other eye. This sort of treatment is usually done in specialised centres.
- *Keratoprosthesis (see Chapter 9):* placing a clear plastic window in the centre of the damaged cornea is the last resort, but may restore some vision at least for the short-term and occasionally in the long term. This is a very specialised procedure (see Figure. 9.31).

Non-penetrating, or blunt injuries to the eyeball

Blunt injuries may occur in many different circumstances such as fights, road accidents or sporting injuries. A blunt injury usually compresses the eye from front to back, which stretches it at the equator (**Figure. 21.7a and b**).

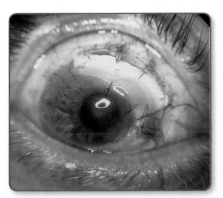

Figure 21.6 Limbal transplant.

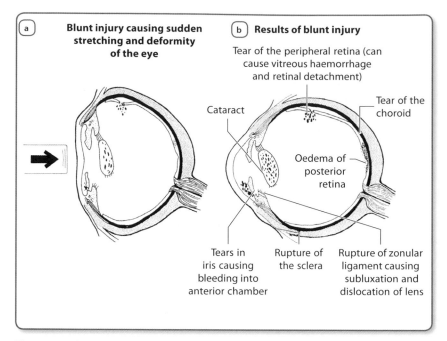

Figure 21.7 Blunt eye injuries. (a) Blunt injury causing sudden stretching and deformity of the eye. (b) Complications of a blunt injury to the eye.

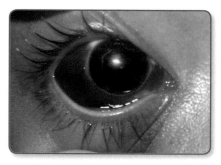

Figure 21.8 Bruised and swollen eyelids, conjunctival haemorrhage and hyphema (blood in the anterior chamber) following a blunt injury. An eye like this must be very carefully examined both at the time and a month later to exclude serious complications.

Complications of blunt injuries

Blunt injures can cause several possible complications:

Bleeding into the anterior chamber (hyphaema)

This is the most common complication. Usually, the blood comes from small blood vessels, which have torn at the base of the iris or in the ciliary body. At first, the red blood cells diffuse throughout the anterior chamber. Later they sink to the bottom of the anterior chamber to form a fluid level (**Figure 21.9a**). They are then gradually absorbed over several days (**Figure 21.9b**). In a very severe hyphaema, the whole of the anterior chamber may be full of blood clot. It will appear as a black opaque mass that obscures the iris and pupil, and is called a 'blackball' hyphaema. The excessive blood may also obstruct the drainage of aqueous fluid, causing secondary glaucoma. A

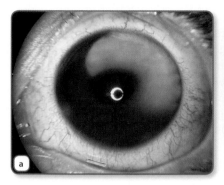 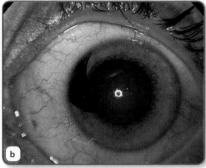

Figure 21.9 Hyphema. This patient suffered blunt trauma to the left eye. (a) Photograph taken 4 hours after the injury. The blood is still settling in the anterior chamber. The patient has been lying on their right hand side and therefore there is more blood on this side of the anterior chamber. (b) The same patient 2 days later. Most of the blood has been absorbed leaving a small clot on the side that the patient sleeps on.

blackball hyphaema together with a rise in intraocular pressure is a very bad sign. If red blood cells and their breakdown products enter the cornea and other eye structures, they leave deposits of blood pigment and cause permanently reduced vision (**Figure 21.10**).

Angle recession

Blunt trauma can cause the iris and ciliary body to become detached or stretched away from the sclera. Although the drainage angle looks wider and deeper on gonioscopic examination (see Chapter 15) it does not function normally and can causes long term pressure changes in the eye: either high pressure (glaucoma) or low pressure (hypotony).

Rupture of the suspensory ligament

The suspensory ligament supports the lens. Minor tears will partially dislocate the lens, causing it to tilt and lies asymmetrically in the eye. This results in refractive changes especially astigmatism and myopia. Severe tears may dislocate the lens completely, so that it falls into the vitreous body.

Delayed cataract

Delayed cataract sometimes follows a blunt injury, and is a result of concussion damage to the lens cells. It may develop months or even years later.

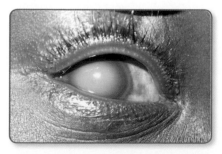

Figure 21.10 Staining of the cornea from a 'black ball' hyphema.

Peripheral retinal tear

A torn retina produces few if any symptoms, but can result in serious eye damage. It may cause a haemorrhage into the vitreous body, or progress later to a retinal detachment. After any blunt injury, the peripheral retina should be examined very carefully for a peripheral tear or dialysis. This is best done either with a slit lamp and a three-mirror contact lens or with an indirect ophthalmoscope, condensing lens and indentation of the peripheral retina. Retinal tears are easily treated, but if they are not detected, a retinal detachment will often develop.

Retinal oedema (commotio retinae)

This can be caused by concussion injury to the retina. The injury damages the blood-retinal barrier causing oedema to collect in the retina. The retina appears white and shiny, and because it cannot function normally, there is blurring of the vision (**Figure 21.11**). Retinal oedema often recovers fully, but if it is near the macula, it may cause some permanent macular scarring or a macular hole.

Choroidal tear

This will cause a choroidal haemorrhage, which will damage the overlying retina (**Figure 21.12**). If the choroidal tear is in the macula the visual acuity will be severely reduced.

Rupture of the eyeball

This is very rare, but if the force of the blunt injury is sufficient, it is possible for the sclera to rupture usually near the equator. A soft eye with a vitreous haemorrhage and a subconjunctival haemorrhage are suspicious signs of a scleral rupture. The prognosis for recovery of sight is usually poor.

Treatment of blunt injuries

Most blunt injuries do not require any special treatment. However, specific complications require treatment:
- *Hyphema:* the patient should rest until the blood settles. Intraocular blood can be quite inflammatory and therefore a topical steroid (e.g.

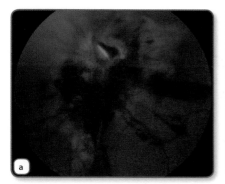 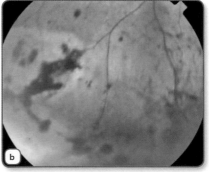

Figure 21.11 Commotio retinae. (a) This fundus has a severe injury with bleeding in the retina, behind the retina and into the vitreous at the posterior pole. The vision will be severely affected. (b) Peripheral commotio retinae. This is a less severe injury that normally resolves without significant problems, but can sometimes result in retinal detachment.

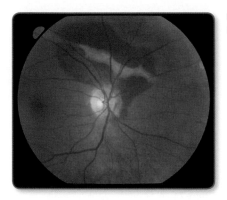

Figure 21.12 Choroidal tear with a haemorrhage on either side of the tear.

dexamethasone 0.1% 4–8 times daily) should be given. A mydriatic can help reduce any discomfort and it is possible it reduces the risk of a secondary bleed, by splinting the damaged blood vessels. If there is both a blackball hyphaema and a rise in intraocular pressure, the anterior chamber should be opened with a small limbal incision. The semi-solid blood clot should be then gently milked or irrigated out of the eye. Many surgeons advise carrying out an emergency trabeculectomy at the same time.

- *High intraocular pressure:* this may be caused by the hyphema, or by inflammation or by iris recession. The pressure should be treated with drops or acetazolamide. The increased pressure caused by hyphema and inflammation will settle as the eye recovers. However, pressure rises from iris recession may be a persistent problem.
- *Scleral rupture:* if this is suspected the patient must be taken to an operating theatre and the conjunctiva incised and the eye explored as far back as the equator to search for any ruptures.
- *Retinal tear or dialysis:* these are treated by laser and/or surgery. This treatment requires a retinal specialist and appropriate equipment.
- *Cataract:* surgical treatment of this may be very difficult if there is zonular weakness.

Penetrating injuries to the eye

Any sharp object or fragment that hits the eye can cause a penetrating injury. In urban communities, industrial and road accidents are the most common causes, but in rural communities, thorns or twigs are a more common cause. Most penetrating eye injuries are fairly easy to recognise (**Figure 21.13**). Occasionally, however, a very small fragment penetrates the eye at great speed, or the penetrating injury occurs through the lid and can be missed, unless the eyeball is carefully examined (**Figure 21.14a–c**). The fragment is usually of metal or stone and comes from grinding, chiselling or hammering. The patient sometimes may not realise that anything even entered the eye. The doctor too may not see either the very small entry wound or the foreign body in the eye.

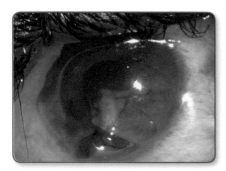

Figure 21.13 Corneal penetrating injury. This eye suffered an injury from a sharp object. The iris can be seen plugging the penetration and therefore the pupil is not round and is dragged towards the site of penetration.

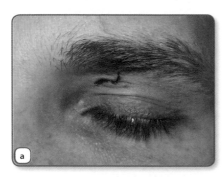

Figure 21.14 Scleral penetrating injury. (a) A small eyelid laceration that is hiding a potentially blinding scleral penetration. (b) The scleral penetration is visible when the lid is gently, but fully, retracted (c) The penetrating injury has been repaired with two sutures.

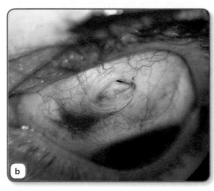

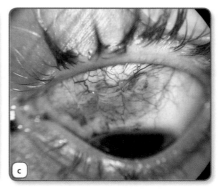

Signs of a corneal or scleral penetration

Penetrating injuries are usually obvious if the eye is carefully examined. However, commonly, injured eyes are not properly examined because of the pain, swelling or light sensitivity. The following signs are clues to the presence of a penetration:

- Uveal tissue prolapse through the wound: iris tissue often comes up to the wound and plugs the defect.
- Pupil distortion, caused by the iris tissue prolapse.
- Anterior chamber shallowing, caused by aqueous leakage. Aqueous leakage is seen by placing a drop of fluorescein dye on the eye, which can be seen flowing away from the site of leakage.
- A defect in the red reflex (**Figure 21.15a and b**)
- Cataract: if the penetrating object touches the lens it usually causes a cataract almost immediately.

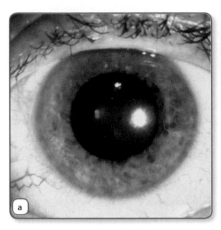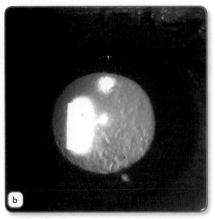

Figure 21.15 A small penetrating injury. (a) The injury is very difficult to see with normal torchlight. (b) The hole in the iris only becomes obvious when it is illuminated by the red reflex from an ophthalmoscope.

- Severe nausea or vomiting: if these are unexpectedly severe, a penetrating injury should be suspected.
- Although it is not a sign, always remember that the mechanism of injury is a very important guide. If the patient was using a sharp instrument or a wire, there is always a risk of a penetrating injury.

Complications of penetrating injuries

There are many possible complications from penetrating eye injuries:
- Corneal scar, from the entry wound.
- Cataract.
- Endophthalmitis (See Figure 12.24): this occurs commonly after penetrating injuries, particularly if a contaminated object enters the eye, such as a twig or other vegetable matter. It usually results in blindness.
- Uveitis and secondary glaucoma.
- Retinal detachment.
- Sympathetic ophthalmitis is a serious but rare complication (see Chapter 11, Figure 11.16).

Treatment of penetrating eye injuries

The visual acuity and the pupil light reflexes must be tested in patients with penetrating injuries. If there is no perception of light at all, it is safe to assume that the eye will never be able to see. However, treatment may still be required to prevent loss of the eyeball and to minimise the risk of sympathetic ophthalmitis. Both surgical and medical treatment may be needed.

Surgical treatment

Surgical treatment is often difficult. In ideal circumstances the aim of surgery is to suture close the cornea and the sclera, and also to replace into the eye any prolapsed uveal tissue. The cornea is sutured with very fine interrupted stitches of 10-0 nylon. The knots must be buried in the cornea and not left on the corneal surface or they will cause great irritation. If 10-0 nylon is not available, virgin silk is the next best suture. For the sclera, the sutures should be slightly less fine (e.g. 8-0), but should be buried under the conjunctiva. There are several factors that will influence the surgical treatment:

How recent was the injury?

If the injury was very recent and very clean it should be treated urgently (ideally the same day, but certainly within 24 hours). If there is a delay in surgical closure of the penetration, there is an increasing risk of endophthalmitis.

If the injury is more than 24 hours old or not so clean, it is probably better to excise any prolapsed uvea rather than try to replace it in the eye. This lessens the risk of infection.

If the injury happened some days previously, it may be best not even to suture it. The tissues will be very soft and friable and will bleed easily. Also there will be a high risk of introducing infection into the eye. In these circumstances it is better to cover the corneal wound by mobilising a flap of conjunctiva. If the corneal epithelium has already covered the wound (this will be shown by the wound not staining with fluorescein dye) it is best to give medical treatment only, and attempt any surgery after some weeks when all inflammation has subsided and the eye is quiet.

How extensive is the injury?

Many penetrating injuries are just puncture wounds and do not require suturing. The need to suture a wound increases as the size of the wound increases. The wound should be sutured if the uvea has prolapsed through the wound, or if aqueous fluid is leaking out preventing the anterior chamber from re-forming.

If the lens has been severely damaged by the injury, it is best to do an extracapsular cataract extraction before repairing the wound. As much of the cortical lens matter as possible should be removed by irrigating and aspirating with physiological saline solution.

If the eye is very severely damaged and there is definitely no perception of light at all, many people would advise surgically removing (eviscerating or enucleating) the eye rather than attempting to repair it. This avoids the slight risk of sympathetic ophthalmitis, and lengthy post-operative treatment. However, if there is any hope of saving any sight at all, it should not be removed. It can always be removed later if it becomes painful and blind.

What facilities and equipment are available?

If very fine sutures, needles and an operating microscope are not available, it is best not to attempt to repair the corneal wound, but just try to cover it with a flap of conjunctiva. Ideally, a general anaesthetic should be given, but a local anaesthetic nerve block is better than just local anaesthetic drops. If possible all penetrating eye injuries should be referred to a specialist, but often this is not possible.

Medical treatment

The medical treatment is important and must not be forgotten. The following measures should be taken:

- *Protection of the eye:* the patient must be clearly and firmly told not to rub the eye. A plastic shield or at very least a pad should be taped over the eye to protect the eye until the penetration is repaired.
- *Antibiotics:* all penetrating injuries have a high risk of causing intraocular infection. Therefore, every patient should receive both topical and systemic antibiotics. If any surgery is performed then a subconjunctival antibiotic and steroid injection is usually given as well immediately after the operation and intravitreal antibiotics (see page 85) should be considered if the penetrating object has a high chance of being contaminated.
- *Steroids:* once the risk of intraocular infection has passed (usually after 3 or 4 days), topical steroid drops or ointment should be given. Steroids help to reduce the inevitable uveitis and lessen the small risk of sympathetic ophthalmitis occurring in the uninjured eye. If the lens capsule has been punctured or the lens has been removed, steroids will suppress the uveitis caused by the leaking of lens protein into the eye. Steroids may also reduce the amount of corneal scarring at the penetration site.
- *Mydriatics:* all penetrating injuries should have mydriatics to stop anterior and posterior synechiae of the iris and to reduce pain.

Treatment of retained foreign bodies

If a small foreign body lodges inside the eye it can cause considerable damage, although the wound is usually self-sealing. Iron and copper particles should be removed, but other materials are best left in the eye. These cases need referral to a specialist centre.

Injuries to the eyelids

The eyelids are exposed. Therefore, injuries are frequent (**Figures 21.16**). However, they have a very good blood supply, and even extensive lacerations will heal well if they are sutured correctly. No knots or suture ends should rub against the cornea. Lacerations at the inner end of the eyelids may cut through the lacrimal canaliculi. Canalicular injuries are difficult to repair and ideally require a microscope and silicon tubes that are left in place for several weeks after the cut ends of the canaliculus are sewn back together. If these are not available, it is best just to suture the lid carefully. Bruising and oedema of the eyelids are very common, but usually subside fairly rapidly.

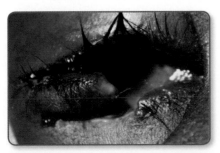

Figure 21.16 Lower eyelid trauma.

Orbital injuries

Orbital margin fractures

The orbital margin is thick, strong bone which protects the eye. It is quite often fractured in facial injuries. Serious fractures can be detected by feeling the orbital rim beneath the skin, and an X-ray will confirm the fracture. Surgical treatment is only necessary if the bones are displaced. In such cases, fractures of other facial bones are very likely, and it is usual for a maxillofacial surgeon to reduce and fix them.

Orbital floor fractures

Sometimes, blunt trauma such as a punch or a ball hitting the eye hard causes a fracture in the very thin floor or medial wall of the orbit. The injury compresses the eyeball into the orbit, and the thin bone gives way (**Figure 21.17**). This is called a *'blow-out' fracture* and the fracture itself is not important. The orbital floor is the most common site of these injuries and sometimes, the orbital fat or extraocular muscles are trapped in the fracture site. This limits the movement of the injured eye especially on looking up, and causes diplopia. There may also be some backward displacement of the eye (enophthalmos). Some damage to the infraorbital nerve usually occurs, causing numbness over the cheek, upper lip and teeth. Because the floor and walls of the orbit are so thin, special X-ray techniques or a CT scan are necessary to demonstrate the fracture. The symptoms of a blow-out fracture usually improve with time, but if the eye movements are severely limited, a surgical exploration of the floor of the orbit may be beneficial. The trapped orbital tissues can be freed and the orbital floor can be repaired.

Cranial nerve injuries

Cranial nerve injuries are quite common after head injuries. The cranial nerves which supply the eye and which are most likely to be damaged in this way are the second (optic), third (oculomotor), fourth (trochlear) and sixth (abducent) nerves.

Damage to the second nerve (optic nerve) is most common after an injury to the temple. It is usually caused by damage to the blood supply of the optic

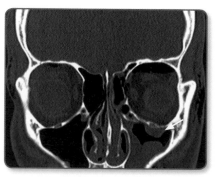

Figure 21.17 CT scan of a left orbital floor fracture. Soft tissue from the orbit has prolapsed into the maxillary sinus through fracture (arrow).

nerve where it enters the orbit through the optic canal. The sight in the eye will be affected, and there is usually no pupil response to light. The damage is usually permanent.

The third, fourth and sixth cranial nerves supply the extraocular muscles, and damage to these will produce diplopia (see Chapter 18). Damage to these nerves may gradually recover after a few months, or may be permanent. A dilated pupil in one eye after a head injury is a very important neurological sign. It may indicate there is raised intracranial pressure from an extradural haemorrhage in the skull pressing on the third nerve. This requires very urgent neurosurgical exploration to save the patient's life.

Prevention of eye injuries

Eye injuries are common and often cause loss of sight. Fortunately, it is unusual for both eyes to be affected in an injury. Therefore, blindness from eye injury is much less common than loss of sight in one eye. Eye injuries appear to be much more common in poor countries for two main reasons:

1. *The environment of a poor country.* Most people live in rural areas and young children often move about and play where there are bushes and trees with thorns and twigs, which may damage or penetrate the eye. Also, home circumstances with children playing near open fires put the eyes at risk.
2. *A lack of concern about safety and protection.* A typical local taxi is overcrowded, poorly maintained, without seat belts and often travelling too fast on poor roads. In construction work camps, people may be seen breaking up stones with a hammer without any eye protection. Sometimes people cannot afford to take the steps necessary to protect their eyes, but road safety and safety in the workplace can be promoted and encouraged. In most countries that have introduced simple laws, such as the wearing of seat belts and crash helmets, and have enforced them, there has been a large reduction in injuries, including eye injuries. Some simple regulations which could greatly reduce the number of eye injuries are:
   a. Regular inspection of the roadworthiness of public service vehicles.
   b. Compulsory fitting and wearing of seat belts in cars.
   c. Banning punishment in schools by slapping the face or the head of the pupil.
   d. Safety officers in factories.

Eye disease and visual impairment in children

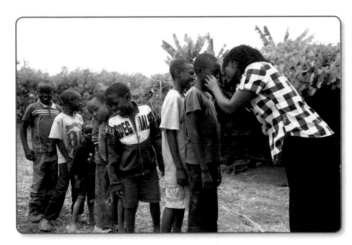

In some countries over half the population is under the age of 16.

The purpose of this chapter is to bring together some of the problems and challenges of children's eye disease and blindness. Many of the diseases have already been described in previous chapters, but here we concentrate on the particular problems of children. The Vision 2020 programme has given high priority to the prevention of blindness in children. There are several fairly obvious reasons for this:

1. Although there are many more blind adults than blind children, a blind child will have their whole life ahead of them rather than just their older years.

2. It is very difficult in poor countries for blind or visually impaired children to receive a satisfactory education.

3. Children are the most vulnerable members of society and need extra protection and care from health services.

4. Most childhood blindness in poor countries is preventable.

The WHO estimates that there are about 19 million visually impaired children in the world and 1.4 million who are irreversibly blind. However, this is almost certainly a serious underestimation of the problem for several reasons:

- Many blinding conditions like xerophthalmia are associated with a high mortality. Therefore, many children do not survive the disease that makes them go blind, but while they are alive they are unlikely to be included in surveys of visual impairment.

- Some statistics are obtained from blind schools. These often underestimate the burden as many blind children never even get to school.
- Children with multiple handicaps, such as blindness and learning delay are often not recorded either, as they may never leave their remote village.

This book has been structured rather like the anatomy of the eye. Most chapters describe the diseases of different parts of the eye like the cornea, the lens and the optic nerve. Most blindness surveys have a similar structure and so give the cause of blindness as corneal scar, cataract, optic nerve atrophy, etc. However, for children we find it more instructive to consider eye disease *according to the time at which the disease first developed.* The advantage of this classification is that it helps focus on what eye disease you might encounter if you see a child of a certain age and what can be done to prevent blindness.

Childhood blindness according to the time of onset

For any child there are four distinct times when a disease may begin:
1. Diseases starting at conception or in the early embryonic stages. These are mostly genetic diseases, and difficult or impossible to prevent. However, their incidence may be reduced by genetic counselling.
2. Diseases starting in the fetus during pregnancy. These are mostly maternal infections, which pass across the placenta to affect the fetus. They are often preventable.
3. Diseases starting at the time of birth. These are mostly preventable.
4. Diseases starting in childhood. These are mostly preventable.

Disease starting at conception or in the embryo

These diseases are caused by genetic mutations and variations. Human have paired genes. Children inherit one gene from the mother and its partner from the father. Therefore, there is the possibility of inheriting a faulty, disease causing gene from either or both parents. Alternatively, the genes can become damaged at conception or in the early embryonic stages of development, even though they were normal when they were inherited from the parents. Faulty genes that are inherited from the parents can be passed on to the child by any of the following genetic patterns:
1. *Autosomal dominant*: the child only needs to inherit one faulty gene (from either parent) in order to develop the disease. If either parent has the faulty gene they will of course also have the disease, and therefore it is often not a surprise that the child develops the same disease.
2. *Autosomal recessive*: the child will only inherit the disease if they inherit a faulty copy of the gene or part of gene from both parents. The parents usually do not know that they are carrying the faulty gene, as they usually have one faulty gene and one normal gene preventing them from having the disease. Therefore, if both parents have one faulty gene and one normal gene, the child has a 25% chance of inheriting both faulty genes and having the disease.

3. *Sex linked*: in these diseases the gene is inherited from the special chromosome that determine whether we are male or female (the X and Y chromosome, which are called the 'sex-chromosomes')
4. *Mitochondrial*: these diseases are very rare. Mitochondria are parts of human cells that produce energy and they have their own DNA. Mitochondrial DNA comes from the mother. Therefore if the child inherits faulty mitochondrial DNA from the mother they are likely to develop the disease.

There are many thousands of genetically inherited diseases. Many of these have some effect on the eye or vision, because the eye has a very special embryological development; it originates very early from the neural tube, the ectoderm, the neural crest and the mesoderm. Therefore, genetic abnormalities of the body have a high chance of affecting one part or another of the eye. Genetically inherited diseases occur more frequently in communities where consanguinity (marrying a close relative, or 'cousin marriage') is common. Such marriages are particularly common in certain cultures and it is only with education and greater understanding that communities will become aware of its problems. It has been estimated that about 10% of births from a cousin marriage will either be stillborn or have a significant congenital abnormality.

A few of the more common (although still very rare) genetically inherited eye diseases are described in **Table 22.1**. At present, most of these genetic conditions cannot be prevented or treated but fortunately they are all very rare. Although the underlying genetic problem cannot be corrected, sometimes, the ocular problem that it causes can be treated, e.g. glaucoma, cataract and retinoblastoma. When eye disease is seen in a young infant, such as cataract or glaucoma, it can be difficult to determine if the disease is genetic or has developed later in the fetus or even very early after birth. For example, a cataract in a 6-month-old baby, can be genetically inherited or can come from maternal rubella during pregnancy, or could be from trauma to the eye (possibly non-accidental injury).

Table 22.1 Some of the more important genetically inherited eye diseases		
Disease	**Inheritance pattern**	**Effect of disease**
Retinitis pigmentosa	Can occur with autosomal recessive, dominant, sex linked and mitochondrial diseases	The retinal pigment epithelium slowly stops functioning normally, causing the retina to stop working. See page 341 for more details
Ocular albinism and oculocutaneous albinism	Mainly X-linked	Lack of pigment in the eyes (oculi) and skin (cutaneous) and sometimes the hair. See page 342 for more details
Retinoblastoma	Autosomal recessive	Intra-ocular tumour of the inside of the eye. This can occur in one or both eyes and if not treated will cause visual loss and then death if not treated. See page 349 for more details
Leber's hereditary optic neuropathy	Mitochondrial	The optic nerve stops functioning normally (optic neuropathy, see Chapter 14) in one eye first and then the other eye soon after. Therefore vision is lost in both eyes.

The science of genetics is advancing very rapidly and it is likely that something can be done for future generations with genetic disease. At present the only means of prevention is to give genetic counselling where there is a family history of hereditary disease, or in communities where 'cousin marriage' is common. Communities which encourage marriage between cousins sometimes do so in the hope of keeping 'bad blood' out of the family when in fact it tends to lead to the opposite.

Disease starting during pregnancy

The growing fetus can be affected in several different ways:
- Infections in the mother may pass across the placenta and damage the fetus (congenital infections).
- Medicines, alcohol, non-medical/illegal drugs and smoking can all affect the fetus. Most of these substances do not specifically cause eye disease, although optic atrophy can be part of foetal alcohol syndrome.
- Some chronic maternal diseases, such as diabetes and hypertension, can affect the fetus
- Severe ill-health or malnutrition of the mother can affect the fetus.

Any of the above can cause generalised developmental abnormalities, which of course may also affect visual development and/or cause squints. However, the most common and most serious problem encountered by the growing fetus is congenital infections.

Congenital infections

The most dangerous time is early pregnancy, particularly around the third month. Many of these infections are very mild in the adult and produce hardly any or no symptoms. But they may cause widespread damage in the fetus because their immune system is not well developed and their embryological development may be disturbed. The more common and serious infections are:

Rubella (German measles)

Maternal rubella infection can cause serious foetal abnormalities. The earlier the infection occurs, the more serious the effects are. The major systemic effects are: learning delay, congenital heart disease, deafness, microcephaly and foetal death. The major ocular effects are: microphthalmos (a very small eye), keratitis, cataract, glaucoma, retinopathy (this is sometimes described as a 'salt and pepper' retinopathy because of its appearance) and optic nerve hypoplasia.

Toxoplasmosis

Toxoplasmosis is a rather confusing disease, because the primary infection and reactivations can occur in humans at different ages causing very different effects. Congenital infection is the most severe, although fortunately most infections do not cause any effect at all. The classic three effects of congenital toxoplasmosis are: hydrocephalus, intracranial calcification and chorioretinitis, although there are numerous other possible effects including myocarditis, encephalitis and in the eye: microphthalmos, panuveitis, cataracts and optic atrophy. The *toxoplasmosis gondii* organism can remain dormant in cysts in the retina and reactivate later in life causing retinal scarring (see Chapter 13).

Human immunodeficiency virus (HIV)

Although this may not cause serious immediate effects in the baby, it is in many ways the most devastating infection to cross the placenta. Unfortunately, in many poor communities, babies born with HIV have little hope of reaching adult life. This is gradually changing with more effective anti-retroviral treatment, but these children are likely to have very short lives with multiple HIV and AIDS related illnesses. The HIV epidemic has also caused a marked increase in other infections like toxoplasmosis and cytomegalovirus.

Other congenital infections

- *Cytomegalovirus*: maternal infection only affects the fetus in approximately 10% of cases. However, it can cause microcephaly, epilepsy, cerebral palsy and deafness. In the eye it can cause chorioretinitis and optic atrophy.
- *Syphilis*: congenital syphilis is rare. It is most damaging in the 2nd and 3rd trimesters. In the eye it can cause interstitial keratitis, uveitis, chorioretinitis and optic atrophy and systemically it causes deafness, and dental abnormalities.

Prevention of congenital infections

- Rubella during pregnancy can be reliably and easily prevented by vaccinating all girls before puberty. This may be done as part of a vaccination package in infancy (MMR: measles, mumps and rubella) or separately later.
- Maternal toxoplasmosis can be reduced by careful preparation of food and cooking of meat and by avoiding touching cat faeces.
- Maternal syphilis can and must be treated with penicillin.
- HIV transmission to the fetus can be reduced by very careful use of antiretroviral treatment in the mother at the time of labour and by not breastfeeding the child.

Diseases starting at birth

The two most important of these are ophthalmia neonatorum (neonatal conjunctivitis) and retinopathy of prematurity.

Ophthalmia neonatorum

This has been discussed in detail in Chapter 7 (Figures 7.9 and 7.10). It should not be a public health problem with good antenatal care to treat vaginal infections in the mother before birth, good asepsis at delivery, and prophylactic treatment for the baby's eyes. In most poor countries, the majority of births are conducted by traditional birth attendants rather than midwives. They perform a vital role and there is a need to give them appropriate training about eye health.

There is quite a high prevalence of vaginal infections, especially of sexually transmitted diseases like gonorrhoea, amongst certain groups and societies. Routine eye prophylaxis should be given for children born to these mothers. Tetracycline 1.0% ointment and/or povidone iodine 5% (remember it normally comes as 10% solution so it will need to be diluted with sterile water) are probably the best treatments as they are effective, cheap and widely available. An additional benefit of povidone iodine is that because it is coloured brown, the nurse or mother can be sure that the drops have gone into the eye. Silver nitrate 1.0% was widely used in the past but is no longer recommended because it may burn the cornea and is not very effective against chlamydial infections.

Retinopathy of prematurity (ROP)

ROP is the abnormal continued development of the retinal blood vessels and the retina in babies who are born very prematurely (**Figure 22.1**). It is one of the unfortunate complications of good medical care. Where medical care is not available, most premature infants who are born before the 30th week of gestation will die. With good care many of these children now survive, but they are at risk of blinding ROP. The retinal vasculature begins to develop at approximately 16 weeks of gestation. The vessels grow out of the optic disc. The nasal vessels are usually complete by about 32 weeks and the whole retina at full term (40–42 weeks). For reasons that are not yet clear, when a baby is born very prematurely the retinal vessels do not always continue to develop normally, i.e. ROP. The more premature and smaller the baby is, the higher the risk. Other risk factors include poor control of oxygen levels and being sick with other medical conditions in the early neonatal period. In very premature children (some babies born at 23 weeks now survive), ROP may even develop in spite of careful monitoring.

Grading of ROP

ROP is classified into four different grades:
- *Stage 1*: the peripheral retina is avascular, in particular the peripheral part of the temporal retina. There is usually a white line separating the normal and the vascular retina.
- *Stage 2*: a ridge develops between the normal retina and the peripheral avascular retina.
- *Stage 3*: new blood vessels and fibrous tissue develop from this ridge into the vitreous. These blood vessels may bleed into the retina or the vitreous.
- *Stage 4*: tractional retinal detachment. This is caused by the activity of the fibroblasts and the blood vessels and is usually untreatable. These children will be blind in the affected eye(s).

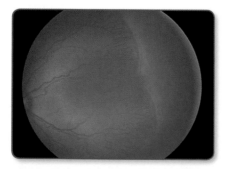

Figure 22.1 Retinopathy of prematurity stage 3 'plus disease'. The vascular ridge in the periphery of the retina has new vessels. The retina beyond the ridge contains no blood vessels. The main retinal vessels are tortuous and very slightly dilated showing early 'plus' disease (the slightly blue colour is an artefact of the camera).

- *Stage 5*: total (funnel-shaped) retinal detachment.
- *Plus disease*: this is increased dilatation and tortuosity of the retinal blood vessels. It can occur in association with any of the five stages and indicates more active disease, i.e. likely to progress to at least stage 3 and much more likely to need to need treatment.

Screening of ROP

The guidelines may vary slightly in different countries, but in general, all babies who are born at age less than 30 weeks should be screened and babies between aged 30 and 32 weeks should be screened if they are of lower than 1500 g of birth-weight. Screening generally starts at 4–5 weeks after birth as ROP does not develop before this time. Screening should continue weekly until a healthy retina has developed.

In order to do the screening, the pupils should be dilated with 0.5% cyclopentolate and 2.5% phenylephrine (not 10%, which must only be used in adults) and if possible the eye examined with an indirect ophthalmoscope as this gives a much better view of the peripheral retina. Using a red free (green) light can make it easier to see the blood vessels.

Who to treat

The most important part of treatment is deciding which babies need treatment. Research has shown that treatment should be given to all babies with stage 3 or higher disease and should be considered for babies with stage 2 with plus disease. Treatment must also be given for all babies whose retinal vessels have not yet grown outside the very central area of the retina (zone 1, which is a circle around the optic nerve with a radius of double the distance between the optic nerve and the fovea). Grade 1 and 2 disease almost never requires treatment unless there is plus disease.

How to treat ROP

The main aim of treating ROP is to scar the areas of peripheral retina that the retinal vessels have failed to reach (areas of avascular retina). The scarring of these areas, stops them releasing chemicals such as vaso-active endothelial growth factor (VEGF) that stimulate the abnormal blood vessel development. The scarring can be done in two ways:

1. Laser, i.e. burning of the retina.
2. Cryotherapy, i.e. freezing of the retina.

Both of these procedures can be very difficult to do in tiny babies, and require ophthalmological expertise as well as support from specialised paediatricians and possibly anaesthetists. It is absolutely essential that the cryotherapy or laser treatment is given at the right time. This 'window' for treatment is quite small, only about 2–4 weeks. Before that time, ROP will not develop and after that time, treatment will be too late. The danger period for the development of ROP is between 5 weeks after birth and 42 weeks gestational age. In the last few years, some people have started treating severe ROP with intravitreal injections of an anti-VEGF agent (Avastin). This does appear to initially stop the disease progressing, but the long-term effects are not known, and there is of course a small risk of serious eye damage from the injection.

Birth injuries

Asphyxia during birth is more common where there are poor obstetric services. The central nervous system is the most sensitive part of the body to anoxia, and there may be damage to the optic nerves or the visual cortex in the brain. Birth injuries directly to the eye are less common, although it is possible for the eyes or eyelids to be damaged during a difficult forceps delivery.

Herpes simplex virus (HSV) keratitis

If a mother has genital HSV infection, the baby is at risk of becoming infected during a vaginal delivery. It does not usually cause severe effects, although occasionally it can cause conjunctivitis, keratitis, cataracts and chorioretinitis, as well as systemic effects including hepatitis, pneumonia and encephalitis.

Diseases starting in infancy and childhood

Refractive error

The most common treatable cause of visual impairment is refractive error. It is often not detected, or correctly prescribed glasses are not available, leaving the children either with poor vision in both eyes or at high risk of developing amblyopia in one eye (see Chapter 18).

Corneal disease

Corneal ulcers are the commonest cause of irreversible visual loss in children in poor countries. The most common causes of these ulcers are:
- Vitamin A deficiency (xerophthalmia). This is described in Chapter 10.
- Measles, which often occurs together with vitamin A deficiency to cause devastating ulcers.
- Toxic traditional eye medicines.
- Herpes simplex keratitis.
- Trachoma: although children are not blinded by trachoma, the long damaging and ultimately blinding process starts in childhood. It is described in Chapter 8.

Optic nerve and cerebral disease

Acute illnesses and fevers in children such as malaria, typhoid and meningitis can damage either the optic nerves causing *optic atrophy* or the visual cortex causing *cortical blindness*.

Trauma

Trauma becomes increasingly common in older children as they play and run around, especially where there is thorny vegetation. Fortunately, trauma nearly always affects only one eye, leaving the other eye intact. In reality it is difficult to prevent young children from playing and putting their eyes at risk to injuries.

Vision testing in children

Ideally, all children should have a sight test and an eye examination before going to primary school or when even younger. Children who cannot go to school also need similar care. Primary and community based health care for eye disease is much more important for pre-school and early school age children than any other age group. In particular, it should be possible to detect and treat the following conditions:

- Xerophthalmia
- Refractive errors and amblyopia
- Trachoma

The global distribution of child blindness

The prevalence of the different causes of child blindness varies greatly from country to country and region to region.

Xerophthalmia is only found where there are extremes of poverty and deprivation. It is always under-reported because so many of these children never receive any medical care at all and many of them will die. Fortunately, several surveys have shown that even in very poor countries corneal blindness is becoming less common, but it still remains the most important cause of child blindness worldwide, and by far the most important cause of preventable child blindness. *Measles vaccination* is usually the single most effective way of reducing corneal blindness in children.

Retinopathy of prematurity is mainly a problem in middle-income communities. In the richest, it can be prevented by careful oxygen monitoring, or treated with cryotherapy or laser. In the poorest countries it is not seen, because very premature children will not usually survive.

Congenital cataract (see Chapter 12) is a major problem in all societies. It can and must be treated, although the vision may never be normal in the treated eye and the surgical and post-operative treatment of childhood cataract is a great challenge and requires high quality paediatric ophthalmic surgical services. Cataract from congenital rubella is preventable by maternal vaccination, but the other genetic and unknown causes of congenital cataract cannot be prevented.

Genetically inherited causes of blindness are extremely varied but their incidence is very much higher where cousin marriage is culturally acceptable, especially in the Middle East and West Asia. The prevalence of congenital cataract is higher in these areas.

Table 22.2 is a summary of what can be done to prevent visual impairment and blindness in children.

Problems and challenges in the clinical care of children with eye disease

The first half of this chapter looked at the community aspect of visual impairment in children. The second half looks at clinical aspects. The clinical care of children with eye disease is more difficult and challenging than for adults at every stage; history taking and visual assessment, clinical examination, diagnosis, refraction and treatment can all be difficult.

Taking the history and assessing the vision

This is much harder with young children and infants. In younger children, the history depends entirely on what the family say about the child and even

Table 22.2 Summary of prevention of blindness in children

Condition	Prevention	Treatment
Genetic disorders	Genetic counselling. Education about the risks of marrying close relatives	Very few genetic diseases can be treated
Congenital rubella*	Maternal vaccination	None
Ophthalmia neonatorum*	Good antenatal care and treatment of maternal genital infection	Urgent treatment of neonates with purulent conjunctivitis
Retinopathy of prematurity	High quality care of premature infants	Retinal laser or cryotherapy. Possibly intravitreal anti-VEGF injection
Congenital cataract	Not preventable except from rubella	Cataract surgery and specialist paediatric ophthalmology care
Congenital glaucoma	Not preventable	Glaucoma surgery and specialist paediatric ophthalmology care
Xerophthalmia*	Vitamin A supplements Nutritional advice	Vitamin A supplements
Measles*	Vaccination	Vitamin A supplements will minimise the extent of measles corneal ulcers if vitamin A deficiency also present
Toxic traditional eye medication (TEM)	Education	Thorough wash out with water or saline if the child is seen soon after the TEM has been used
Amblyopia*	Treat causative pathology, e.g. cataract, ptosis, large chalazions	Patching or atropine for better eye
Refractive error*	Not possible	Carefully prescribed glasses

* Should be fairly easily treated and it is a great failing of governance and health systems if they are not.

older children might find it difficult to give a clear history. The younger the child, the more difficult it is to assess the vision (see page 50). Patience and encouragement, and the correct use of simple equipment, are the best ways to assess the vision of young children, and it is surprising how in the right circumstances very young children will co-operate if encouraged.

Examining the eyes of children

This is also difficult, and the most important thing is to gain the child's confidence so they are not frightened or tearful. Techniques are described on page 73 to restrain either neonates, who are too young to co-operate, or older children who refuse to co-operate, but wherever possible restraint should not be used. Patience, by allowing a child to run around and make themselves at home in a busy clinic, may well be rewarded by a co-operative patient. Sometimes a nervous or frightened child will be encouraged by examining older children or a sibling first, and if there are drops to put in a child's eye, for instance to dilate the pupil, it may be best to get the mother to apply the drops. A child who has a happy experience in the eye clinic will be happy to return. However, a child who is scared and needs to be restrained may be reluctant to attend any clinic in future years. Sometimes either sedation or general anaesthetic is needed to carry out a complete examination in a child. Ketamine is an extremely useful, safe and quick-acting drug for providing anaesthesia for eye examination in children, but it does not prevent eye movements.

Making the diagnosis

Diagnosis can be difficult for several reasons:
- A thorough examination and vision assessment may not have been possible.
- Health practitioners are often not familiar with the common causes of visual loss in children, which are different from adults.
- There are often many rare and unusual causes of blindness and visual loss in children.

The single most useful test in trying to make a diagnosis is the pupil light reflex. Retinal or optic nerve disease will always have a diminished or absent pupil light reflex. Diseases of the ocular media like cataract, and also amblyopia and cortical blindness have normal pupil light reflexes. The second most useful test is the corneal light reflex to see if there is a squint. Nearly all children who are blind will squint; although, not all children who squint are blind. Young children who are blind in one eye only do not usually complain of poor vision. Even if the disease can be treated, the eye is probably amblyopic, and treatment will not greatly improve the sight.

Refracting young children

This is also harder in young children than in adults. Refractive errors are common in children, but because accommodation is so active in children, the ciliary muscle must be paralysed with cycloplegic drops in order to do an objective refraction. A subjective refraction alone (see page 109) is not good enough for young children but may be possible in older children.

Treatment

One of the particular problems in caring for children's eye disease is the difficulty and complexity of the treatment, especially surgical treatment. Furthermore the medical and surgical treatment of childhood eye disease usually requires many years of follow-up. Some examples of this are:
- *Cataract in childhood*: the surgical treatment of cataract in childhood is both much more difficult and much more controversial than in adults. Most experts advise intraocular lens implants nowadays for children, but the operation is technically harder, and the posterior capsule will always opacify. For those without special training it is safer to just wash out the cataract with a two way syringe and carry out a posterior capsulotomy later, and prescribe aphakic glasses. These children will need refractive assessments and appropriate treatment for many years as well as, treatment (possibly several times) of the posterior capsular opacification.
- *Childhood glaucoma*: medical treatment is of little value. The only possible treatment is surgical which is technically much harder than the surgical treatment of glaucoma in adults. These children will require pressure measurements for many years, and may need several surgical procedures and pressure lowering drops.

The eye in systemic disease

There are certain systemic diseases of children where a careful eye examination can give essential information. The most important two conditions are miliary tuberculosis and malaria.

Cerebral malaria

Cerebral malaria is an extremely dangerous condition with a high mortality rate. Very urgent and intensive treatment is required. The retinal changes of cerebral malaria have only recently been properly recognised and described. However, they are fairly distinctive and so very helpful in both diagnosing and treating this lethal disease. About 40% of children with cerebral malaria will have changes in the retina, and often the extent of these changes will indicate the severity of the cerebral malaria, i.e. extensive retinal changes indicates a very severely ill child who is near to death but can still recover with prompt and effective treatment. If the retina is normal, then the prognosis is better. The changes are mainly caused by the large number of red blood cells that contain malarial parasites. These stick to the walls of the fine blood vessels causing a loss of blood supply and oxygenation of the tissues. The following changes may be seen (**Figure 22.2**):

- The smaller vessels may be very pale or white because of the poor blood flow. Sometimes they may look orange in colour from the appearance of the red blood cells that are damaged by the malarial parasites and sticking to the vessel wall. The larger retinal blood vessels usually appear normal.
- Parts of the retina may look white. These white patches may be caused by retinal oedema due to poor blood supply.
- There may be scattered round haemorrhages in the retina.

Miliary tuberculosis

Miliary tuberculosis is often a difficult diagnosis to make, but untreated the child will die. One of the earliest and most reliable signs is to detect the lesions of miliary tuberculosis in the choroid (Figure 11.27). It is also a good way of checking the progress of the disease by seeing if the lesions are healing.

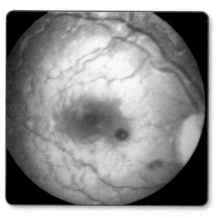

Figure 22.2 Malarial retinopathy. The main vessels appear normal but the smaller vessels are pale. Large areas of the retina are white and there is an obvious round retinal haemorrhage.

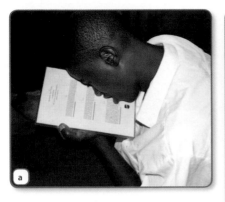

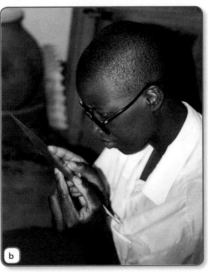

Figure 22.3 The benefits of appropriate refractive correction. (a) This visually impaired boy can just read with his eye right next to the card.(b) With corrective glasses, the child can read at a normal distance and therefore is much more likely to progress in school.

Low visual aids education and rehabilitation

Most 'blind' children do not have a visual acuity of 'no perception of light' but have some vision. Visual aids or even just the correct glasses (**Figure 22.3**) (See Chapter 5) enable the child to make the best use of that vision, and often with a visual aid and assistance a child can be taught by sighted methods rather than Braille. Unfortunately, in countries where it is difficult for a child with normal vision to receive an education, it is even more of a struggle for a visually impaired child. Where education for the blind is good, many blind people progress to university degrees and play a full part in all aspects of life.

23 Diagnosis of common eye conditions

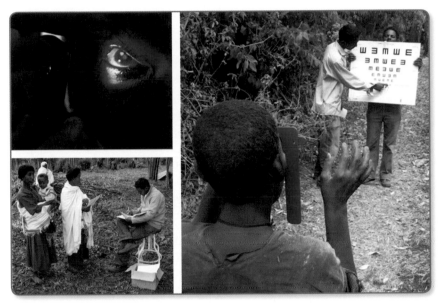

Take a good history, test the vision carefully with and without a pinhole, and examine the patient thoroughly. You are likely to be rewarded with the correct diagnosis and the patient can receive the correct treatment.

Diagnosis is the most important step in the care of an individual patient. The purpose of the history and examination is to make the diagnosis, and having made the diagnosis the correct treatment can then be given (**Figure 23.1**). If the diagnosis is wrong, then the treatment will also probably be wrong. The individual eye conditions are discussed in the other chapters of the book; the purpose of this chapter is to look at how to make the right diagnosis.

Diagnosis is sometimes difficult even for the specialist. It is not surprising that the non-specialist, the nurse or the pimary health worker finds diagnosis of eye diseases to be a great challenge. The equipment may seem daunting, complicated and difficult to use and the names used in ophthalmology are frequently confusing. However, a short and clear history, an assessment of the vision and a careful examination with a few basic instruments should provide enough information to diagnose most eye patients correctly.

Diagnosis is more difficult in the early stages of a disease, but becomes easier as the signs and symptoms become more obvious. This means that di-

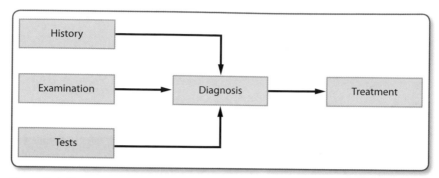

Figure 23.1 How investigations allow a diagnosis to be made and correct treatment to be given.

agnosis is usually easier in areas where medical facilities are poor and where patients usually come at an advanced stage of the disease. But of course this means that for some eye conditions there is less hope for treatment and recovery of vision.

By far the two most important problems in ophthalmology are firstly, loss of vision and secondly, a painful or inflamed eye.

Loss of vision

Loss of vision is the most important symptom of eye disease. The major causes of visual loss can be divided into five groups (**Table 23.1**):
1. *Refractive errors.* The patient needs spectacles.
2. *Opacities in the ocular media.* These prevent the light rays reaching the retina. These patients will have painless loss of vision. An examination with an ophthalmoscope will show either an absent or a poor red fundus reflex.
3. *Retinal or optic nerve diseases.* These patients also have painless loss of vision, but the red reflex is clearly visible with an ophthalmoscope.
4. *Acute inflammatory eye disease and acute glaucoma.* This causes loss of vision and a painful red eye.
5. Conditions in which the eye appears normal but the patient can't see properly. The problem may be in the brain (e.g. stroke or cortical blindness page 368), in visual development (amblyopia page 438) or functional visual loss/hysteria/malingering (i.e. the patient is pretending to have visual loss).

Refractive errors

The patient has painless, reduced vision. However, the patient's vision improves with a pinhole (see page 50). The pinhole test is very simple and one of the most important tests in ophthalmology; if the reduced vision improves through the pinhole, it usually means that the vision can be corrected with glasses and if the vision is normal through the pinhole it almost always means that there is not significant or advanced eye disease. There are some exceptions to the pinhole test for refractive error: in particular the vision

Table 23.1 The four major groups of diseases causing visual loss

Group of Diseases	Common diagnoses	Characteristic signs and symptoms	Treatment
Refractive errors	Myopia Hypermetropia Presbyopia Astigmatism	Vision improves with pinhole	Spectacles
Ocular media opacities	Lens opacities Corneal scars/opacities Vitreous opacities	No pain 'White' (not inflamed) eye Reduced or altered red reflex	• Cataract: elective treatment • Cornea: prevent further scarring • Vitreous: no treatment
Retina and optic nerve	Retinal disease: – Degeneration – Vascular disease – Retinal detachment – Chorioretinitis Optic nerve disease: – Optic atrophy – Optic neuritis – Open-angle glaucoma	No pain 'White' (not inflamed) eye Normal red reflex	• Very urgent treatment for some diseases, e.g. retinal detachment, nutritional optic neuropathy • Glaucoma: chronic treatment • Other diseases not treatable, e.g. optic atrophy, retinal dystrophy
Acute inflammatory eye disease and acute glaucoma	Corneal ulcer Acute anterior uveitis Acute glaucoma	Pain 'Red' (inflamed) eye Light sensitivity (photophobia)	Emergency medical treatment and sometimes surgical treatment

may improve with a pinhole in patients who have an early cataract or some irregularity in the cornea such as scarring or keratoconus. Often, patients with refractive errors screw up their eyelids to make their own pinhole, and they usually see better in bright light when the pupil constricts.

Refractive errors start at different ages:

- Hypermetropia and astigmatism are present from birth, but young children can overcome hypermetropia by accommodating.
- Myopia usually starts between 5 and 15 years, but very rarely it is present at birth.
- Presbyopia starts at 40 years, and progresses until 60 years.

Most eyes with refractive errors are otherwise normal, although the following associated conditions should be looked for:

- Children with refractive error in one eye are very likely to develop amblyopia in that eye. This is irreversible and therefore the refractive error must be treated (Chapter 18)
- Some diseases cause refractive changes, e.g. early nuclear sclerotic cataract causes an increase in myopia and corneal scars can cause irregular astigmatism. Pressure on the back of the eye from tumours and swelling in the orbit can cause hypermetropic change.
- Adults with very myopic eyes (approximately worse than -10) can develop degenerative changes at the macula with wet macular degeneration and have a higher risk of retinal detachment.

- Quickly progressing myopia and astigmatism is suggestive of keratoconus, which is a disease in which the cornea gradually develops an abnormal shape (see Chapter 9).

Opacities in the ocular media

Opacities are very common in the lens, quite common in the cornea, and less common in the vitreous. Dense cataracts and large or dense corneal ulcers can usually be seen without any specialised equipment. However, the best way to assess the density and position of an opacity anywhere in the ocular media is to dilate the pupil and examine the red fundus reflex with an ophthalmoscope, and if the condition is unilateral, to compare it with the other eye:

- An absent or much reduced red reflex indicates a dense opacity.
- A shadow or irregularity in the red reflex indicates a slight opacity.

Small opacities that only cast a shadow in the red reflex may be difficult to locate. The best way to locate them is to bring them into focus using a positive lens in the ophthalmoscope:

- Opacity in front of the plane of the iris is probably in the cornea.
- Opacity behind the plane of the iris is probably in the lens.
- An opacity behind the plane of the iris that moves when the eye moves is probably in the vitreous.

Lens opacities can be treated with cataract extraction, as long as the retina and optic nerve are healthy. Corneal opacities can sometimes be treated, but this requires highly specialised surgery that is rarely available in poor countries and has very variable outcomes.

One common diagnostic problem is to assess whether there is retinal or optic nerve disease when opacities in the ocular media obscure the fundus. The light projection test is a simple test of a normal retina and optic nerve (see page 49). The pupil reflexes are also a good test (see page 69). A brisk pupil reflex indicates a healthy retina and optic nerve, and an absent pupil reflex indicates a diseased optic nerve or retina. However, there are exceptions:

- Dilating drops: if the patient or the health worker has put dilating drops in the eye, it will not react. However the relative afferent pupillary defect test will still be normal.
- Adhesions between the iris and lens: these prevent the iris reacting and constricting.
- There are a few rare diseases that prevent the pupil reacting to light, even though the retina and optic nerve are normal.

A fixed, dilated pupil in a patient who has definitely not had mydriatics is a sign that serious retinal, optic nerve or oculomotor nerve disease is very likely.

Diseases of the retina and optic nerve

Loss of vision together with a clear red fundus reflex indicates disease of the retina or optic nerve. If the visual loss comes on very suddenly (or the patient wakes up with the visual loss) it usually means there is a vascular disease of the retina or optic nerve. If the visual loss comes on quite quickly (over a few days) it might indicate a retinal detachment, inflammatory optic nerve disease or wet macular degeneration.

The pupil must be dilated for a proper examination of the retina and optic nerve, but before dilating the pupil light reflexes must be checked. An afferent pupil defect (see page 69) is a simple and extremely reliable test for optic nerve or extensive retinal disease.

Unfortunately, it requires some experience to recognise many of the different fundus disorders. However, many of the diseases of the retina and optic nerve are untreatable. This means that making the correct diagnosis is often more important in theory than in practice. Most retinal diseases are recognised by their appearance. Therefore, it is very difficult to make a logical system for diagnosis. However, the following hints may help to identify the more important diseases of the retina and optic nerve:

- Retinal diseases usually produce fairly obvious changes in the appearance of the fundus, but may still leave some useful vision. Very extensive retinal disease will produce a 'severe' afferent pupillary defect (APD), moderate disease will produce a more subtle or relative (RAPD) one and more localised retinal disease will not produce any defect at all.
- Hypertension and diabetes are both common causes of retinal vascular disease. Haemorrhages and exudates are likely to be seen. Always measure the blood pressure, and test the urine for sugar.
- Macular degeneration is the most common retinal disease of older people. The changes are only in the macula and the rest of the retina looks normal. If the patient reports a rapid change in vision, possibly with distortion (straight lines look bent) it is likely that they have wet macular degeneration, which may be treatable (see page 337)
- The retina has no pain fibres. If the eye is uncomfortable and does not appear red or inflamed then choroiditis or optic neuritis are possible causes of the loss of vision. Choroiditis is often difficult to recognise clinically, but it is usually treatable.
- Retinal detachments are not common. However, the need for surgical treatment is urgent. Therefore, it is very important to recognise them. It helps to remember the three predisposing factors: aphakia, myopia and trauma. Remember the three warning signs of a retinal detachment: floaters, flashing lights and field defects.
- Optic nerve diseases, especially in the acute stage, may produce minimal or no change in appearance of the optic disc but cause severe loss of vision and a severe afferent pupil defect.
- The most important optic nerve disease to detect is glaucomatous optic atrophy. This is because glaucoma is very common, and early treatment should stop the progress of the disease. Unfortunately, it is difficult for both patient and doctor to recognise glaucoma in its early stages (see Chapter 15). Advanced glaucoma is much easier to detect, but by then it is too late to save any useful sight. However, although one eye might be blind, the other eye may have useful vision, which can be saved with treatment.
- If a careful examination of the eye can still not find any cause for the visual loss, there may be damage to the visual pathways in the brain

(see page 368). This will usually cause bitemporal visual field defects if the lesion is at the optic chiasm or a homonymous hemianopia if it is behind the chiasm.

The irritable or painful red eye

Numerous conditions can cause a painful red eye, and some of these are serious and sight-threatening. It is very important to identify these correctly. The three most common serious conditions are corneal ulcers, anterior uveitis and acute glaucoma (**Table 23.2**). The common non-serious conditions are corneal abrasions, conjunctivitis and superficial corneal and conjunctival foreign bodies. There are several symptoms that will help to determine the nature and severity of the condition: pain, photophobia (severe light sensitivity), reduced vision and discharge.

Pain and photophobia

The cornea has a very rich nerve supply. Therefore corneal disease, such as corneal ulcers and corneal abrasions causes severe pain. The iris also has a nerve supply. Therefore, inflammation in the eye and acute high pressure in the eye (acute glaucoma) usually cause severe pain headache and even nausea. However, acute glaucoma does sometimes present less severely with little or no pain, particularly in black patients. The conjunctiva does not have a very rich nerve supply, and therefore conjunctivitis may cause irritation but not significant pain. Disease of the cornea causes light rays to be reflected around the eye instead of being directed towards the retina, which causes light sensitivity. Disease of the conjunctiva obviously does not have this effect on light rays. Occasionally, conjunctivitis (and particularly when caused by adenovirus) causes inflammation of the superficial epithelial cells of the cornea and therefore causes some pain and photophobia.

Vision

Corneal disease usually affects the vision unless the corneal lesion is very peripheral. The amount of visual impairment depends on the size, density and exact location of the lesion. The visual loss caused by iritis varies greatly with the severity of the disease. Angle closure glaucoma causes severe loss of vision, except in very early or less acute cases. Conjunctivitis does not affect the vision unless the cornea is also involved. However, it may be necessary to wipe away discharge and mucus from the eyelids and conjunctival sac before checking the vision.

Redness

Redness means that the blood vessels of the conjunctiva and/or episclera and/or sclera are dilated. The type of 'redness' can help diagnose the disease. In conjunctivitis, the superficial conjunctival blood vessels become dilated. The conjunctiva appears pink or red all over, but this redness is often most noticeable towards the fornices and away from the limbus. Corneal ulcers, iritis and angle closure glaucoma all cause the anterior ciliary vessels to dilate. Therefore, the redness is most noticeable near to the cornea.

Table 23.2 The common causes of a red, irritable or painful eye				
	Conjunctivitis	Corneal ulcer	Iritis	Acute intraocular pressure rise (acute glaucoma)
Pain and photophobia	Irritation, grittiness, mild pain, itchiness if allergic	Moderate/ severe pain and photophobia	Moderate pain and photophobia	Severe pain and photophobia and can cause nausea, vomiting and severe headache
Vision	Normal except intermittent blurring from discharge which can be blinked away	Variable visual loss depending on size and location of ulcer	Variable visual loss depending on severity	Severe visual loss
Redness	Diffuse and especially in the fornices	Mainly around limbus ('ciliary injection')	Mainly around limbus ('ciliary injection')	Around corneal limbus
Corneal appearance	Normal Occasionally multiple small superficial opacities (typically adenoviral infection)	Staining of ulcer with fluorescein	Keratic precipitates seen with magnification or against red reflex	Oedematous and hazy all over
Pupil	Normal	Normal or slightly constricted	Constricted, irregular, poorly reacting	Half-dilated, vertically oval, non-reactive (fixed)
Anterior chamber	Normal	Normal or some inflammatory exudate	Inflammatory exudate	Shallow
Other features	Discharge: – Purulent: likely bacterial infection – More watery: likely viral infection – Stringy: likely allergic		Often recurrent. Can occur in either eye, but rarely both at same time May be systemic/ autoimmune disease	Very raised pressure detectable by pressing on eye ('stony hard') More common in South East Asians, Eskimos, American Indians. Rare in Africans
Treatment	• Bacterial: topical antibiotics • Viral: none, unless persistent, then consider topical steroids • Allergic: mast cell stabilisers and consider steroid drops	Antibacterials, antifungals, antivirals as per causative organism Mydriatics NOT steroids (can be disastrous)	Topical steroids and mydriatics	Urgent pressure reduction with acetazolamide, topical steroids, miotics and then surgery or laser

When the patient is examined, there are specific signs that need to be looked for to make the definite diagnosis. They are discussed in detail in the relevant chapter. Some of the tests for these signs require a lot of experience and practice, while others are relatively simple (and very important) for non-eye care practitioners to be able to do. We will discuss a few of the most important signs here, which should be looked for in all patients with a red, painful eye.

Fluorescein staining of the cornea

Corneal lesions that damage the corneal epithelium, such as abrasions and corneal ulcers and the epithelial spots that sometimes develop after adenoviral conjunctivitis stain with fluorescein (see Figures 9.2 and 9.7).

Anterior chamber inflammation and keratic precipitates

It requires a slit lamp and a lot of practice to see anterior chamber inflammatory cells (see Figure 11.3). However, sometimes clumps of these cells settle on the endothelium forming keratic precipitates, which may be seen standing out against the red reflex with an ophthalmoscope (see Figure 11.7).

Corneal haziness

Most corneal conditions cause localised opacities and damage. A few conditions cause the whole cornea to become hazy, of which acute glaucoma is the most serious. In angle closure glaucoma, the whole cornea becomes hazy, because the rise in intraocular pressure makes it oedematous. When there is a lot of oedema it can be seen with the naked eye. In acute glaucoma the high pressure also makes the eye feel stony hard if pressed on through the lid with fingers.

The pupil

In conjunctivitis, the pupil is normal, and the anterior chamber is clear. In a corneal ulcer, the pupil may be slightly constricted. In iridocyclitis, the pupil appears constricted and irregular to the naked eye and may not react to light as it is stuck to the lens behind it (see Figure 11.6). In angle closure glaucoma, the pupil is always half-dilated and non-reactive and sometimes slightly vertically oval in shape.

Discharge

Conjunctivitis causes discharge to be produced. Therefore, discharge is suggestive that there is not severe or sight-threatening disease. However, uveitis, acute glaucoma and corneal disease cause photophobia which can cause excessive tearing.

One or both eyes affected

Most sight-threatening diseases, such as corneal ulcer and uveitis occur in one eye, although acute glaucoma occasionally presents in both eyes at the same time. Conjunctivitis typically occurs bilaterally. *Therefore, always suspect that a diagnosis of unilateral conjunctivitis might be wrong.*

Disorders at the limbus

The limbus is a common site for pathological changes. Most of these are fairly distinctive, and many of them do not require treatment, but there is often some confusion and delay in making the diagnosis.

Limbal inflammation

Inflammation of the limbus is quite common. It is usually the result of an immune reaction rather than a specific infection, and so usually responds to steroid drops. Some examples are:

- A phlycten (see Figure 9.13)
- Marginal corneal infiltrates (see Figure 9.12)
- Vernal conjunctivitis (see Figures 7.15–7.18)
- Mooren's ulcer (see Figure. 9.16).

Excessive limbal pigmentation

This is a sign of various different conditions in adults and children.

- In adults it is often a sign of previous inflammation. It is also common in severe onchocerciasis and superior limbal pigmentation occurs in patients who have had chronic trachoma (Herbert's pits).
- In children, vitamin A deficiency and vernal conjunctivitis both produce excessive limbal pigmentation. Vitamin A deficiency can cause a pigmented area at the limbus (Bitot spot, Figure 10.8). Vernal conjunctivitis often causes pigmented inflammatory nodules of the limbus.

Degenerative changes

These often occur at the limbus in older people

- A pinguecula is a sub-conjunctival fatty deposit (Figure 7.28b).
- A pterygium is a wedge-shaped opacity that grows over the cornea from the limbus (see Figures. 9.24 and 9.25).
- Arcus senilis is another very common degenerative change at the limbus (see Figure 9.19).

Other disorders located at the limbus

- Foreign bodies often come to rest in the shallow groove between the cornea and the sclera.
- Scarring at the limbus will follow any previous inflammation.
- Most conjunctival tumours start at the limbus.

Functional visual loss (hysterical/malingering)

Functional visual loss (i.e. the patient pretending not to be able to see) should be considered if the clinical history and the signs do not match the apparent level of visual loss. Usually this can be detected with some simple methods or tests:

- Does the patient's visual behaviour match the visual loss? For example if their vision can only count fingers, then you might expect them to have difficulty finding their way around the examination room or to the chair.
- Check the vision at the correct distance. Then move the patient 3 metres closer. Often, patients with functional loss will read exactly the same line, when in fact more lines should be read when closer

- Other techniques exist but require more equipment or expertise, for example looking for spiralling visual fields on a Goldman visual field test or using lenses to fog one eye without the patient being aware that they are then only looking through the apparently bad eye.

APPENDIX

Further Resources

Eye care and eye disease information and training materials

1. The International Centre for Eye Health (ICEH):
   http://iceh.lshtm.ac.uk/
   Contains a wide range of training guides, manuals and reports covering many eye care subjects.
2. Community Eye Health Journal: http://www.cehjournal.org/
   A free journal produced by ICEH that has covered and continues to cover all the major eye diseases and related issues in poor countries.
3. The Kilimanjaro Centre for Community Ophthalmology (KCCO):
   http://www.kcco.net/
   Contains a variety of training guides, manuals and reports covering a wide range of eye care subjects.
4. The World Health Organization: http://www.who.int/en/
   Contains information about vision impairment epidemiology, Vision 2020/Universal Eye Health, educational materials on specific diseases such as vitamin A deficiency, cataract, trachoma and onchocerciasis and numerous training manuals and guides.
5. International Council of Ophthalmology: Icoph.org
   Contains a range of educational resources for eye care and ophthalmic education.
6. Global Sight: www.globalsight.org
   Website of a network of individuals and organisations working in global eye health. It contains global eye health news, educational materials and surgical videos on a range of ophthalmic procedures.

Books, teaching aids and tools for clinical and surgical ophthalmology

1. Dean WH, Sandford-Smith J. Eye Surgery in Hot Climates, 4th Edition. London; JP Medical, 2015. ISBN: 9781909836235
   This book describes the surgical management of all common eye diseases that are seen in hot and poor countries, such as cataract, trachoma and glaucoma.
2. Williams C, Waddell K, Sandford-Smith J, O'Callaghan C. Ophthalmology, a global multimedia guide.
   This is an educational DVD about all aspects of ophthalmology, but in particular describing in detail clinical examination, the diagnosis and management of common eye diseases and how to prescribe glasses. It is targeted for Africa, but it would be relevant for anywhere in the

world where eye care is not well developed. It is available from TALC (Teaching Aids at Low Cost) and the material is also online at http://www.ocbmedia.com/Ophthalmology/

3. Peek vision

A mobile phone application and lens adaptor that allows you to use a mobile phone for eye examinations such as fundoscopy, visual acuity, visual fields, colour vision and cataract imaging. http://www.peekvision.org

4. The Arc light

A very small, very cheap, lightweight solar powered ophthalmoscope and magnifying loupe.

a.   Website: http://arclightscope.com

b.   How to use the Arclight low cost ophthalmoscope: http://vimeo.com/50923766 and http://arclightscope.com/videos/

5. Trachomatous Trichiasis Surgery Training DVD

A Step-By-Step Guide to Trachoma Surgery. Saul Rajak and Matthew Burton. DVD widely available in English and French in trachoma endemic settings, or on request from The International Centre for Eye Health, The London School of Hygiene and Tropical Medicine. Full DVD online: http://vimeo.com/channels/trachomasurgery

Index

Note: Page numbers in italic refer to figures.

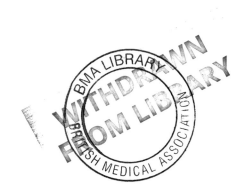